MILITARY PSYCHIATRY
PREPARING IN PEACE FOR WAR

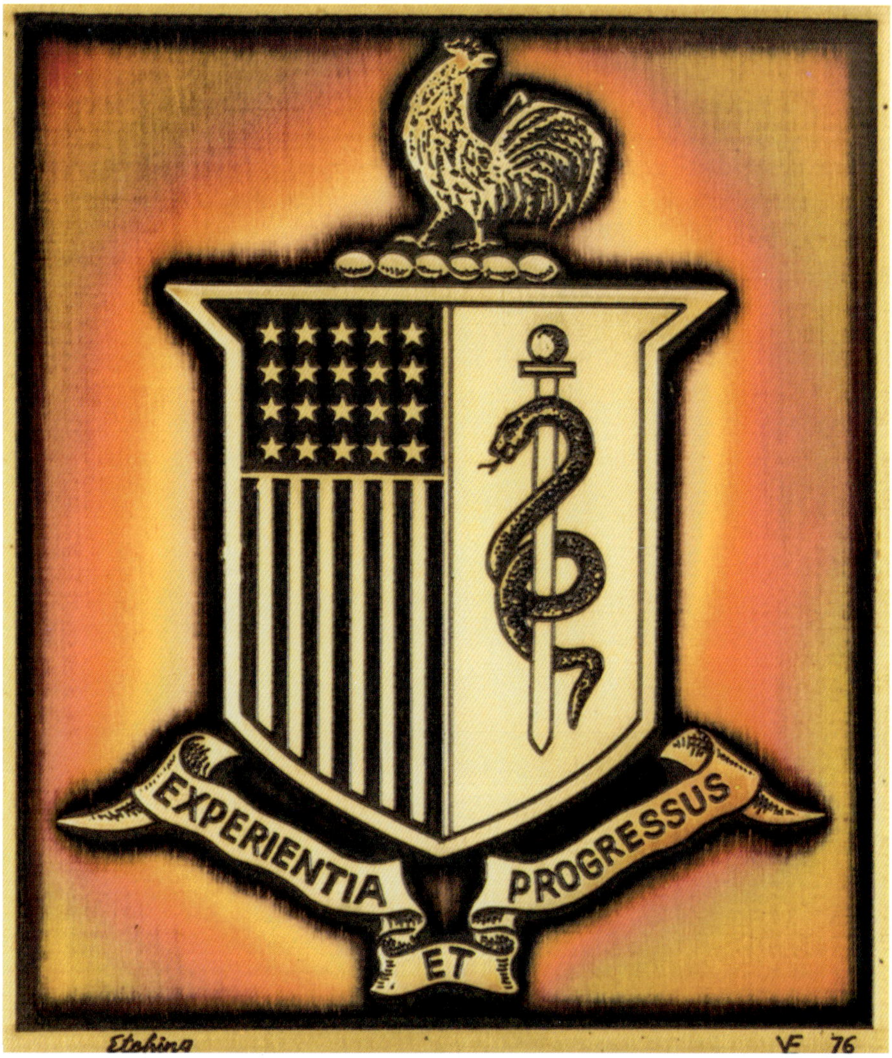

The Coat of Arms
1818
Medical Department of the Army

A 1976 etching by Vassil Ekimov of an original color print that appeared in *The Military Surgeon*, Vol XLI, No 2, 1917

The first line of medical defense in wartime is the combat medic. Although in ancient times medics carried the caduceus into battle to signify the neutral, humanitarian nature of their tasks, they have never been immune to the perils of war. They have made the highest sacrifices to save the lives of others, and their dedication to the wounded soldier is the foundation of military medical care.

Textbook of Military Medicine

Published by the

Office of The Surgeon General
Department of the Army, United States of America

Editor in Chief
Brigadier General Russ Zajtchuk, MC, U.S. Army
Director, Borden Institute
Commanding General
U.S. Army Medical Research and Materiel Command
Professor of Surgery
F. Edward Hebért School of Medicine
Uniformed Services University of the Health Sciences

Officer in Charge and Managing Editor
Colonel Ronald F. Bellamy, MC, U.S. Army
Borden Institute
Associate Professor of Military Medicine,
Associate Professor of Surgery,
F. Edward Hebért School of Medicine
Uniformed Services University of the Health Sciences

Scientific Advisor
Donald P. Jenkins, Ph.D.
Deputy Director for Healthcare
Advanced Research Projects Agency
Department of Defense
Adjunct Associate Professor of Surgery
Georgetown University
Visiting Associate Professor of Anatomy,
F. Edward Hebért School of Medicine
Uniformed Services University of the Health Sciences

The TMM Series

Part I. *Warfare, Weaponry, and the Casualty*

Medical Consequences of Nuclear Warfare (1989)

Conventional Warfare: Ballistic, Blast, and Burn Injuries (1991)

Military Psychiatry: Preparing in Peace for War (1994)

War Psychiatry

Medical Aspects of Chemical and Biological Warfare

Military Medical Ethics

Part II. *Principles of Medical Command and Support*

Medicine and War

Medicine in Low-Intensity Conflict

Part III. *Disease and the Environment*

Occupational Health: The Soldier and the Industrial Base (1993)

Military Dermatology (1994)

Mobilization and Deployment

Environmental Hazards and Military Operations

Part IV. *Surgical Combat Casualty Care*

Anesthesia and Perioperative Care of the Combat Casualty

Combat Injuries to the Head, Face, and Neck

Combat Injuries to the Trunk

Combat Injuries to the Extremities and Spine

Rehabilitation of the Injured Soldier

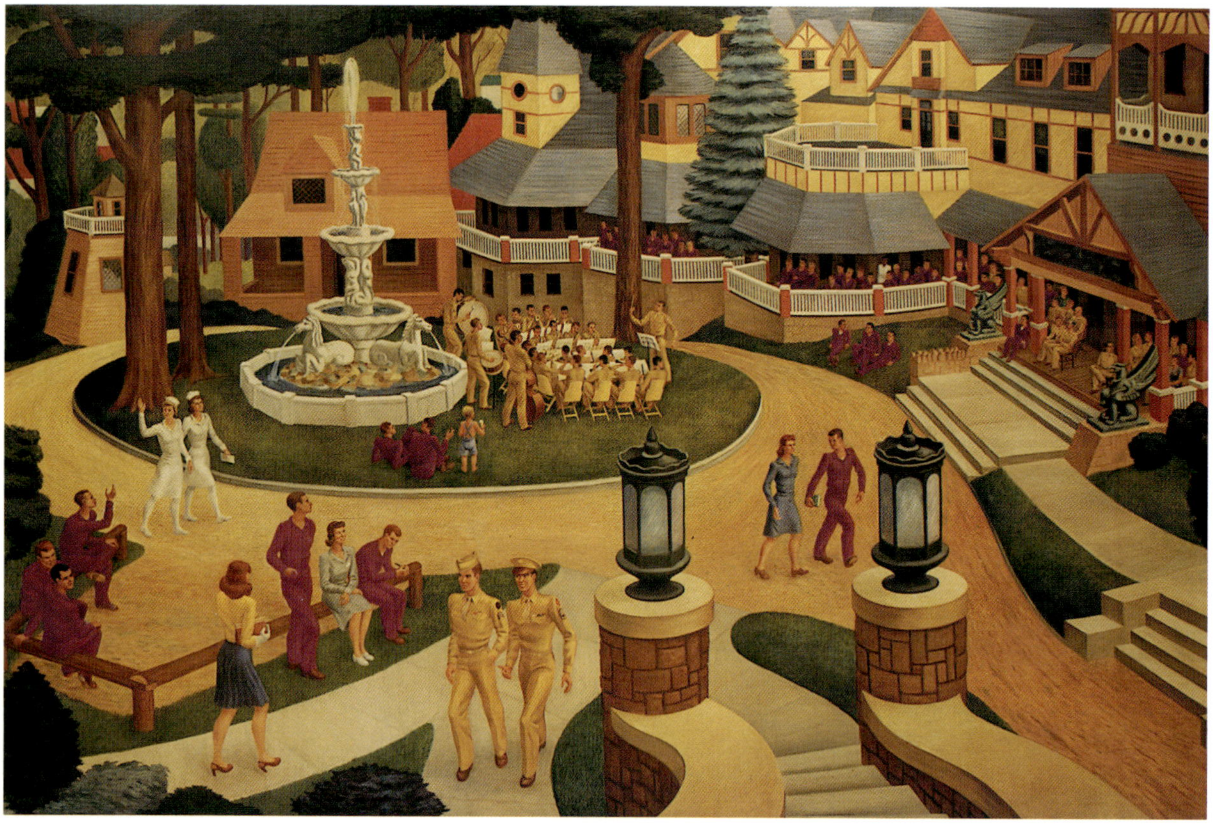

This 1944 painting by Jack McMillen was commissioned by the U.S. government for Walter Reed Army Medical Center as part of the Works Projects Administration (WPA) artists' program of World War II. It illustrates the historical function of the Forest Glen annex of the Walter Reed Army Medical Center as a holding and rehabilitation unit for medical patients, including psychiatric patients, during World War II. This is a role the Forest Glen annex also played in subsequent wars. Psychiatric patients were identified, and to an extent stigmatized, by wearing maroon hospital clothing. For many years this painting was on display at the Forest Glen annex in Silver Spring, Maryland.

MILITARY PSYCHIATRY
PREPARING IN PEACE FOR WAR

Specialty Editors

FRANKLIN D. JONES, M.D., F.A.P.A.
LINETTE R. SPARACINO, M.A.
VICTORIA L. WILCOX, Ph.D.
JOSEPH M. ROTHBERG, Ph.D.

Office of The Surgeon General
U.S. Department of the Army
Falls Church, Virginia

Walter Reed Army Institute of Research
Washington, D.C.

Uniformed Services University of the Health Sciences
Bethesda, Maryland

Armed Forces Institute of Pathology
Washington, D.C.

1994

Editorial Staff: Lorraine B. Davis
Senior Editor

Colleen Mathews Quick
Associate Editor/Writer

Scott E. Siegel, M.D.
Copy Editor

This volume was prepared for military medical educational use. The focus of the information is to foster discussion that may form the basis of doctrine and policy. The volume does not constitute official policy of the United States Department of Defense.

Dosage Selection:

The authors and publisher have made every effort to ensure the accuracy of dosages cited herein. However, it is the responsibility of every practitioner to consult appropriate information sources to ascertain correct dosages for each clinical situation, especially for new or unfamiliar drugs and procedures. The authors, editors, publisher, and the Department of Defense cannot be held responsible for any errors found in this book.

Use of Trade or Brand Names:

Use of trade or brand names in this publication is for illustrative purposes only and does not imply endorsement by the Department of Defense.

Neutral Language:

Unless this publication states otherwise, masculine nouns and pronouns do not refer exclusively to men

Published by the Office of The Surgeon General at TMM Publications
Borden Institute
Walter Reed Army Medical Center
Washington, DC 20307-5001

Library of Congress Cataloging–in–Publication Data

Military psychiatry : preparing in peace for war / specialty editors,
Franklin D. Jones . . . [et al.].
p. cm. -- (Textbook of military medicine. Part I, Warfare, weaponry, and the casualty)
Includes bibliographical references and index.
1. Military psychiatry--United States. 2. Military psychiatry.
I. Jones, Franklin D., 1935- . II. Series.
[DNLM: 1. Military Psychiatry. 2. Military Personnel--psychology.
3. Psychology, Military. UH 390 T355 Pt 1 1994]
UH629.3.M55 1994
616.89'008'80355--dc20
DNLM/DLC
for Library of Congress 94-33532
CIP

PRINTED IN THE UNITED STATES OF AMERICA

03 5 4 3 2 1

Contents

Foreword

This volume of the *Textbook of Military Medicine* addresses the multiple mental health services provided by the military during peacetime. Although military psychiatrists and other mental health professionals must view soldiers as they function within the larger organization and contribute to, or detract from, success of the combat mission, we must remember that soldiers and their families are also subject to mental and emotional stresses during peacetime. The U.S. Army's mental health services' peacetime roles include but are not limited to supporting soldiers and commanders as they participate in rescue missions with combat potential as occurred in Grenada and Somalia, peace-keeping roles as in the Sinai and Macedonia, combating terrorists and hostage takers, interdiction of traffickers in drugs and illegal aliens, providing assistance in handling large influxes of refugees, assisting civilian officials in the aftermath of large-scale civilian disturbances such as rioting and environmental disasters, and assistance following certain stressful human experiences such as accidents and deaths. What is not always recognized is that soldiers' families also require the services of military mental health professionals during these operations.

Disasters and other mass civilian disturbances, such as influxes of refugees, are opportunities not only for medical officers to sharpen our surgical and medical skills but also for commanders to use our military organizational and leadership skills, and our mental health professionals, to contain and ameliorate the mental and emotional sequelae of such disturbances. Disaster victims often exhibit symptoms similar to those of combat stress casualties (ie, disaster fatigue) and respond to the simple interventions and expectancy that are therapeutic for combat fatigue casualties. After disasters, some of these victims may develop chronic post-traumatic stress disorder. Early, appropriate treatment of acute post-traumatic stress disorder may be an important preventive measure for chronic post-traumatic stress disorder.

I strongly recommend that all commanders and medical officers heed the central theme of this book: the stresses of military life can be significant, and it is the responsibility of the commander to assure that appropriate, timely prophylaxis, psychiatric intervention, and other mental health services are delivered to the entire military family.

Lieutenant General Alcide M. LaNoue
The Surgeon General
U.S. Army

August 1994
Washington, D.C.

Preface

The stresses of the peacetime military environment range from the traditional (garrison life, training, deployment), to the contemporary (disaster relief, peace-keeping, hostage situations, civil disturbances). Soldier's families are also subjected to these stresses. Soldiers who are worried about the emotional stability of their family members can be distracted from performing their duties.

One of the cardinal lessons relearned during the Vietnam War is that unit cohesion and morale are essential to conserving fighting strength. The integrity of a fighting unit depends not only on the quality of its materiel, training, and public support but also on the emotional well-being of its individual members. Although soldiers are generally young and physically healthy, they are at risk—both for the fear and anxiety that accompany battle, and for the same psychiatric and emotional disorders that are seen in their civilian cohort.

A forthcoming volume, *War Psychiatry*, covers the psychiatric and emotional problems of soldiers in combat. This volume of the *Textbook of Military Medicine* deals with the full spectrum of mental health in the peacetime military community. However, the principles of military psychiatry that have proven successful in managing combat stress have been successfully adapted to noncombat settings. For example, mental health professionals and commanders use these principles—centrality, proximity, immediacy, simplicity, expectancy—to enable soldiers to use their own strengths to recognize that anxiety is a normal, not a pathological, phenomenon, and that recovery is not only possible but also expected. The soldier's treatment is enhanced by the mental health professional's intense familiarity with the soldier's unit. Avoiding hospitalization and keeping soldiers in geographic proximity to their own units enable the soldier to return to work rapidly, with follow-up at the working level rather than the clinic.

From malaria to sexually transmitted diseases, prophylaxis is a command responsibility. Medical officers and other mental health professionals must strive to educate and reeducate their commanders so they will understand that, in psychiatry as in other medical specialties, effective prophylaxis is vastly more cost- and time-effective than treatment.

Brigadier General Russ Zajtchuk
Medical Corps, U.S. Army

August 1994
Washington, D.C.

The current medical system to support the U.S. Army at war is a continuum from the forward line of troops through the continental United States; it serves as a primary source of trained replacements during the early stages of a major conflict. The system is designed to optimize the return to duty of the maximum number of trained combat soldiers at the lowest possible level. Far-forward stabilization helps to maintain the physiology of injured soldiers who are unlikely to return to duty and allows for their rapid evacuation from the battlefield without needless sacrifice of life or function.

Medical Force 2000 (MF2K)
PATIENT FLOW IN A THEATER OF OPERATIONS

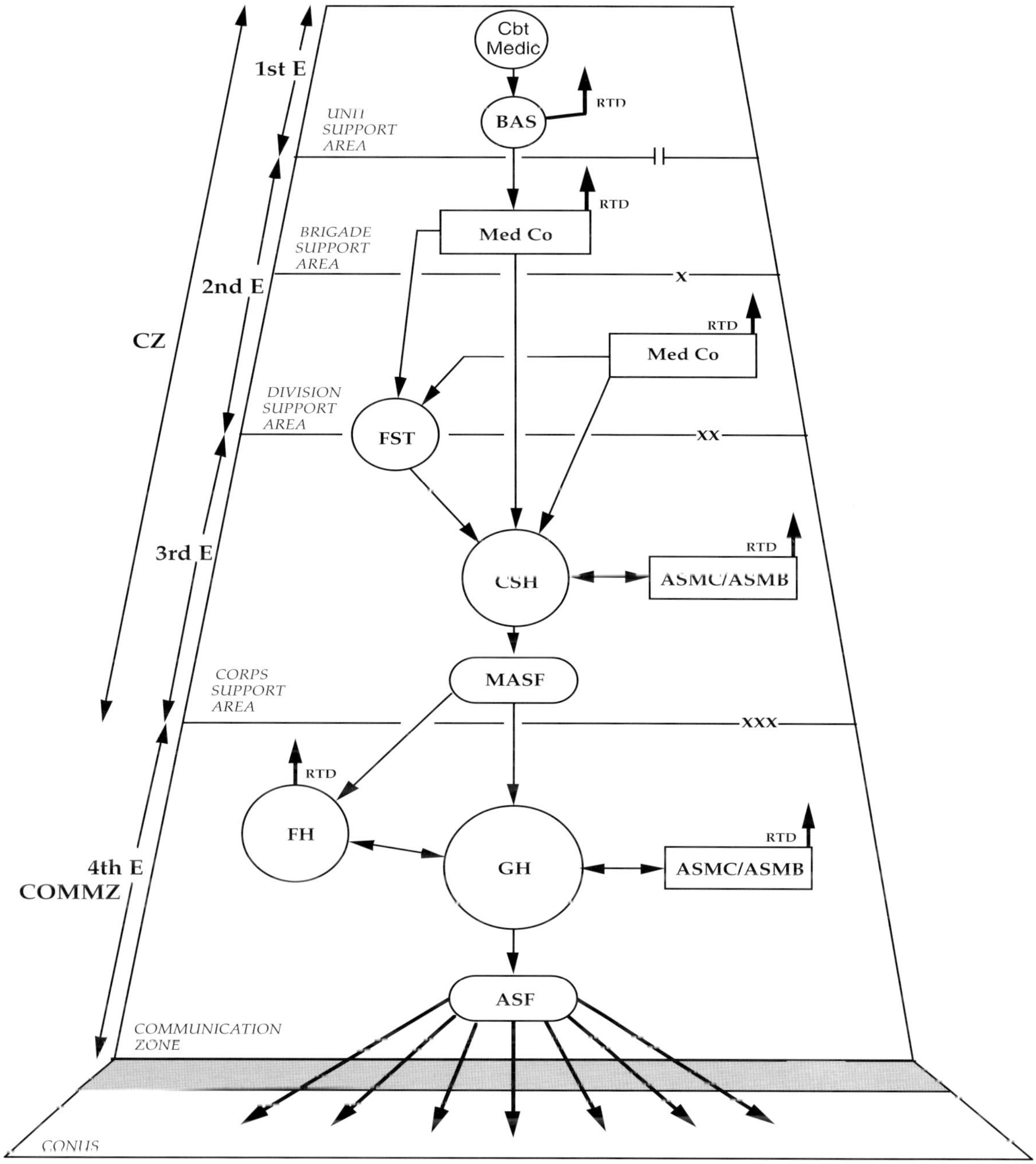

ASF:	Aeromedical Staging Facility, USAF	E:	Echelon
ASMB:	Area Support Medical Battalion	FH:	Field Hospital
ASMC:	Area Support Medical Company	FST:	Forward Surgical Team
BAS:	Battalion Aid Station	GH:	General Hospital
Cbt Medic:	Combat Medic	MASF:	Mobile Aeromedical Staging Facility, USAF
CSH:	Combat Support Hospital	Med Co:	Medical Company
COMMZ:	Communication Zone	RTD:	Return to Duty
CZ:	Combat Zone		

Chapter 1

MORALE AND COHESION IN MILITARY PSYCHIATRY

FREDERICK J. MANNING, Ph.D.*

*Senior Program Officer, Institute of Medicine, National Academy of Sciences, 2101 Constitution Ave., N.W., Washington, D.C. 20418; Colonel (ret), Medical Service Corps; U.S. Army, formerly, Director, Division of Neuropsychiatry, Walter Reed Army Institute of Research, Washington, D.C.

INTRODUCTION

One of the enduring legacies of World War II military psychiatry was the recognition that the incidence of psychiatric casualties in various units had more to do with characteristics of the unit than with characteristics of the casualties themselves.[1] Present day writers might use the term *social support* instead of *group identification, group cohesiveness,* or *group bonds,* but nowhere in civilian life is the social group of such major and crucial importance in the life of the individual as it is for the soldier in combat.

This was apparent to Spiegel,[2] a psychiatrist inadvertently assigned as an infantry battalion medical officer during the very first American combat action in North Africa in World War II. It did not take much first-hand experience for Spiegel to puzzle not about why some men broke, but how so many could push on for so long in such miserable conditions. He rejected the notion that these men were peculiarly tough characters who loved to fight, and he noted that they expressed very little real hate for the enemy. Instead, Spiegel suggested that it was regard for comrades, respect for leaders, concern for their reputation with both of those groups, and an urge to contribute to the success of the unit that kept them fighting. These cohesive forces, which Spiegel called the basis for the X factor underlying good morale, were "something that often decided whether or not a man became a psychiatric casualty."[2(p116)]

Other psychiatrists came to similar conclusions from their experiences with casualties. Weinstein for example described the typical "combat-induced neurosis" case as "a frightened, lonely, helpless person whose interpersonal relationships have become disrupted. . . . He had lost the feeling that he was part of a powerful group and had become instead a lonely and frightened person whose efforts to protect himself were doomed to failure."[3(p307)] A special commission of civilian psychiatrists headed by Menninger pointed to the nature of precipitating incidents as confirmation of the critical importance of "the soldier's position in the constellation of his social group, the combat team."[4(p369)] The actual events that finally overwhelmed the psychiatric casualty's defenses varied widely, but the common denominator, according to the commission, was not so much that they were the last straw in any quantitative way, but rather that they involved a sudden change in the soldier's relation to his group. Somehow he had lost his place as a member of the team, whether it was he who changed or the team. In either case, alone, he was overwhelmed and disorganized.

Additional support for the assertion of Glass[1] that began this chapter came from some of the many pioneering survey studies of Stouffer and colleagues[5] in the Research Branch of the War Department's Information and Education Division. They questioned men from over 100 companies undergoing pre–D-day training and compared the subsequent nonbattle casualty (all medical losses except wounded in action and killed in action) rates of these same companies in Normandy. Their data showed a correlation of -0.33 between nonbattle casualties and preinvasion morale. For heavy weapons companies, the correlation was -0.41. A division commander could in fact have used preinvasion morale scores to sort his rifle companies into thirds. The lowest scoring third ultimately suffered 62% more nonbattle casualties than the highest scoring third.

As a result of these World War II observations, morale and group identification suddenly emerged as concepts of great importance to military medicine, but practitioners and students of warfare have known for more than 2,000 years that ". . . not numbers or strength bring victory in war; but whichever army goes into battle stronger in soul, their enemies generally cannot withstand them."[6(p3)] Tolstoy, like Spiegel, used the term "an unknown quantity, x" to indicate ". . . the spirit of the army, the greater or less desire to fight and face dangers on the part of all the men composing the army. . . ."[7(p198)] *Morale, cohesion,* and *esprit de corps* are the terms that this century's military have given to this unknown X, and it is these terms that provide the frame of reference for this chapter.

The first part of this chapter will lay out in some detail the ways in which influential authors, civilian and military, have used these terms, provide consensus definitions, and propose a set of relations among them. The next part of the chapter deals with the individual and organizational determinants of morale, and the final part of the chapter deals with methods of assessing morale in military units. Most of the examples and evidence are focused on land warfare, but the general principles involved are applicable to sailors and airmen as well. Last, the chapter is predominantly descriptive rather than prescriptive. This is a consequence of my faith in the ability of my military mental health colleagues of the U.S. Army, Navy and Air Force to deduce specific advice appropriate to their particular situations from a comprehensive description of general truths.

KEY CONCEPTS

The Meaning of Morale

The term *morale* is one that has appeared in an ever-growing number of contexts—industrial, educational, and medical as well as military. Unfortunately, the term seems to have sharply different meanings in each of these contexts. In more recent applications, it often seems to refer primarily to a person's sense of well-being, happiness, and job or life satisfaction. The U.S. Army, for example, provides such a definition of morale in its *Field Manual on Leadership:*

> Morale is defined as the mental, emotional, and spiritual state of the individual. It is how he feels—happy, hopeful, confident, appreciated, worthless, sad, unrecognized, or depressed.[8(p228)]

Bartone[9] has argued persuasively that if morale is just a synonym for happiness or mood, then it probably serves no useful purpose. Earlier conceptions of morale, both military and industrial, included an element of mood or emotional state, but tied it closely to a goal-oriented group. Munson, for example, organized the Morale Branch of the U.S. Army General Staff during World War I, defining morale as the "determination to succeed in the purpose for which the individual is trained, or for which the group exists."[10(p97)] In his classic study of the Second Scottish Rifles, Baynes devoted 16 pages to the definition of morale, which he called "the most important single factor in war."[11(p1)] He concluded with the following definition:

> A confident, resolute, willing, often self-sacrificing and courageous attitude of an individual to the functions or tasks demanded or expected of him by a group of which he is a part that is based upon such factors as pride in the achievements and aims of the group, faith in its leadership and ultimate success, a sense of fruitful participation in its work, and a devotion and loyalty to the other members of the group.[11(p108)]

Others are more succinct. Grinker and Spiegel, for example, defined morale simply as "the psychological forces within a combat group which impel its members to get into the fight."[12(p37)] Leighton[13] maintained that morale is the capacity of any group of people to pull together consistently for a common purpose. Moran described morale as "the ability to do a job under any circumstances to the limit of one's capacity."[14(p95)] He contrasted the soldier with high morale, who does his duty without the constant threat of punishment, to those of the Peninsular War, who did their job "because the fear of flogging was greater than the fear of death."[14(p162)]

Shibutani[15] provided a picture of a military unit with high morale in his study:

> An organized group is characterized as having high morale when it performs consistently at a high level of efficiency, when the tasks assigned to it are carried out promptly and effectively. In such units each member is likely to contribute his share willingly doing what he believes to be worthwhile and assuming that his associates will do their part. When necessary, the men help one another without even being asked. Mutual encouragement is commonplace, and those whose zeal is exemplary are singled out for praise. The few who do not share the prevailing orientation feel pressures to comply: those who fail repeatedly to live up to expectations are scorned as "slackers," and efforts may be made to expel them from the group. The successful completion of each transaction occasions no surprise; it is the expected thing. Members of such groups usually place a high evaluation on themselves. They often develop a strong sense of identification with each other; they develop pride in their unit, become conscious of its reputation, and take pleasure in displaying emblems of belonging to it.[15(p4)]

Motowidlo et al [16] attempted to summarize definitions of both industrial psychologists and military writers by arguing that most definitions include some aspects of satisfaction, motivation, and group membership. While the industrial model has certainly become relevant for peacetime garrison armies,[17] job satisfaction must be taken in a very relativistic way in the wartime situation. Evonic[18] also provided a tripartite view of morale similar to that of Motowidlo et al[16] but more easily applicable to armies in combat as well as armies in garrison. Evonic's three dimensions are concern for the organizational aim, commitment to the group's identity, and personal factors related to self-confidence.

Smith[19] and Gal and Manning[20] came to similar three-component views, with the former relying on interviews of Australian infantrymen, and the latter relying on factor analyses of survey data from Israeli and American combat arms soldiers. Motowidlo et al[16], Evonic[18], Smith[19], and Gal and Manning[20] also have in common a view of morale as an individual-level attribute, rather than something that is characteristic only of groups, as the quotations from Leighton[13] and from Grinker and Spiegel[12] might imply. It is this view I adopt in this chapter, considering morale as a characteristic of individuals, albeit only individuals in goal-oriented groups. Groups with high morale would then simply be groups a large proportion of whose members have high morale. We thus arrive at a working definition of morale applicable in both wartime and peacetime, emphasizing membership in a group and willing participation in the group's work: *Morale is the enthusiasm and persistence with which a member of a group engages in the prescribed activities of that group.*

In this chapter, I identify morale, so defined, with Spiegel's[2] X factor. Two other concepts, cohesion and esprit, often used uncritically as synonyms of morale, I view as major contributors to morale, but distinct from it and from each other. In the next two sections of this chapter, I will clarify these distinctions before turning to a wider ranging discussion of morale's determinants, in which cohesion and esprit are subsumed under the category of *group factors*.

The Meaning of Cohesion

The importance of group solidarity for effective military performance has been a staple of military doctrine for 2,500 years. For most of this time, it has been reflected in the elevation of close-order drill to near sacramental status; that is, physical unity was the explicit goal. As weaponry improved to the point where time-honored battle formations like the phalanx, the infantry square, and the line had to give way to dispersion, cover, and concealment, the need for psychological unity became more apparent. DuPicq called this psychological unity *moral cohesion* and claimed that "As the ranks become more open, and the material cohesion of the ranks not giving confidence, it must spring from a knowledge of comrades, and a trust in officers. . . ."[21(p115)] He is more explicit in another place, where he says that which makes a soldier capable of obedience and direction in action includes: "Respect for and confidence in his chiefs; confidence in his comrades and fear of their reproaches and retaliation if he abandons them in danger; his desire to go where others do without trembling more than they."[21(p122)]

America's great combat historian Marshall made much the same observation in his summary of his World War II experiences: "I hold it to be one of the simplest truths of war that the thing which enables an infantry soldier to keep going with his weapons is the presence or near-presence of a comrade."[22(p42)] Later, Marshall answers the question of what makes a soldier face death bravely: "Largely the same things that induce him to face life bravely—friendship, loyalty to responsibility and the knowledge that he is a repository of the faith and confidence of others."[22(p161)]

Military psychiatrists grappling with the "neuropsychiatric casualties" of World War II came to a conclusion remarkably close to Marshall's. The war forced them from a view of such casualties as unfortunate aberrations best explained by their own weakness and an unusually stressful incident, to seeing battle fatigue as a normal and natural consequence of extended combat, staved off by some better than others only by virtue of supportive relations to their unit and leaders. Little's[23] work on the buddy relationships of Korean conflict soldiers, Marlowe's[24] study of basic training, and Moskos'[17] observations in Vietnam have put more emphasis on the instrumental, pragmatic, and situational specific aspects of primary group bonding but nevertheless reinforced the central role of these interpersonal relationships for both psychological well-being and military performance.

In the 1980s, the U.S. Army recognized the risk of leaving cohesion development to the hardships of war and made an explicit and unprecedented attempt to foster cohesion. The most visible effort in this regard has been the Unit Manning System, which has shifted the whole basis of assigning and moving soldiers from an individual basis to one based on units of up to company size. This attempt to provide sufficient stability in interpersonal relationships for cohesion to flourish stemmed from then Chief of Staff, Edward Meyer, who defined unit cohesion as: ". . . the bonding together of soldiers in such a way as to sustain their will and commitment to each other, the unit, and mission accomplishment, despite combat or mission stress."[25(p2)]

Like the military definitions of morale, this definition makes no mention of satisfaction or well-being and explicitly includes commitment to mission accomplishment as well as commitment to the unit. Unit cohesion should thus be seen as a contributor to morale, albeit a very important one, rather than a synonym or a related but independent concept. A second implication of this definition and the reason that the word *unit* was appended are that most of the academic literature on cohesion is based on a definition of cohesion entirely focused on interpersonal attraction, with no consideration of the member's enthusiasm for chosen or assigned tasks.[26] Adding unit to cohesion directs attention to a group focused on a task.

A third noteworthy aspect of unit cohesion, not so obvious in Meyer's definition, concerns the size of the unit involved. Little's[23] observations on the predominance of a two-person buddy system in the Korean conflict suggests that having just one other soldier to rely on goes a long way, and the seminal World War II papers[1,2,3,4,12,22] repeatedly use the term *primary group,* defined as one characterized by intimate face-to-face association and cooperation. As Ingraham[27] has shown, even for the peacetime soldier, at least the single barracks dweller, this pretty much draws the upper bound at the company level.

None of this approach denies that soldiers may take great pride in, draw great strength from, and on occasion give their lives for organizations far larger than the 80-to-160 man company that makes up their everyday world. It is in fact just such feelings and actions that are the referents of the term *esprit*.

The Meaning of Esprit de Corps

Effective combat performance requires not only the existence of cohesive primary groups, but also that these primary groups be articulated with the larger military organization and thereby with the larger society. The Crusades, Imperial Japan, and revolutionary Iran provide examples where soldiers apparently fought because of a strong belief in the rightness of their country's cause or simply a belief in their country, right or wrong. By and large, however, observers have agreed that patriotism, ideology, and politics may be important, like high pay, in inducing modern Western youth to join the service, to remain in a peacetime force, and even to volunteer for combat, but are generally far from mind when the bullets start to fly.[5,11,22,23]

Soldiers, nevertheless, in Kellett's[28] words, need to have some justification, however inchoate, to stimulate them to do something that so obviously conflicts with the urge of self-preservation. The enemy, of course, often provides some justification. As an anonymous soldier said to Parks, "Nobody that fires at me ain't my friend."[29(p49)] Ashworth's[30] study of the ubiquitous live-and-let-live system that sprang up in the trenches of World War I suggests, however, that additional factors are at work in an aggressive hard-fighting unit.

Vertical or hierarchical cohesion is one such factor. That is, soldiers bond not only with peers (horizontal cohesion), but also with the leaders they see every day. They identify with these small unit leaders and, in the process, come to accept these leaders' aims and goals as their own. By virtue of their additional membership in groups beyond the squad, platoon, or company (eg, the battalion, regiment, division, or corps), the leaders are, of course, subject to the same process of identification and, thus, in theory pass on to their subordinates the aims and goals of the service's higher leaders.

Armies enlarge the boundaries of this tacit and imperfect contract between soldier and primary group leader by the creation of a larger secondary group, still small enough to serve as a focus of identity yet large enough to escape sudden catastrophe at the hands of an enemy (or gradual enervation in the hands of a faint-hearted leader). The bond between soldier and this secondary group, in many armies a regiment, is an impersonal one, relating soldier to institution rather than soldier to soldier, as in the case of unit cohesion. Secondary groups provide a smaller cause, free of conventional politics and ideology, between the soldier and the great national cause.

By establishing relatively demanding expectations of combat behavior and by linking the soldiers' self-esteem to the reputation of the unit, the secondary group provides additional motivation for enthusiastic participation in combat by its members. A regiment (or a brigade, division, squadron, or wing) that does this successfully is said to have esprit. *Esprit* then is a higher order concept, paralleling cohesion at the primary group level, implying above all pride in and devotion to the reputation of a formal organization beyond the primary group and, along with cohesion, necessary for sustained effective performance of soldiers in combat.

Related Concepts

To this point my discussion of morale, cohesion, and esprit has relied heavily on the use of such terms by military writers. The use of the term and concept of *morale* by industrial and organizational psychologists was noted but, in large measure, dismissed because of its heavy emphasis on job satisfaction versus my heavy emphasis on sustained performance in combat, where job satisfaction has a very limited and relative meaning.

Similarly, in discussing unit cohesion, great care was taken to point out that the *cohesion* studied at some length by academic psychologists was quite different from the *cohesion* of military writers. *Esprit* seems to be a purely military concept, used in civilian contexts as a more or less explicit analogy to military esprit de corps. This is not to say that the civilian psychological literature has nothing to offer the military mental health professional interested in morale, cohesion, and esprit. In fact, two relatively recent concepts, *organizational commitment* and *social support,* bear a marked resemblance to morale and cohesion despite very different pedigrees.

Mowday and associates[31] never use the term *morale* in their extensive review of "Employee-Organization Linkages," but their definition of organizational commitment distilled from 10 different studies of civilian organizations is similar to my earlier definition of morale in both denotation and connotation. *Organizational commitment,* they say, is the relative strength of an individual's identification with and involvement in a particular organization. They go on to say that this involves something beyond mere passive loyalty to an organization and mere desire to maintain membership; it involves, in addition, a strong belief in the organization's goals and values and a willingness to exert considerable effort on behalf of the organization.

Commitment is differentiated from job satisfaction in several ways: it is more global and thus more stable in the face of day-to-day work experiences; it develops more slowly and dissipates more slowly. Mowday and associates[31] also find it useful to discuss the determinants and consequences of organizational commitment on three levels: personal, work group, and organizational. A similar approach has been used in the next section of this chapter.

A second civilian concept of considerable value to the military mental health professional is that of *social support*. Perhaps ultimately traceable to the observations by Durkheim[32] and others[33,34,35] on the role of industrialization in the transformation of the dominant social order from one of *Gemeinschaft* (a highly personal community) to one of *Gesellschaft* (an impersonal, bureaucratic community), *social support* refers to the ways in which people's interactions with others in some way affect their vulnerability to physical and mental illness. On the one hand, the socially marginal person, or one who has lost his circle of intimates to death or dispersion, becomes substantially more prone to illness in all forms.[36] Conversely, membership in a network of significant others seems to provide far more protection from stress and illness than a purely mechanical summation of resources would predict.[37]

The nature, meaning, and measurement of social support are still subjects of some debate, but there appears to be some consensus that it involves both problem-solving and emotionally sustaining behaviors on the part of the supporters.[38] House[39] further splits these behaviors into instrumental support and informational support, depending on the nature of the help provided, and emotional support and appraisal support. (The former involves expressions of care and empathy; the latter involves feedback on personal performance.)

The receiver of such support approaches life crises armed with confidence that he is cared for and loved, that he is esteemed and valued as an individual, that he is embedded in a network of mutual obligation.[40] The parallel with the soldier's overwhelming dependence on his primary group is too obvious to require much elaboration. (See the quotes of Spiegel[2] and Marshall[22] above, as well as Bartemeir et al[4] and Shils and Janowitz.[41]) I would suggest, as has Griffith,[42] in fact that it is precisely this social support literature that the military mental health professional should turn to in advising commanders on improving primary group relations.

DETERMINANTS OF MORALE

Munson began the U.S. Army General Staff's Morale Branch by providing himself an extremely large area in which to work: "Every physical thing entering into the environment of the soldier, and the expressed state of mind of every person with whom he comes in contact, affects his morale."[10(p51)] The essential truth of this assertion should not discourage the reader, the practicing military mental health professional, or the military leader interested in enhancing that precious commodity because, clearly, some things affect morale to a greater extent than others and some are easier to change. In this section, I will describe some of the most important determinants of morale, organize them in a rational framework, and illustrate their action with historical examples.

Individual Factors

Individual factors include both biological and psychological needs. Good health, good food, adequate rest and sleep, clean dry clothes, washing facilities, and protection from the elements are examples of the former and are regularly cited as causes of high morale.[6(p171),11(p101)] Satisfaction of these rather elementary needs is more the exception than the rule for combat soldiers. Holmes cites a World War I account as representative of 20th century soldiering: "For most of the time the average private was tired. Fairly often he was so tired as no man at home ever is in the common run of his work."[43(p115)]

Complaints about food are also a common denominator among soldiers over the ages and around the world. Napoleon allegedly said that an army marches on its stomach, and British Brigadier Fergusson opined that "lack of food constitutes the single biggest assault upon morale."[44(p99)] It is not merely quantity of food that is so important to morale, but quality. Variety is an important consideration—within limits because unfamiliar food will generate its own list of gripes—and the preparation and consumption of food provide a momentary diversion from the grim business of war. A hot meal in the company of comrades can work wonders for morale. In fact, a hot meal in a relatively safe environment has been high on the list of treatments for battle stress casualties ever since mental health professionals recognized the psychological nature of shell shock in World War I.

Bugs and dirt are staples of warfare in all but the coldest climes, and as a result, a bath and clean clothes are among the most effective morale raisers. World War II infantry company commander McDonald summed it up: "It had never occurred to me that I could derive so much pleasure from a bath."[45(p119)]

If combat is so generally a dirty business fought by chronically tired, hungry soldiers, it is difficult to put much credence in the assertion that rest, food, and clean dry clothes are important for morale, above some minimum, because the wide range of morale among units in every war is undeniable. Stouffer and colleagues[5] answered this paradox with the concept of relative deprivation. It is not so much the absolute level of physical discomfort that controls morale, they argued, as the relation of a soldier's discomfort to that of those around him, or more generally, to the level he has been led to expect.

No one disputes that war is hell, but one of the front-line soldier's dearest beliefs is that war should also be the great leveler. Perceived violations of this tenet are sources of very bitter feelings, for example the well-documented[5,46] friction between "tooth" (frontline combat) and "tail" (rear echelon support). Although the delineation of front line and rear echelon depends a great deal on who is doing the talking, every war seems to produce an abusive epithet for support personnel, for whom the frontliners envision a life of luxury amidst all the amenities they themselves are denied (and perhaps even amenities originally destined for soldiers further forward).

Beyond the physical factors involved in morale, but still primarily at the individual level, are a number of psychological needs, the fulfillment of which plays a substantial role in the soldier's morale. In contrast to the physical needs, mere equality of deprivation will not suffice. High morale demands, for each soldier, a goal, a role, and reasons for self-confidence.

Conventional wisdom in the social sciences of the 1960s and 1970s was that, in Baynes' words, "the writer or speaker about war has more faith in causes than those who actually fight."[11(p99)] Pre–World War I views, on the contrary, held that patriotism, or an equally grand and glorious cause, was the sine qua non of effective military performance. Disillusioned World War I citizen-soldier-writers such as Sassoon[47] began the assault on this view, which ultimately collapsed at the hands of the psychiatrists and social scientists of World War II. Even Dollard,[48] studying perhaps the most idealistic Western soldiers of the 20th century, the International Brigade of the Spanish Civil War, concluded that the soldier in battle is too busy to be constantly whispering, "My cause, my cause." He further noted that ideology serves mostly to get soldiers into battle.

The post–World War II emphasis on primary groups and interpersonal obligations in the small combat unit served a useful purpose in countering an unrealistic belief in the "Great Cause" as motivator, but America's Vietnam experience in the 1970s (and perhaps that of the Israelis in the Lebanon War of the 1980s) suggests that the pendulum may have swung a bit too far. Without the widespread agreement on the necessity for and the value of the war effort that underlies American involvement in the two world wars, morale plunged among U.S. soldiers in Vietnam.

Before 1969, morale in Vietnam was generally high, and local variations occurred against a background of widely shared if not universal acceptance of a latent ideology. Moskos[17] used this term to describe general acceptance of the worth of the social system for which the soldiers were fighting. Early in the war, U.S. soldiers shared a more or less firm belief in the American way of life and the need to stop communism.[17]

After 1969, despite a steadily diminishing role in the actual fighting, morale steadily declined as antiwar sentiment in the United States eliminated consensus on at least the first of these two very general beliefs. U.S. troops characterized themselves with the graffiti initials U.U.U.U.—the unwilling, led by the unqualified, doing the unnecessary for the ungrateful.[49] The counter-insurgency, nonterritorial nature of that war denied them even short-term goals—such as capture of a particular piece of terrain—that could have had a salutary effect.

Every bit as important as an objective or a goal is a role. Holmes quotes a fellow Briton to the effect that "many a man behaves as a hero or coward, according as he is expected to behave."[43(p314)] Indeed, Gal's[50,51] studies of heroes in the Israeli Defence Forces are in full agreement, finding four distinct combat situations far more useful in explaining heroic battlefield behavior than any inborn or acquired characteristics of the heroes, with the exception of officer status—also an acquired role. Civilian studies of job satisfaction are relevant here also because they consistently emphasize the importance of seeing oneself as a valued member of the workforce (ie, having an important role).[16] Suggested[16] cures for low worker commitment are increasing job scope or challenge or eliminating role conflict or role ambiguity.

Closely linked with the previous two factors, goal and role, is a sense of progress or at least a sense that the goal is attainable and the role is one that can be carried out. Malone[52] in fact argues that because of the importance of confidence, the key to building will (or morale) is building skill. Training thus has a central role in morale. The wise leader will ensure not only that training is realistic, but also that his soldiers grow accustomed to success because nothing succeeds like success in building confidence.

Group Factors

As indicated in the introductory portion of this chapter, much of the combat soldier's ability to endure the stress of combat depends not so much on the enemy as on the soldier's relationships with those around him. Grinker and Spiegel assert that "the ability to identify with a group and the past history of such identification are probably the most important . . . components of good motivation for combat."[12(p41)] Out of the soldier's relationships with those in his primary face-to-face group grows what military writers have traditionally called unit cohesion and social scientists have lately called social support. The soldier's relationships with others in his organization, but outside his primary group, provide the basis of esprit de corps. Both unit cohesion and esprit de corps can be powerful influences on morale. The following sections describe the determinants or components of cohesion and esprit.

Cohesion

Stephen Crane referred to the comradeship of the small combat unit as a "mysterious fraternity born out of smoke and the danger of death."[53(p31)] In this definition, he will find few dissenters, but convinced of the importance of cohesion, both to mission accomplishment and individual survival, one might reasonably search for ways of fostering cohesion before battle itself (at least ensuring by conscientious preparations that smoke and danger will be effective in creating it). For example, George[54] points out that a common social background assists soldiers in developing close personal relationships, and conversely, heterogeneous ethnic, racial, class, and even regional origins tend to inhibit the development of unit cohesion. Similarity in more personal characteristics (like age, personality traits, upbringing, and values) also plays a role, perhaps a much larger one.

Few if any modern armies make much of an effort to create homogeneous units around any of these variables. The traditionally regional recruiting of regiments in European armies often created distinctly homogenous units, but shifting demographics and population centers have largely rendered this practice a thing of the past. American forces have also become more heterogeneous since 1917, in part for the same reasons, but in large measure as a result of deliberate attempts to avoid inequities in the risks and benefits of military service to segments of the population.

Shared experiences while in the military thus become the glue that holds the work group together. Combat experience itself has, of course, long been recognized as a primary force in bonding soldiers. The presence of an enemy with the capacity and intent to kill or injure produces strong pressure to unite in a common effort. As Grinker and Spiegel describe it:

> Friendships are easily made by those who might never have been compatible at home, and are cemented under fire. . . . Such powerful forces as antisemitism, anticatholicism or differences between Northerners and Southerners are not likely to disturb interpersonal relationships in a combat crew. . . . The camaraderie is so effective that even the arbitrary distinctions imposed by the military caste system, probably one of the most rigid social devices in the world, are noticeably weakened.[12(p22)]

What can the division mental health staff do to facilitate this process of bonding that the enemy accomplishes so readily (but so painfully)? To begin with the obvious, the first prerequisite for cohesion is opportunities for interaction (eg, the primary group must remain intact and in close contact long enough to accumulate a significant body of common experience). Until very recently, the U.S. Army's replacement system, which achieved relatively stable unit strength at the cost of stable personal relationships, was a serious impediment in this regard.

The supersession of the assembly-line-style individual replacement system with a unit system similar to that of most other Western armies seems to have reversed this trend.[42,55,56] The more time people are together, the greater the chance they will discover, invent, and experience commonalities, including a shared understanding of the group's history. This occurrence is a natural phenomenon of groups and increases with the number of roles and settings in which members know each other and feel comfortable interacting. The activities are not as important as who participates—the more people, the more varied the settings, and the longer the group remains stable, the more the members have in common and the higher the resulting cohesion.

An important consideration here, however, is the distinctiveness of the group's common experiences. Being in the army is of course an experience common to all the members of any platoon, but because it is not an experience unique to the squad, it is not as effective in inducing cohesion as more limited experiences—for example, having gone through basic training together, won the company basketball title, or simply survived a bitter night together "downrange." Establishing a "them" also helps in defining an "us" so that threats from outside the group, even in friendly competition, are particularly effective common experiences.

The examples given above also illustrate two other important aspects of cohesion-enhancing experiences: (1) The unit must derive some feeling of success or accomplishment, and (2) the more interdependence among the members that is necessary for success, the greater the payoff in cohesion. Malone argues that successful mission accomplishment leads to high morale more often than vice versa. In his words, "Practice doesn't make perfect. What makes perfect is perfect practice."[52(p89)]

Malone[52] also differentiates three kinds of teamwork, illustrating each with a sports analogy, in encouraging military leaders to train for interdependence. The simplest kind of teamwork he says is like a bowling team—individual scores are simply added together. A relay team is slightly more complicated—there is a necessary sequence involved, and there is a brief moment at the start of each leg when team members must interact. The battlefield, Malone contends, requires above all teamwork of the sort displayed by a successful football team, in which every member has a different job, but each is dependent on everyone else.

Common experiences do not have to take place only in officially sanctioned military activities to build cohesion (although I would argue that leaders as well as followers have to be involved if unit cohesion is to result). Ingraham in fact points out that drug use and heavy drinking "facilitate the bonding between isolated individuals who find themselves living together largely by chance rather than choice and who are held in place by a number of specific environmental structures, both physical and social."[27(pxviii)] Sanctioned alcohol-centered events have long been a military custom precisely because they are felt to enhance unit cohesion. Ingraham provided an explanation of how this happens, at the same time extending it to the nonsanctioned abuse of both drugs and alcohol by off-duty soldiers:

> Alcohol is particularly helpful in generating distinctive, memorable episodes involving brawls, "broads," and bad news that the participants can recall and recount as evidence for the meaningfulness of their relationship and what they have been through together. . . . Illicit drug use creates two large superordinate oppositional categories: user and nonuser, or "we" and "they." These explicitly defined categories cut across cliques, build stable perimeters despite unstable personnel, and engender a sense of group identity.[27(p65)]

Drinking bouts and drug use are certainly not being suggested here as useful techniques for promoting unit cohesion. On the contrary, because unit leaders are seldom included in the "we" generated by such activity, unit cohesion is in fact decreased, even while interpersonal bonding among junior soldiers is increased. I cite alcohol and drug use here primarily as evidence for the importance of creating distinctive and memorable experiences for all unit members; sense of membership in an accepting and protective group is a strong enough need so that they will build their own if the organization does not provide it.

Whatever the nature of the common experiences that build unit cohesion, they are successful in doing so only to the extent that they provide soldiers with confidence in the ability and determination of their peers and their leaders to protect them in combat. This concept is related to my earlier argument that the cohesion so widely cited by World War II and Korean conflict observers as crucial to soldier endurance bears a very strong resemblance to what the mental health field now calls social support. Central to this concept is the individual's conviction that he is firmly embedded in a network of mutual obligation. This confidence that in times of difficulty one has someone who is willing and able to help is at the heart of unit cohesion. Indeed, I would argue that confidence that others *can* help (that is, have the ability and training to provide effective assistance, for example in staying alive) is at the heart of what Gross and Martin[57] call instrumental cohesion.

Affective cohesion, on the other hand, is based on confidence that others in the group *will* help if the need arises. Moskos,[17] for example, argued from his observations in Vietnam that it is not altruism born of intrinsic interpersonal attraction that leads a soldier to risk his life for another but a recognition that his own self-interest, his own survival, depends on his ability to make others willing to help him in his own time of need. The strong interpersonal ties characteristic of the small combat group, in the words of Kviz, "develop secondarily to the collective pursuit of survival in a highly stressful situation."[58(p219)]

A Korean conflict study by Clark (as noted by Watson[59]) suggests that soldiers can and do distinguish between likability and military dependability, choosing different colleagues with whom to perform a risky mission and to go on leave. More recently, Tziner and Vardi[60] reported on an Israeli armor corps experiment in constructing tank crews at the end of basic armor training on the basis of sociometry. It quickly became clear that high-ability soldiers were selected far too frequently and low-ability soldiers far too infrequently to maintain the program.

A reasonable conclusion is that soldiers are well aware of their dependence on others for survival in combat. Their attraction to their combat group is very much dependent not only on the willingness of the group to help them survive but also on their ability to do so. A perception that the group is short of either one will lead the soldier to devalue membership in the group and participation in the group's activities (ie, low morale).

Leaders, even more than peers, must generate this double dose of confidence because in combat it is the leader more than anyone else who can spell the difference between certain death and the rush of victory. Being technically and tactically proficient is a value that is drummed into leaders incessantly, although they are not told as often how important it is for their soldiers to see and know their leader's talents. If they doubt his knowledge they will hesitate to commit their lives to his judgment—they will not act as a cohesive unit. They may be willing to die if they must, but no one wants to sacrifice his life to ignorance.

Yet it is not enough that a leader merely be technically proficient. If he is to inspire confidence, his subordinates must see not only that he will not waste their lives through incompetence but also that he will not waste them through indifference. As Grinker and Spiegel put it, combat soldiers:

> . . . have given up most of their selfish interests for the sake of their group. But they do this for their buddies and for the leaders on a personal basis, out of affection and loyalty. They can only be paid back on a personal basis. The leaders must return the loyalty and affection in kind.[12(p46)]

Two Israeli studies[51,61] have confirmed these World War II views. Solomon and colleagues[61] found that although lack of affective support from officers or peers was associated with feelings of loneliness, only lack of such support from officers was related to combat stress reactions. Gal[51] showed that soldiers' trust in their commanders depended on three qualities: (1) professional capability (technical competence), (2) credibility as a source of information, and (3) the amount of care and attention that commanders pay to their men. The last of these qualities need not imply a popularity contest, nor is it incompatible with fair but firm discipline. In fact, soldiers most often view discipline as does Oldenquist who points out, "If a social group does not impose its rules on me and hold me responsible to it, I know it does not accept me as a member."[62(p9)]

Care and attention, including explicit acknowledgement of one's skills, abilities, and accomplishments, are of vital importance to the morale of others. Napoleon is said to have counted on soldiers fighting "long and hard for a bit of ribbon."[63(p255)] Medals, promotions, a mention in the dispatches—all have become common since plundering ceased to be acceptable military behavior (although gallantry awards were well-known even in Roman times). Like any selective reward, the distribution of medals will produce complaints of inequity. Few soldiers ever turn them down, however, because in Mauldin's words, "Civilians may think it's a little juvenile to worry about ribbons, but a civilian has a house and a bankroll to show what he's done for the past four years."[64(p113)]

Medals are of course only one form of recognition and, as Mauldin's words imply, are likely to be more important when looking back on military service than as an incentive to heroic action. (Medal hunters are frequently very unpopular with their peers and subordinates, who occasionally murdered them with fragmentation grenades ["fraggings"] in Vietnam.[65]) Less dramatic forms of recognition often have immediate effects on morale however because they reassure the soldier that he is valued as a person, a person whose life will not be thoughtlessly expended.

The last component of unit cohesion I will discuss is the need for clear and meaningful group missions. In some ways this component is simply another way in which good leaders can demonstrate to their units that they care—by seeing that their efforts and the risks (and losses) they incur are for something undeniably worthwhile. Certainly, the discipline problems, wholesale drug abuse, and fraggings of the U.S. Army in Vietnam came primarily in the latter years of the war when it was clear that America had made the judgment that its task was not worth pursuing. Interpersonal bonding at the small unit level could not overcome the quite rational desire not to be the last one killed in an effort without glory or thanks.

On a lesser scale, in the interests of "security," leaders will sometimes fail to provide their soldiers with the whys and wherefores of an operation, expecting them to undertake it because they are well-trained or well-disciplined. If the leader has had ample opportunity to prove to his men that he would not ask what was not important, he may succeed. If not, he may find he has quite unnecessarily brought on a crisis in command.

Esprit de Corps

Leaders are also links by which primary groups are integrated into a larger, secondary group and by which values and directions of that larger group and the parent organization are impressed on the primary group.[66] High levels of esprit mean that soldiers' loyalties go beyond their primary face-to-face peers and immediate leaders. This is an important step if morale is to be maintained in combat because hard fighting will result in losses, no matter how good the unit.

If the will to fight depends solely on personal loyalties, it will wither as ties are severed by death and wounds, despite the bitterness toward the enemy initially produced by the loss of buddies. For this reason, most Western armed forces have attempted to instill loyalties to a secondary group larger than the company but smaller than, for example, the army. For navies, this is often a ship or a type of ship (eg, submarines). In the more technical branches, it is often a profession (eg, the medical corps). For the combat arms soldier, it is most often a regiment.

The United States has been a notable exception in this regard, at least since World War II, although it has of late revived the idea, at least on paper, in concert with efforts to change the replacement system focus from individual to small "packages." Other Western armies, ironically, have been fighting a losing battle with cost-conscious governments to maintain their regimental systems. Admittedly not the cheapest way to fill an organizational structure, these systems are designed to assure that replacements arriving at any small combat group already share a significant body of common yet distinctive experiences with those they are joining. With luck, these commonalities serve as a skeleton on which cohesion-building small group experiences can build.

Although no longer tactical units in combined arms armies, regiments are both symbolic and administrative. Significant features of such systems have been distinctive names, colors, "messes" and dress, territorial affiliation, and recruitment. The Royal Welsh Fusiliers, the Gordon Highlanders, and the second Scottish Rifles are familiar names even to Americans, whose units Bidwell decried as "soulless things known by letters and numbers."[67(p139)] Other features have included fixed home bases, unit training (even basic entry-level training), unit rotation (to the regiment's overseas area of responsibility), long service, and return assignments. Museums, bands, veterans associations, honorary ranks, and publications are other frequent props, the effect of which, ultimately, is to link the soldier's self-esteem to the reputation and expectations of the regiment.

Military mental health professionals are admittedly not in position to modify most of these esprit-producing activities, structures, and policies, which prevent potential stress casualties in combat. Psychiatrists are important beneficiaries, however, and should thus be knowledgeable and vocal opponents of the ever more frequent attempts to replace these old-fashioned customs with more modern, centralized, and less expensive practices that mistakenly trade off peacetime economy for combat effectiveness. They can also be alert for ways to incorporate these esprit-building regimental trappings into available secondary groups like army divisions.

ASSESSING MORALE AND COHESION

Most leaders know a great deal about the status of their unit and its cohesiveness. They gather impressions, talk, listen, observe, and monitor the kinds of problems unit members are having and can pretty well gauge whether their unit is militarily cohesive and effective. However, even the best leader can be blindsided, communications systems may fail, the press of other work may lead to inattention to danger signals, and the actual status of unit military cohesion may be misrepresented or misinterpreted. For these reasons, the good unit leader should have the same kind of checklist for cohesion and cohesion-related issues that he uses for his weapons system, supplies, and combat gear. As a prime beneficiary of good morale and cohesion, mental health professionals can and should provide advice and assist the leaders both in drawing up such a list and in periodically using it to assess their unit.

The definition of military unit cohesion was presented earlier in this chapter: the bonding together of soldiers in such a way as to sustain their will and commitment to each other, the unit, and mission accomplishment. This definition clearly has three major components, each potentially independent of the others and requiring attention in the assessment process: (1) horizontal bonding, binding members of the same leadership level (ie, soldiers with soldiers, noncommissioned officer (NCO) with NCO, officer with officer); (2) vertical bonding, binding unit members of different ranks (soldier to squad and platoon leaders, commanding officer to soldiers and NCOs); and (3) personal commitment to unit and army missions and values. Leaders at all levels have three major means of gathering information about these three facets of unit cohesion: personal observations, traditional morale indicators, and outside observers. Each facet has its pluses and minuses, but together they can provide a reasonably accurate snapshot of unit cohesion to the leader who wants to know.

Horizontal Bonding

Key questions to be answered in any assessment of horizontal bonding are:

1. Do unit members (NCOs and officers as well as junior enlisted) have confidence in their peers?

2. Do unit members have a sense of loyalty or commitment to their peers?

A good leader (note that none of the actions discussed are meant to be restricted to company commanders) finds the answers to these questions by making first-hand observations, asking unit members (and members of other collocated units), and checking official records. The sort of things he looks for and asks about are:

- Formal and informal requests for transfers out or into the unit. (Do not forget the most informal request of all—the absent without leave.)
- Reenlistments and the reasons for reenlisting or not reenlisting.
- Incidents of vandalism, theft of personal belongings, or fights in the barracks or work areas.
- Large numbers at daily sick call, especially when disposition is return to duty.
- Off duty friendship patterns. (Do members choose to play with the same people they work with? Do race, language, gender, or other common features count for more than assignment when it comes to choosing friends? Do the sides in informal ball games reflect work units? Do squads, sections, platoons have social get-togethers? [fishing or hunting trips? volksmarches? concerts? ballgames? and so forth]).

- Unit collections for soldiers in the hospital, with a death in family, a new baby, a new spouse, or birthdays.
- Personal assistance. (Do unit members with personal difficulties, ranging from having debts to being out of shape, get any help from peers? Do peers feel any sense of responsibility to help?)
- Personal socialization. (Do unit members know each other's families, or do they view this as a silly question?)
- Attempts by unit members, or subunit members, to make their work group special in some way (nicknames, attire, rituals, and jargon).
- "Initiation rites" or spur-winning requirements for newcomers.
- Humor. (Are unit members able to laugh at themselves and their difficulties, or is work a grim struggle?)

Vertical Bonding

Key questions for vertical bonding are similar to those in the preceding section, except we are now talking across rank groups rather than strictly about peers:

1. Do the unit's soldiers have *confidence* in their NCOs and commissioned officers? Similarly, do the officers and NCOs have confidence in each other and in their soldiers?
2. Do the unit's soldiers have a sense of *loyalty* or commitment to their NCOs and officers? Do the NCOs and officers have similar feelings of loyalty and commitment to their soldiers?

Finding the answers to these questions is generally much harder than assessing horizontal cohesion because the leader's own relationships with his unit members are a central issue. In most cases, however, relationships between subunit leaders and followers are not only easier to assess objectively, but also tend to reflect the leader's own situation as well because he sets the example. Once again he must make first-hand observations (in fact, the very act of making them tends to increase vertical cohesion!); solicit the opinions of others, both inside and outside the unit; and pay attention to the unit's own records. He should be looking for:

- Technical competence in leaders. Soldiers will not have confidence in leaders who are not themselves experts in the subjects they teach. NCOs should be leading the way on skills qualification tests, as well as setting the example for fitness and appearance.
- Put-downs. Rarely will a unit member make disparaging remarks about a higher ranking unit member (in his presence), but in low-cohesion units, many in the chain of command will freely and frequently put down those under their supervision.
- Communication flow. In a high-cohesion unit, the commanding officer will hear about problems, gripes, and snafus from those involved, not outsiders. Likewise, information that he puts out to subordinate leaders will get all the way down to the newest private.
- Personal data. Platoon leaders and platoon sergeants will know at least all their squad leaders well enough to tell you their first names, their wives' names, whether they have kids, their hobbies and interests, and so forth. Squad leaders will be able to tell you these things about their squad members. The commanding officer should know this information about at least the platoon leaders and platoon sergeants. Do the privates know his name and the names of those in their chain of command?
- Social interaction. How often do the unit's leaders, including the commanding officer, simply chat with subordinates about their lives, in and out of the workplace?
- Availability. How busy is the commanding officer's office during "open door" hours? Lots of traffic may mean the junior leaders are not generating the same trust and confidence in their subordinates that he is.
- Inspector General complaints, congressional inquiries, and so forth. By definition, these actions indicate lack of trust in the chain of command.
- Language. Who are junior enlisted talking about when they say "we"? When subordinate leaders bring problems to the commanding officer for advice and help, do they say "we have a problem in our unit" or "Private ______ has a problem in my unit"?
- Spouse and family member contact with unit leaders. Do spouses see leaders as a source of help in time of need? Do they even know who the unit leaders are, or how to contact them? Conversely, are there any attempts being made to keep families in-

formed about unit activities, post or Army benefits, opportunities, and so on?

- Outside activities of unit leaders. Are unit leaders so busy being students, teachers, coaches, club members, moonlighting, and so forth that unit members have a hard time seeing themselves as top priority?
- Decision sharing. Do unit leaders solicit input from their subunits when they have a decision to make that affects them (ie, does the leader attempt to make the decision "ours" rather than "his"?)

Commitment

The U.S. Army has long recognized the significance of instilling in its soldiers *values* it holds in esteem, (eg, readiness, loyalty, discipline, punctuality, courage, physical fitness, and above all mission accomplishment). Military unit cohesion implies widespread success in this process so that every unit member holds a similar set of values and behaves accordingly. These behaviors, which all members of the unit exhibit and expect of others in the unit, are the unit *standards*. Although it is the commanding officer who most often makes these standards explicit, a highly cohesive military unit requires some degree of personal commitment to them by every unit member. Important questions for the leader are:

- Do unit members (all ranks) know what the leader's values and priorities are?
- Do the members of the unit act as if they share the values and priorities?

In practice, the extent of vertical bonding in the company will play a large role in the personal commitment of lower ranking unit members to unit and army ideals and goals. The following are checks on vertical bonding as well as on personal commitment:

- Can unit members (all ranks) state the unit's general mission and, more important, the missions and goals of upcoming exercises and other unit actions? A good starting place is the commanding officer himself.
- Can unit members tell you why their own job is important to unit success?
- Do unit members show pride in being in the army and in this unit in particular? Do they wear the uniform and unit crest properly? Do they rush to take it off as soon and as frequently as possible? Is there antiarmy graffiti in the unit areas? Are salutes and greetings rendered freely and with enthusiasm (in both directions)?
- What kind of a reputation does the unit have around the post? Do members have respect and status because of membership? Do they realize this?
- Are disciplinary actions increasing, decreasing, or higher than sister units? Are they for military infractions or criminal infractions (ie, acts punishable in civilian courts as well as in military courts)?
- Do unit members know anything about the unit's history? Do they hold onto any myths about the unit's recent or distant past?

Command Climate

No action takes place in a vacuum, and many good intentions never result in actions at all because of circumstances beyond the control of the parties involved. Leaders at every level of the army can have a powerful effect, for better or worse, on the ability of their subordinate leaders to build militarily cohesive teams. They thus have the obligation to ask themselves, in any assessment of unit cohesion, whether they are encouraging, or even allowing, subordinate leaders to follow the advice they get in their manuals on leadership and team building. Indeed, unless the leaders lose sight of the fact that they themselves are central figures in the vertical bonding process, they will have largely answered this question in their assessment of the unit's vertical bonding. There are, nonetheless, a few items that deserve close inspection by themselves because they may on occasion conflict with other worthwhile activities or goals:

- Intraunit turbulence. Reducing the frequency of permanent change of station moves or restricting the range of units to which a soldier might be reassigned is perhaps necessary for cohesion, but it is not sufficient. It is stability in face-to-face relationships that is most important in this regard. Continual cross-leveling and reshuffling of junior leaders thus makes team building just as difficult as continual permanent changes of station.
- Unit goals, priorities, values, and standards. Making these clear and consistent across levels of authority is every leader's responsibility. Remember that what the boss checks on is what is important as far as subordi-

nates are concerned, regardless of what is said or published. Are there standing operating procedures, directives, guidelines, and so forth that conflict with stated priorities or values?

- Loyalty. Does the boss reward subordinate leaders for being loyal to their soldiers? Or is his idea of a team player one who gives an enthusiastic yes to all his ideas?
- Equitable benefits. Does the boss see to it that accomplishment of unit objectives results in benefits for all even when the contributions of some are clearly greater than others?
- Subordinate's credit. Is the boss careful to ensure that subunit leaders get proper (or maybe more than proper) credit from their men when rewards are handed out or even when simple snafus are straightened out.
- Success. Does the boss actively seek out tasks on which his unit can succeed? Does he fight off unreasonable demands from higher headquarters?
- Unit individuality. Does the boss allow subunits to differentiate themselves? Is standardization so important to him that he prevents subunits from developing their own identities?
- Perceived lack of organization. How often do plans get changed? Are sufficient reasons provided for subunit leaders to dispel perceptions of disorder? Does the benefit always justify the price, which is the undermining of unit members trust and confidence in their leaders?

Like everybody else, leaders tend to see their world as they would like it to be, not always as it is. Therefore, it becomes especially important for them to check their views constantly against those of others they respect and trust. These might include fellow commanders, the sergeant major, respected senior NCOs outside the unit, chaplains, or medics. Some of these folks will know of questionnaires and other team-building techniques that may be of additional help. One example, found in the *Unit Climate Profile Commander's Handbook*,[68] is an 82-item questionnaire designed for use by unit commanders in assessing their unit's psychological readiness. It comes with directions for scoring and some guides to interpreting the 21 "climate areas" assessed.

SUMMARY AND CONCLUSION

One constant in the ever-changing nature of warfare over the centuries has been the recognition that success on the battlefield involves more than the appropriate disposition of men and weapons. Whether this unknown X factor be called soul, spirit, heart, or morale, it refers to the enthusiasm and persistence with which soldiers carry out the prescribed activities of their unit. Since World War II, we have known that it is crucial not only to success, but also to survival itself. Determinants of morale include both individual and group factors. Among the former are biological needs such as adequate food, sleep, and protection from the elements, although most frequently it is the relative rather than the absolute satisfaction of these needs that is important for morale. Other individual needs are psychological and not so negotiable as the physical. High morale demands a goal, a role, and a reason for self-confidence.

Perhaps the most critical determinants of individual morale are group factors, unit cohesion, and esprit de corps. Confidence in the ability and willingness of peers and leaders to protect in combat and a feeling of obligation to do the same for them are the heart of unit cohesion. Military activities, field exercises especially, provide opportunities to observe the abilities of the unit, but other shared experiences, including the purely recreational, can confirm for the soldier that his comrades are willing to stick by him. A perception that the group is short on either ability or willingness puts the soldier at risk to become a stress casualty.

When soldiers' loyalties and confidence go beyond their immediate work group, we speak of their esprit de corps. This impersonal sort of bonding is important because combat means casualties, and if the will to push on depends solely on personal loyalties, it will wither as casualties mount. To the extent that small unit leaders are seen as typical of the larger organization, some of the confidence and loyalty they generate will accrue to the organization as well. However, most Western armies have made deliberate efforts to instill loyalty to a secondary group large enough so that its members do not all know each other, but small enough that all can share a body of distinctive experiences. The regiment is the best example. By extending this network of mutual obligation in which the soldier functions, his morale can withstand better the loss of close friends because replacements are already in the network. The military mental health professional must form a strong partnership with unit leaders in maximizing these elusive qualities well before the first battle or soldiers will pay the price in combat casualties.

REFERENCES

1. Glass AJ. Lessons learned. In: *Neuropsychiatry in World War II*. Vol 2. In: Mullens WS, Glass AJ, eds. *Overseas Theaters*. Washington, DC: GPO; 1973. GPO Stock No. 0832–00047, 989–1027.

2. Spiegel HX. Psychiatry with an infantry battalion in North Africa. In: *Neuropsychiatry in World War II*. Vol 2. In: Mullens WS, Glass AJ, eds. *Overseas Theaters*. Washington, DC: GPO; 1973. GPO Stock No. 0832–00047, 111–126.

3. Weinstein EA. The function of interpersonal relations in the neurosis of combat. *Psychiatry*. 1947;10:307–314.

4. Bartemeir LH, Kubie LS, Menninger KA, Romano J, Whitehorn JC. Combat exhaustion. *J Nerv Ment Disease*. 1946;104:358–389.

5. Stouffer SA, Lumsdaine AA, Lumsdaine MH, et al. *The American Soldier*. Princeton, NJ: Princeton University Press; 1949.

6. Richardson FM. *Fighting Spirit*. London: Leo Cooper; 1978.

7. Tolstoy L. *War and Peace*. Translated by Constance Garnett. New York: McClure, Phillips; 1904.

8. US Department of the Army. *Field Manual on Leadership*. Washington, DC: GPO; October 1983. GPO Stock No. 466–680. Field Manual 22–100.

9. Bartone P. Fighting morale and comfort morale. Presented at the Expert Panel on Sustained Operations; January 27, 1988; US Army Aeromedical Command, Atlanta, Ga.

10. Munson EL. *The Management of Men*. New York: Holt; 1921.

11. Baynes JC. *Morale*. New York: Praeger; 1967.

12. Grinker RR, Spiegel JP. Men Under stress. Philadelphia: Blakiston; 1945.

13. Leighton AH. A working concept of morale for flight surgeons. *Milit Surgeon*. 1943;92:601–609.

14. Moran L. *The Anatomy of Courage*. 3rd ed. New York: Avery; 1966.

15. Shibutani TI. *The Derelicts of Company K: A Sociological Study of Demoralization*. Berkeley, Calif: California Press; 1978.

16. Motowidlo SJ, Dowell BE, Hopp MA, Borman WC, Johnson PD, Dunnette MD. *Motivation, Satisfaction, and Morale in Army Careers: A Review of Theory and Measurement*. Arlington, Va: US Army Research Institute for the Behavioral and Social Sciences; 1976. ARI Technical Report TR–76–A7.

17. Moskos C. *The American Enlisted Man*. New York: Russell Sage; 1970.

18. Evonic IN. Motivation and morale in military noncombat organizations. In: *Proceedings of the NATO Panel VIII Symposium on Motivation and Morale in NATO Force*. Brussels, Belgium; 1980: 173–210.

19. Smith KR. Understanding morale: With special reference to the morale of the Australian infantryman in Vietnam. *Def Force J*. 1985;52:53–62.

20. Gal R, Manning FJ. Morale and its components: A cross-national comparison. *J Applied Soc Psychol.* 1987;17:369–391.

21. DuPicq A. *Battle Studies.* 1865. Reprint. Harrisburg, Pa: Stackpole; 1958.

22. Marshall SLA. *Men Against Fire.* New York: William Morrow; 1947.

23. Little R. Buddy relations and combat performance. In: Janowitz M, ed. *The New Military.* New York: Russell Sage Foundation; 1964: 195–224.

24. Marlowe DH. The basic training process. In: Artiss KL, ed. *The Symptom as Communication in Schizophrenia.* New York: Grune and Stratton; 1959: 75–98.

25. Meyer EC. The unit. *Defense.* 1982;82(February):1–9.

26. Zander A. The psychology of group processes. *Annu Rev Psychol.* 1979;30:417–451.

27. Ingraham LH. *The Boys in the Barracks.* Philadelphia, Pa: Institute for the Study of Human Issues; 1983.

28. Kellett NA. *Combat Motivation.* Boston: Kluwer; 1982.

29. Parks D. *GI Diary.* Washington, DC: Howard University Press; 1968.

30. Ashworth T. *Trench Warfare, 1914–18: The Live and Let Live System.* New York: Holmes and Meier; 1980.

31. Mowday RT, Porter LW, Steers RM. *Employee-Organization Linkages.* New York: Academic Press; 1982.

32. Durkheim E. *The Division of Labor in Society.* 1893. Reprint. New York: Free Press; 1933.

33. Spencer H. *The Principles of Sociology.* New York: Appleton; 1895.

34. Park RE, Burgess EW. *Introduction to the Science of Sociology.* Chicago: University of Chicago Press; 1921.

35. Paris REL. *Chicago Sociology, 1920–1932.* Chicago: University of Chicago Press; 1967.

36. Cassell J. The contribution of the social environment to host resistance. *Am J Epidemiol.* 1974;104:107–123.

37. Caplan G. *Support Systems and Community Mental Health.* New York: Behavioral Publications; 1974.

38. Gottlieb BH. The development and application of a classification scheme of informal helping behaviors. *Can J Behav Sci.* 1978;10:105–115.

39. House JS. *Work Stress and Social Support.* Reading, Mass: Addison-Wesley; 1981.

40. Cobb S. Social support as a moderator of life stress. *Psychoso Med.* 1976;38:300–314.

41. Shils FA, Janowitz M. Cohesion and disintegration in the Wehrmacht in World War II. *Public Opinion Q.* 1948;12:280–315.

42. Griffith J. The Army's new unit personnel replacement and its relationship to unit cohesion and social support. *Milit Psychol.* 1989;1:17–34.

43. Holmes R. *Acts of War.* New York: Free Press; 1985.

44. Fergusson B. *The Wild Green Earth.* London: Cassell; 1946.

45. McDonald CB. *Company Commander*. New York: Bantam; 1978.

46. Ellis J. *The Sharp End*. New York: Charles Scribner's Sons; 1980.

47. Sassoon S. *Memoirs of an Infantry Officer*. London: Coward-McCann; 1930.

48. Dollard J. Fear in Battle. Washington, DC: *Infantry J*. 1944.

49. Camp NM, Carney CM. *Painful Memories and Crushing Burdens: U.S. Army Psychiatrists in the Vietnam War*. Westport, Conn: Greenwood Press; 1989.

50. Gal R. Courage under stress. In: Breznitz S, ed. *Stress in Israel*. New York: Van Nostrand Rheinhold; 1983: 65–91.

51. Gal R. Unit morale: From a theoretical puzzle to an empirical illustration—an Israeli example. *J Appl Soc Psychol*. 1986;16:549–564.

52. Malone DM. *Small Unit Leadership*, Novato, Calif: Presidio; 1983.

53. Crane S. *The Red Badge of Courage*. New York: W.W. Norton; 1976.

54. George AL. Primary groups, organization, and military performance. In: Little RW, ed. *Handbook of Military Institutions*. Beverly Hills, Calif: Sage; 1971: 293–318.

55. Marlowe DH, ed. *New Manning System Field Evaluation*. Washington, DC: Walter Reed Army Institute of Research; 1985. Technical Report 1.

56. Marlowe DH, ed. *New Manning System Field Evaluation*. Washington, DC: Walter Reed Army Institute of Research; 1986. Technical Report 2.

57. Gross N, Martin WT. On group cohesiveness. *Am J Sociol*. 1952;57:546–554.

58. Kviz FJ. Survival in combat as a collective exchange process. *J Polit Milit Sociol*. 1978;6:219–232.

59. Watson P. *War on the Mind: The Military Uses and Abuses of Psychology*. London: Hutchinson; 1978.

60. Tziner A, Vardi Y. Ability as a moderator between cohesiveness and tank crew performance. *J Occup Behav*. 1983;4:137–143.

61. Solomon Z, Mikulincer M, Hobfill SE. Effects of social support and battle intensity on loneliness and breakdown during combat. *J Pers Soc Psychol*. 1986;51:1269–1276.

62. Oldenquist A. On belonging to tribes. *Newsweek*. 1982;(April 5):9.

63. Heinl RD, Jr. *Dictionary of Military and Naval Quotations*. Annapolis, Md: US Naval Institute; 1967.

64. Mauldin W. *Up Front*. New York: Holt and Company; 1945.

65. Bond TC. The why of fragging. *Am J Psychiatry*. 1976;133(11):1328–1331.

66. Ingraham LH, Manning FJ. Cohesion: Who needs it, what is it, and how do we get it to them? *Milit Rev*. 1981;61(6):2–12.

67. Bidwell S. *Modern Warfare*. London: Allen Lane; 1973.

68. US Department of the Army. *Unit Climate Profile Commander's Handbook*. Washington, DC:DA;1986. DA PAM 600–69.

Chapter 2

MILITARY FAMILIES AND COMBAT READINESS

ROBERT J. SCHNEIDER, Ph.D.* AND JAMES A. MARTIN, Ph.D.†

*Lieutenant Colonel (ret), Medical Service Corps, U.S. Army; Guest Scientist, Department of Military Psychiatry, Division of Neuropsychiatry, Walter Reed Army Institute of Research, Washington, D.C. 20307-5100

†Colonel, Medical Service Corps, U.S. Army; Executive Assistant to the U.S. Army Assistant Surgeon General for Medical Research, Development, and Acquisition, Fort Detrick, Maryland 21702-5012; formerly Commander, U.S. Army Medical Research Unit—Europe; formerly Deputy Director, Department of Military Psychiatry, Division of Neuropsychiatry, Walter Reed Army Institute of Research, Washington, D.C.

INTRODUCTION

This chapter examines military family issues associated with combat readiness. It includes a description of the history of the still-evolving relation between the military and its families. Discussion of military culture is included to enhance understanding of current military beliefs, customs, and actions. Both military history and military culture have shaped and determined how the military and its families interact and affect one another. Their inclusion is necessary to understand the military-family interface in the modern armed forces. It is within this interface that families can affect military readiness. Finally, the chapter highlights the importance of institutional efforts to build and sustain healthy, self-reliant families as a factor in promoting military readiness. The information in this chapter is important for all operational mental health personnel supporting divisions and corps, including mental health teams and hospital sections. It is also important for garrison mental health and human services agencies and even has value for local social service agencies supporting military families. The active-duty U.S. Army is the primary focus of this chapter. However, the issues discussed are relevant to the other U.S. military services (Navy, Marine Corps, and Air Force). Some of the issues also apply to Reserve and National Guard component service members and their families.

Historically, military families were not included in the discussion of organizational prevention of combat stress casualties or any other aspect of military readiness. The military family was simply not considered a part of military readiness. This is not surprising because until fairly recently (circa 1967), our enlisted military force comprised mostly single men (61%).[1] Among units that actually face the enemy on the battlefield (combat and combat support units), it was unusual to find married soldiers in the enlisted ranks. Wives were primarily associated with higher ranking servicemen (who have generally adequate pay and good support groups), who had the time and experience to have adjusted to military life. This ensured that there was no historical precedent for considering family effects on readiness. This situation changed during the past 20 years (1970–1990). The change was due to the accumulation of data from a number of sources[2,3,4] that unequivocally demonstrated that families can and do affect military readiness.

Military unit readiness is assessed routinely. It is based on a numerical score determined by comparing the actual availability of personnel and material with a published description of what the unit requires (at 100% strength). This measure is not fully relevant to discuss organizational factors affecting soldier functioning because an important aspect of our discussion concerns psychological readiness. Therefore, in this chapter, *unit readiness* is defined to comprise additional (but inherently more difficult to measure) attributes. We define *readiness* as a combination of a soldier's willingness and ability to do his job and cope in peacetime and during combat, and the army's ability to retain trained service members during peacetime. Obviously this definition involves much more than a simple manpower count.

We now know that family life affects a service member's military performance during peacetime and during combat. Families play a major role in the army's retention of personnel and also affect the service member's well-being. The military has its own set of regulations, cultural norms, and behavioral proscriptions. These affect military families, especially when they are not congruent with behaviors acceptable to the larger society. At the same time, the service member's duties and military situation can have an important effect on family life and family member well-being. The dynamic and reciprocal relations between these institutions (military and family) vary across the family life cycle and the soldier's career.

Before the creation of an all-volunteer U.S. Army in 1973, less than one-fourth of junior enlisted soldiers were married, although the majority (80%) of older officers and noncommissioned officers (NCOs) were married.[1] This adoption of the all-volunteer military established the pattern for the current married career military force. It is important to remember that the composition of army families is not static. Every year large numbers of families leave the military and return to civilian life, while other new families join (or are established in) the army.

The timing of this change also coincided with numerous changes in U.S. society's views and expectations about family composition and family member roles. Today, the employed husband-father and his homemaker wife-mother no longer reflect the normative U.S. family. Like society at large, the military services also have a wide variety of family types, including dual-career families, single-parent families, and families where the wife is the military member and the husband is a civilian dependent. Despite this variety, the career component of the military, especially the army, is still composed almost exclusively of stable, two-parent families,[5] and traditional family values remain the institutional norm.

In 1983, the U.S. Army formally embraced the family when the then Army Chief of Staff, General John A. Wickham, Jr., issued a white paper stating that "A partnership exists between the Army and Army families. . . . Towards the goal of building a strong partnership, the Army remains committed to assuring adequate support to families in order to promote wellness; to develop a sense of community; and to strengthen the mutually reinforcing bonds between the Army and its families."[6] Underlying this partnership was a clear sense of its import to the mission: The Army recruits soldiers but retains families.[6] Headquarters, Department of the Army, proclaimed 1984 as the Year of the Army Family. During 1984, the first in a series of Army Action Plans was developed, and the army established the U.S. Army Community and Family Support Center, a major headquarters office, to oversee the development and operation of all army-family policies and programs. In 1988, this center became a Department of Defense organization.

While there are some demographic differences between services, the major difference in family demographics (and especially family lifestyle) is in the comparison between military and civilian populations. The vast majority of today's military families are young couples with small children. When compared to their civilian age cohorts, military members marry earlier, bear children at an earlier age, and have somewhat more children than their civilian counterparts. There are also proportionally fewer single parent families in the Army than in the similar-aged civilian population.[7] From an economic perspective, all army families have at least the income of one parent and access to a range of health and social service resources sometimes not available to civilian families.

CHANGING EXPECTATIONS AND CHANGING CULTURE

During the most recent 20-year period (1970s to 1990s), all the military services have been confronted by society's increased expectations for benefits, services, and employment accommodations for spouses and for expectations for a range of family-related services, such as programs for the handicapped, special needs children, and recently dependent elderly parents. In addition, adoption of the all-volunteer force resulted in a current force that is predominantly married and contains a stable but small minority of alternate family types (eg, single-parent families, dual-career families, and so forth). The dramatic increase in the number of young enlisted families led to a corresponding need to expand and enhance a variety of family support services designed to ease some of the stressors associated with military life. In response to this need, the Department of Defense developed a variety of programs and administrative services such as the child care centers and volunteer-based community service programs to support and manage the needs of military families. The stressors can be categorized into two major areas: (1) cultural, based on organizational norms developed over the years; and (2) military life, based on unit demands on the service member.

Cultural Norms and Family Stress

Until the 1980s, all family members were referred to by the term *dependent*. Military regulations reflected the fact that the spouse (typically the wife) and children were dependent on the military member (typically the male) for all support, including access to military benefits and services. The term *dependent* is now considered to be pejorative in nature; the term *family member* is currently the acceptable way to refer to a spouse or child of a military member. This change was fostered in part by effective women advocates pressing military leaders for change, including a change in overall status as a military spouse (Wickham's concept of partnership referred to earlier). However, the term *dependent* is still well entrenched in the minds and vocabulary of the active military forces today.

Before the increases in the number of married enlisted soldiers, military families were predominantly wives of NCOs and officers. There was an expectation that these wives would support their husband's military careers by performing various service or charitable activities. Senior enlisted and officers' families were implicitly made part of the military, but they received little formal recognition and no compensation.

Today, however, military spouses are increasingly likely to be employed outside the home. The spouses of career military members may also be trying to establish their independent careers. In spite of these trends, military spouses often feel that they should not work, and they are sometimes even made to feel that it is their duty to volunteer for post community activities. Not long ago, complaints by a group of U.S. Air Force wives led to a letter by the Secretary of Defense banning such pressure in all services.[8] However, military culture based on the traditional premise that wives are dependents will undoubtedly continue to foster these competing roles and competing demands. It is easy to see how the stress normally associated with such expectations is exacerbated in a marriage where one partner is often unavailable for "domestic duty" because of the priority attached to military duties and where frequent separations are considered the norm.

Military spouses are subjected to the demands of a number of competing, overlapping, and sometimes mutually exclusive roles. The military spouse is often idealized as a competent homemaker, mother, and volunteer. While the number of single parents, male spouses of service members, and the number of dual-career couples are relatively small in comparison with the traditional male service member (female family member, military family), the issues of balancing the requirements of military duty and family life are even more complicated and often more stressful for these families. The military has historically supported rank-based wives clubs (generally for officers and NCOs wives) that perform both social and charitable functions. Today's unit-based family support groups did not evolve until the 1980s. Although their precise purpose varies by military command and facility, the most common functions of these sanctioned spouse groups are to enhance communication between the unit and wives and to encourage development of social supports to help buffer against stress commonly associated with military life. In particular, they are to help families cope during lengthy unit training or operational deployments. Today's family support group generally mimics the military chain of command, and the commander's wife is usually the leader. This hierarchy is sometimes referred to as a "chain of concern." Members serve as an important communication link between the military unit and spouses connected with it and ensure that spouses have a support group when their active duty partners are deployed.

Spouses of all ranks are supposedly able to, and are even expected to (by the military), associate freely and work together. After all, the spouse has no military rank, but many wives "wear" the rank of their soldier husbands. Especially among the spouses of higher ranking service members, many expect status benefits to accrue from their own years of marital association with the military. These contrary expectations led to the presumption that wives of different rank soldiers must not socialize; this presumption is firmly embedded in the military's traditional culture. This implicit norm is occasionally asserted explicitly; it is tacitly understood by seasoned military husbands and wives alike. Indeed, such interspouse socialization is labeled as a form of fraternization and is often alleged to be "against the regulations." (Fraternization is a military term for inappropriate interrank relationships). Although no such regulation concerning spouses has ever existed, the myth of a spousal fraternization ban exerts great influence on family-to-family relationships in military communities and within units. The effect can be to decrease social integration and social support, isolate those lower ranking families who most need help, and reduce familial support for the service member to remain on active duty.

Some family members remain out of the reach of unit family support programs. For example, a wife who elects (or is required) to remain in the United States when her husband is assigned overseas is usually not carried as a member of any military family support group even if she has remained in the vicinity of an army installation. Army-sponsored support programs for these "waiting" spouses are typically weak or nonexistent. These waiting families are full-fledged military families with all the rights and privileges due any family member, but practically and administratively they are treated quite differently (ie, they are often ignored). As the U.S. Army downsizes and reduces the number of soldiers stationed overseas, short-term, unaccompanied tours of duty and long training deployments will become the norm. As a result, more families will find themselves in this difficult and sometimes ambiguous waiting category.

Single parents are officially recognized as military heads of households and provided the same financial and service benefits as married soldiers. However, within the Army's very traditional culture they are sometimes not well tolerated by unit leaders and are usually ignored by formal spouse organizations. Soldiers who are single parents usually are not included in formal unit family activities such as support groups. Single parents are also not usually included in unit mailings to military families.

In many cases, these cultural aspects of the military work against the adjustment of the young military family. It is the young family with a low income that is at greatest risk for coping problems. The U.S. Army has a large number of such families, many with very small children. Regardless of the nature of their extended family relationships, these families often lack the immediate availability of extended family support during some of the most difficult and challenging phases of both marital and military life. The increased stress this places on the soldier can certainly decrease his effectiveness on the job during peacetime training and wartime combat. To the extent that spouses are dissatisfied with family life in the military, they will not support further active duty by the service member.

The marital and parenting issues associated with these family responsibilities may distract or physically impede the soldier from participating in unit training activities, and when severe, these family-life difficulties (eg, a spouse's severe illness or injury) may make the soldier nondeployable for combat. In this sense, family problems present serious readiness challenges for small unit commanders and military service care providers, for example, social workers, family counselors, drug and alcohol counselors, and other specialists.

Military Life and Stress

Unit factors, especially the attitude and behaviors of small unit leaders, have a tremendous effect on soldier well-being and, in turn, on the well-being of the soldier's family. When leadership and morale in the unit suffer, the problem is often transferred to home and family. Army policy and policies made at division, brigade, and battalion levels affect the soldier in a general way. But the day-to-day coping and adjustment of the typical soldier and his family are determined by the attitudes and behaviors of the soldier's company commander, first sergeant, platoon sergeant, and squad leader. This is one of the reasons why small unit leadership is such a critical dimension of military readiness, and it provides a model for understanding the reciprocal relation between the army and its families.

In spite of the change in the official attitude, unit leader attitudes and practices often betray a contrary belief that does not include family members as full-fledged partners in the military mission. For example, we have observed rules against wives telephoning the military unit, expectations that wives must join affiliated wives' clubs, ignorance of spouses' and children's needs for a reasonably predictable time off-duty, and the need for reasonable duty schedules with sufficient time off to meet family needs. Such practices contribute to negative attitudes toward further military service. On the other hand, when unit leaders attend to the issue in a positive way, enhanced family adjustment and commitment to the military can result.

There is a common belief[5] among military family advocates that family life in the military is more stressful than civilian family life. This assertion is based on factors like frequent, prolonged, or unannounced absences; "lockins"; long and often irregular duty hours with a corresponding inability to share domestic and child care responsibilities; frequent family moves; legal constraints and requirements of military service; and stress associated with training with modern weapons and the real possibility of deployment to a combat zone. Frequent reassignment and relocations may have a negative impact on the military family member's personal well-being, employment, and career opportunities. These beliefs are supported by research. For example, Lewis[9] reported that U.S. Air Force wives viewed their lives as more stressful than their civilian counterparts, and Pierce and Luchsinger[10] found that U.S. Air Force wives reported greater psychological stress than comparable civilian wives. Vernez[11] concluded that the U.S. Army environment is yet more stressful for families than is that of the other services.

Many of these military life stressors impact on children. Father (and now, mother) absence can have a profound negative impact on children's social and psychological development.[12,13] Furthermore, family relocations require children to change schools and disrupt their social networks of friends, teachers, and other important sources of developmental support. The developmental problems to which this mobility can contribute were reported by Shaw and Pangman.[14] While some civilian families experience similar stressors, no one group in American society is so institutionally bound to an organization for all aspects of life as is the military family.

For most soldiers, worries about the home front can be a source of severe distress, can jeopardize the individual soldier's ability to adequately participate in training activities, and most important can interfere with the soldier's ability to adequately perform his combat role. Worry or preoccupation with home-front issues jeopardizes self and other unit members, risks the success of the mission, and places the soldier at risk for psychological breakdown. In modern combat, these problems can be more severe than ever before. Deployed soldiers may be engaged in combat within hours or days of arrival into the theater of operations. They may have little if any time to shift their mental focus from family to the events at hand. Even in the remotest parts of the world, current technology allows soldiers instantaneous telephone communication with their families. While this contact can be comforting to soldiers and their families, it also means that there is no buffer (of time and psychological distance) between the soldier and family. Loneliness and immediate concerns about well-being are brought into the present in a situation where the soldier and family are relatively helpless to effect any change or provide real comfort. This situation presents a tremendous challenge for all small unit leaders.

Across a typical military career, families face a variety of life-cycle issues. These issues include marriage, birth of children, raising and educating children, moving households, career decisions of civilian spouses, and so forth. Various life stages will be stressful for some families and most families will experience some type of family or individual member physical, psychological, or social crisis during one or more of these periods. Such personal or family crises inevitably have at least a temporary impact on the service member's military performance. This impact means that military leaders must be able to manage soldiers' experiencing family difficulties and at the same time to ensure that the unit's mission is accomplished. Leaders require the skill and knowledge to direct the soldier to seek and make use of appropriate military and civilian services designed to correct or ameliorate family-related stress. Otherwise, family issues will adversely affect the soldier's performance and reenlistment and, in turn, unit readiness.

While military families may experience unique stressors associated with their military lifestyle, some unique aspects of social and emotional support distinguish military from civilian family life. By the nature of their transient lifestyle, career military families find that other military family members and various unit and military community-based organizations become over time their primary source of tangible and emotional support. This is particularly true for soldiers in the combat arms and soldiers associated with combat units. Regardless of the strength of their initial extended family ties, across the time and distance of a military career these ties usually diminish (at least as sources of everyday tangible support). If they are replaced, it is usually by ties to other military families that they have come to know across the experiences of shared time and military-related hardships.

Military families typically develop strong relationships with other military families based on their shared experiences, proximity, and similar life circumstances. Frequent relocations force military families to continually re-create local friendships. A shared military identity and daily activities involving the use of common installation programs and services facilitate relationship development in this somewhat nomadic lifestyle. Regardless of rank, most military families use the post (base) exchange and the commissary. Most also use the military medical facilities as needed, and many live in military housing. Specific stressors, such as spouse absence due to training requirements, or stressors associated with an actual combat deployment serve to facilitate bonding among military families.

Military families also have access to a wealth of support agencies; few of these agencies are available to the public at large or from other civilian employers. It is this institutional commitment to family well-being, especially during a deployment, that provides soldiers the psychological capacity to leave family and place their lives in danger.

There are also many myths about military family life. One of these is that military families are bonded together in close knit military communities. While some military families live in the all-encompassing confines of a military installation, most military families live offpost, and much of their life (religious activities, education of their children, family recreation, and shopping) centers on activities in the civilian sector, not on the military installation. Even for military families who do live on post, most typically perceive their sense of community in terms of their neighborhood—the area comprising the houses and apartments on a few streets around them.[15] This operational face-to-face level organizes important daily aspects of their family life.[16] However, military families living overseas are increasingly likely to live on a military installation and to use military facilities and services. As the number of military families overseas continues to decline and as the monetary exchange rates in these host countries diminish the value of the dollar, these trends will continue.

FAMILY ISSUES AND READINESS

Retention

Military readiness includes the retention of trained service members. The link between family issues and retention has been well documented. Moghadam,[17] in a study across time, found that wives' attitudes towards reenlistment were as important as soldiers' intent in predicting soldiers later actual reenlistment behavior. Lewis[9] found that wives' attitudes toward reenlistment in the U.S. Air Force predicted career intent of their airman husbands. Dansby and Hightower[18] reported job-related satisfaction and retention were related to spouses' attitude toward and commitment to the military. Two studies of retention in the Navy reported similar conclusions. Sehoda and Szoa[19] and Bruce[20] found that wives' attitudes related significantly to their husband's career intent. The former study included follow-up and confirmed that career intent predicts retention behavior fairly accurately.

The implication that the military must attend to family needs to maintain force levels is clear. This issue will become more critical in the future if current demographic trends continue. Thus, the personnel pool of young men and women is predicted to shrink. At the same time, job complexity with its increased training costs and costs to replace skilled workers will continue to rise. Unfortunately, military leaders and those responsible for family programs do not always agree on priorities for resources, programs, and demands on troop time. Military leaders typically give priority to the immediate mission; family program managers give priority to family needs. Long-term consequences (eg, spouses might not support continued military service) are rarely considered by local military leaders. Nichols[21] pointed out that family issues need to be integrated into the broader concerns of military operations and military management. A report by the Army Science Board (an independent advisory group to the Secretary of the Army) concluded. "Recognition of the powerful impacts of the family on readiness, retention, morale and motivation must be instilled in every soldier from the soldier's date of entry-to-service through each succeeding promotion."[22(p5)]

Military Performance

The link between family issues and military performance is supported primarily by assertion and belief and only somewhat by empirical research. A bibliography of military research prepared by the Military Family Resource Center in 1984[2] illustrates this point. Of the more than 200 references listed, none involve an empirical study of the influence of families on military readiness. At the same time, military leaders need to know more about the military life factors that are known to influence family member well-being, general life satisfaction, and support of a spouse's decision to remain in the military. These factors include length and predictability of duty hours, training absences, deployments, family relocation, unit communication with families, and unit support during temporary family difficulties. Many of these factors are controlled or influenced by local commanders and are likely to have variable impacts depending on factors such as the service member's military and family life stage.

While there are only a limited number of empirical studies linking readiness and family issues, there are considerable data[4,23,24] from which one can infer a family impact on readiness. For example, domestic problems in the home are believed to translate into decreased combat effectiveness and increased risk for death on the battlefield. Data from the Israeli Defence Force (IDF) show that 30% of their casualties in the Lebanon War were due to combat stress reaction, a temporary breakdown due to accumulated stress. It renders the soldier dysfunctional and unable to effectively carry on. The IDF found that soldiers who had experienced certain marital discord or stress in personal relationships (parents or girl-friend) were at especially high risk to suffer a combat stress reaction.[25,26]

U.S. Army medical personnel have frequently reported[27,28] that both military sick call and family member outpatient visits increase just before a deployment, probably due in part to an increase in family stress. Knudson and colleagues[27] demonstrated negative changes in the general well-being of wives associated with their husbands' deployment. In 1979, a major study[29] of the relation between unit deployment and various associated health problems was begun at the Walter Reed Army Institute of Research. This study was among the first to detail the reciprocal relation between family life stress and soldier adaptation. A similar military–family life reciprocal relation was demonstrated by Schneider and coworkers[30] in a report showing that wives' adjustment is related to morale in their husbands' military unit (and unit morale is a commonly accepted readiness factor).

Other investigators[4,31] reported that individual performance and combat efficiency are in part dependent on marital and family issues. For example, Dooms[32] reported on a U.S. Air Force–Europe study that identified broadly defined personal and family factors related to air crew stress as figuring in 7 of the command's 10 aircraft crashes during the study period. Although these last results were based on expert opinion (rather than on quantitative data), they point out a dramatic and important relation between family issues and military performance.

The Present

While there are still family issues that need to be addressed, the Persian Gulf War resulted in a number of changes in policies and programs and represents a high-water mark in the relation between the U.S. Army and the U.S. Army family. (The same is true for each of the other services and, to a lesser degree, the U.S. Army Reserve Components.) When U.S. military forces began their deployment to Southwest Asia, senior Department of Defense officials spoke publicly about our nation's commitment to our military families. National and local news media described the stress experienced by military families and showed stories about family courage and commitment. For army leaders in the United States and Germany taking care of the families of deployed soldiers was a primary mission.

Military installations, often with the support of the surrounding civilian communities, became a focal point for making certain that the deployed soldier's family was enmeshed in a social support safety net. An array of programs and services were set in place to cover a range of contingencies from normal life stressors such as the car breaking down to the crisis posed by the potential of mass combat casualties. No military service in history ever devoted more resources to sustaining its military families.[33]

The Persian Gulf War provided an extensive test of the various components of the military's family support system. For the most part, family support efforts worked well. Overall, only a small percentage of active duty soldiers were not able to deploy because of severe family problems, and few soldiers had to return early due to family problems. Even the army families already deployed in Europe weathered this deployment without large numbers of families returning to the United States. However, the Persian Gulf War demonstrated that the U.S. military, and particularly the Army, cannot deploy a major force into combat without the reserve components. The Persian Gulf War was a convincing demonstration that being a member of the military reserves requires being prepared to put civilian life aside for an extended period of active duty, possibly in a combat zone. Many reservists, their spouses, and their children were not adequately prepared for this reality, and as a result, they experienced significant distress during the deployment. A U.S. Army review[34] of these experiences highlights the need to substantially enhance reserve component family support services and benefits.

The Persian Gulf War deployment, particularly of an already forward deployed force in Europe and large numbers of Reserve and National Guard personnel, demonstrated a depth and range of family needs that sometimes exceeded institutional plans, capabilities, and leadership expectations. As a result, a new era has emerged. The leadership focus has shifted from taking care of families to promoting family readiness. By family readiness, leaders mean enhancing family self-sufficiency so that the family supports and sustains the soldier in peacetime and during war and does not become an additional source of stress for the deployed soldier to carry onto the battlefield. The Persian Gulf War provided a powerful example of the important relation between the military family and the army. This is a relation that exists at the level of the soldier's unit, the installation where the family resides, and the senior levels of the army where family policy is developed and managed.

Survey and interview data[33] suggest that the most important sources of support for most of these military families were their relationships with immediate friends, neighbors, and especially the families of other unit members. Unit-based family support groups, facilitated by assistance from the unit rear detachment, were primary sources of information, practical assistance with day-to-day family life problems, and personal social support. Just knowing that there was a family support group available to assist in an emergency provided the spouses of deployed soldiers a sense of comfort and security.

The Future

The rest of the 1990s presents enormous challenges for the U.S. Army and the other military services. The demise of the Soviet Union and the birth of democracy in eastern Europe shifts the focus of military readiness from the threat of global war with the now defunct Warsaw Pact to rapid response to regional confrontations, such as the invasion of Panama, the Persian Gulf War, and the humanitarian relief effort in Somalia. At the same time, Europe is evolving beyond the post-World War II structure that has dominated United States-European relations for the past 40 years. There has also been marked flux in the relation between North Korea and South Korea. Overall, the direct outcome of these changes will be a much smaller U.S. military. Army forces will be primarily based in the United States yet will be required to be constantly ready for rapid deployment for a range of worldwide contingencies. In terms of reduction in size and relocation of personnel from overseas back to the United States, the army has borne the brunt of these changes. The other services and the reserve components have been affected, but to a lesser degree.

It is possible that the 1991 army's 750,000 members will be reduced in size by 1995 to a force of about 450,000 soldiers. This reduction is a very stressful process for soldiers and families and creates an extended period of uncertainty for everyone. For those leaving the army as a result of force reduction, the move back to areas in the United States with weak economies and high unemployment rates makes the transition all the more difficult. Some individual and family problems and conditions (eg, a child with a severe physical handicap requiring lifelong specialized care) may also require a decision to leave military service. (This decision may come voluntarily or be directed by the army if the condition prevents the soldier from meeting his military duty requirements.) These are often questions of individual and family values and lifestyle choices and / or an official recognition that for a variety of reasons, the individual does not meet retention standards. Individuals faced with such decisions need counseling and institutional support. Family members may also benefit from professional advice and counseling to ease the difficulties associated with transition back to civilian life. Organizations that have a climate of caring provide employees with outplacement counseling and transition assistance. The recent implementation of the Army Career and Alumni Program (ACAP) to assist soldiers' (and family members') transition back into civilian life demonstrates this enlightened attitude.

The all-volunteer force means that the majority of service members, especially in the career grades, will continue to be married. If there are any substantial demographic changes in the composition of the force, they are likely to be changes among those family types (single parents and dual-career couples) who face the greatest challenge maintaining their ability to meet family demands, the increased requirement for extensive training absences, and the need to be available for immediate worldwide deployment. For example, the Persian Gulf War demonstrated that family care plans (for single and dual-career military parents) have to be realistic and take into consideration extended absences and the possibility of combat. The Persian Gulf War made it clear that the requirement to deploy involves everyone in uniform including those in the reserves. These are all readiness requirements that cannot be taken lightly.

Downsizing the military, returning forces to the United States, and in particular maintaining a worldwide rapid deployment capability will have an enormous impact on military family life. Retaining only the best will add pressure to the perceived greedy relation that already exists between duty and family life demands.[15] While an army based primarily in a small number of U.S. installations may provide an opportunity for longer periods between family moves, the focus on readiness for rapid deployment and contingency operations requirements will likely mean frequent training deployments, including extended 3-, 6-, or 12-month overseas unit-training exercises. These deployments bring with them added stress for the soldiers, the spouses, and especially the children who have to shoulder this readiness burden.

In addition, there is always the possibility of military involvement in what appears to be a growing array of regional, ethnic-based conflicts, as well as the likelihood of our using military personnel to assist in a variety of worldwide humanitarian relief efforts. For an army that is composed primarily of soldiers who have significant family responsibilities, the relation between the stress of a military lifestyle and family life remains a critically important topic. The fact that the majority of these military families will continue to be young and inexperienced and without a readily available extended family support system heightens these concerns.

CONCLUSION

A paucity of married soldiers and cultural values established in the all male military in which wives were "dependents" delayed recognition of the vital role families play in readiness. Today, military family policy is one element of a national defense policy. Military families play an important role in recruitment, retention, and commitment to the combat mission. Even good soldiers distracted by family concerns do not make effective soldiers. Family issues affect individual and unit readiness and function as a protective factor in preventing combat stress reactions. The U.S. military services have made a substantial commitment to family wellness. These efforts view family members as true partners in a military that is seen as a way of life, not simply a job. The family's responsibility in this partnership is to support the service member and other unit families and to participate in building and sustaining healthy, supportive military organizations. The military's responsibility is to create an environment where families and family members can prosper and realize their potential.

The future has many implications for this partnership. The structure of the military, the way it trains and operates, and the demands that it will make as an institution on service members and their families will continue. What is not changing is the basic premise that the volunteer force concept will continue to be the way the United States staffs its armed forces. The force will continue to be composed primarily of married personnel, especially in the career ranks but increasingly among newer and younger service members. Family life will continue to be an important source of strength and support for soldiers, and family life stress will remain an important readiness issue for all the military services.

REFERENCES

1. Military Family Clearinghouse. *Military Family Demographics: Profile of the Military Family.* Arlington, Va: Military Family Clearinghouse; June 1992.

2. Military Family Resource Center. *Review of Military Family Research and Literature: Annotated Bibliography.* Washington, DC: Military Family Resource Center; 1984.

3. Burnam MA, Meredith LS, Sherbourne CD, Valdez RB, Vernez G. *Army Families and Soldier Readiness.* Santa Monica, Calif: Rand Corporation; 1992.

4. Kirkland FR, Katz P. Combat readiness and the Army family. *Milit Rev.* 1989;69:64–74.

5. Segal MW, Harris JJ. *What We Know About Army Families.* Alexandria, Va: US Army Research Institute for the Behavioral and Social Sciences; 1993. Special report 21.

6. Wickham JA, Jr. *The Army Family.* Washington, DC: Chief of Staff, Headquarters, US Department of the Army. 15 August 1983. White Paper.

7. Vernez G, Zellman GL. *Families and Mission: A Review of the Effects of Family Factors on Army Attrition, Retention, and Readiness.* Santa Monica, Calif: Rand Corporation; 1987.

8. Willis G. DOD letter affirms spouses' right to work. *Army Times.* 1987;48(12):3.

9. Lewis PM. *Family Factors and Career Intent of Air Force Enlisted Personnel.* Maxwell Air Force Base: Leadership and Management Development Center; 1985. Report LMDC–TR–85–9.

10. Pierce MM, Luchsinger ML. Psychological distress among air force wives. In: *Proceedings of the 10th Symposium on Psychology in the Department of Defense*. Colorado Springs, Colo: US Air Force Academy; 1986. 643–648.

11. Vernez G. *Enhancing the Effectiveness of Army Family Programs. Overview and Status Report*. Washington, DC: Rand Corporation; 1988.

12. Baker S, Fagan S, Fischer E, Janda E, Cove L. Impact of father absence on personality factors of boys: An evaluation of the family's adjustment. *Am J Orthopsychiatry*. 1967;37:269.

13. Schneider RJ, Kojac G, Ressdorf H. Father distance and drug abuse in young men. *J Nerv Ment Dis*. 1977;165:269–274.

14. Shaw JA, Pangman J. Geographic mobility and the military child. *Milit Med*. 1975;140(6):413–416.

15. Segal M. The military and the family as greedy institutions. *Armed Forces Society*. 1986;13:9–38.

16. Schneider RJ, Gilley M, Family adjustment in USAREUR. Washington, DC: Walter Reed Army Institute of Research; 1984. Unpublished technical report.

17. Moghadam LL. *The Reciprocal Nature of Work and Family: Perception of the Work/Family Interface and Its Impact on Army Reenlistment Behavior*. College Park, Md: University of Maryland; 1989. Thesis.

18. Dansby MR, Hightower JM. *Family and Work in the Air Force*. 1984. Alexandria, Va: Defense Technical Information Center Report AD–P003324.

19. Seboda BL, Szoa R. *Family Factors Critical to the Retention of Naval Personnel: The Link Between Retention Intention and Retention Behavior*. 1984. Alexandria, Va: Defense Technical Information Center Report AD–A144–492.

20. Bruce RA. The family separation catchall. *Naval Institute Proceedings*. 1986;(October):110–111.

21. Nichols RS. The military family/military organization interface: A discussion. In: Hunter EJ, Nice S, eds. *The Military Family and Military Organization*. New York: Praeger Publishers; 1978.

22. Army Science Board. *The Army Community and Their Families*. Washington, DC: Office of the Secretary of the Army; Research, Development, and Acquisition; 1989.

23. Rosen LN. Human factors in Operation Desert Shield: The role of family factors. Presented at the Department of Defense Operation Desert Shield Task Force Meeting; 8 November 1990; Alexandria, Va.

24. Sadacca R, Stawarski C, DiFazio A. *Preliminary Analysis of the Impact of Army and Family Factors on Individual Readiness*. Alexandria, Va: US Army Research Institute for the Behavioral and Social Sciences; 1993. Technical report 967 (AD A139–803).

25. Noy S. Stress and personality as factors in the causality and prognosis of combat reactions. Presented at the Second International Conference on Psychological Stress and Adjustment in War and Peace; 19–23 June 1978; Jerusalem, Israel.

26. Neumann M, Levy A. A specific military installation for treatment of combat reactions during the war in Lebanon. *Milit Med*. 1984;149:196–199.

27. Knudson KHM, Jellen LK, Harris J, Schneider RJ. Health and family problems related to short term army deployments. Presented at the annual meeting of the American Psychological Association; August 1982; Washington, DC.

28. Rothberg JM, Harris JJ, Jellen LK, Pickle R. Illness and health of the U.S. battalion in the Sinai MFO deployment. *Armed Forces Soc*. 1985;11:413–426.

29. Van Vranken EW, Jellen LK, Knudson KH, et al. *The Impact of Deployment Separation on Army Families*. Washington, DC: Walter Reed Army Institute of Research; August 1984. Technical Report NP–84–6.

30. Schneider R, Vaitkus M, Hoover E. Military unit climate and spouse adjustment. Washington, DC: Department of Military Psychiatry, Walter Reed Army Institute of Research; 1987. Unpublished paper.

31. Griffith JD, Helms RF. *Unit Demands on Soldiers and Families*. Alexandria, Va: US Army Research Institute for the Behavioral and Social Sciences; 1993. Technical report 985.

32. Dooms C. USAFE study ties stress to air crashes. *Stars and Stripes*. 1983;41(280):1.

33. Teitelbaum JM. Unit level spouse support and generic family assistance at major Army posts during Operation Desert Shield/Storm. Presented at the Inter-University Seminar on Armed Forces and Society, Biennial International Conference; 12 October 1991; Baltimore, Md.

34. US Army Combined Arms Command. *The Yellow Ribbon: Army Lessons Learned From the Home Front*. Fort Leavenworth, Kans: Center for Army Lessons Learned; 1991.

Chapter 3

BURNOUT IN MILITARY PERSONNEL

VICTORIA L. WILCOX, Ph.D.*

**Assistant Professor, Department of Community Health, Brown University, Providence, Rhode Island 02912; former Postdoctoral Fellow, Department of Epidemiology and Public Health, Yale University School of Medicine, New Haven, Connecticut; Guest Scientist, Division of Neuropsychiatry, Walter Reed Army Institute of Research, Washington, D.C.*

INTRODUCTION

In 1947, Sobel[1] described soldiers who were "burnt out" and "worn out." These were highly dedicated, previously very efficient soldiers who, after prolonged, continuous exposure to combat, became reluctant to accept responsibility for others, began to show difficulty in making decisions, and came to prefer routine, simple tasks over more challenging ones. They had difficulty making new friends and instead tended to be viewed as "callous, cold task masters, and slave drivers." [1(p316)] They exhibited symptoms of mild depression and a loss of self-confidence, as manifested in a tendency to make self-deprecatory remarks. Their ability to carry out their duties deteriorated to the point that they became unfit for combat and a handicap to their units. In spite of these changes, their motivation to carry out the mission remained steadfast. Because they were often noncommissioned officers (NCOs), the term *old sergeant syndrome* was coined. In many respects, old sergeant syndrome is similar to the phenomenon of *burnout* as the term has since evolved in the civilian literature.

Despite Sobel's early use of the term *burnt out*, Freudenberger[2] is generally credited with writing the first published paper on burnout. He described a constellation of symptoms occurring among highly dedicated civilians working in the free clinic movement. He noted that a number of physical and behavioral symptoms typically appeared in individuals after they had worked at the same institution for about 1 year. Like soldiers suffering from old sergeant syndrome, burned-out clinic workers appear depressed and emotionally exhausted. They become anxious and irritable. They become cynical and suspicious of the people with whom they work. Their thinking becomes rigid and inflexible. They resist change, however warranted, viewing anything new as a further drain on their already overwhelmed coping resources. They experience physical symptoms such as fatigue, headaches, gastrointestinal disturbances, and sleeplessness. Burned-out people spend an increasing amount of time at work but accomplish less and less. They spend time just "hanging around" at work as if they have nowhere else to go. They may in fact have few social activities outside of the workplace because routinely working overtime may have negatively affected their relationships with people outside of work.

Since Freudenberger's[2] description of burnout, numerous accounts have appeared describing a similar syndrome among individuals in a variety of occupations, including nurses,[3,4] physicians,[5] emergency medical technicians,[6] mental health workers,[7] social service workers,[8,9] police officers,[10] teachers,[11] and employees of a commercial manufacturing firm.[12]

Despite the initial use of the term *burnt out* to describe a military population, only a few studies[3,13,14] have examined burnout in military personnel. Nonetheless, military duty is fraught with stressful experiences that are conducive to the development of burnout. In fact, stress may be an integral part of military training:

> Basic training is designed to place the trainee under various forms of stress, both physical and psychological. While some trainees are in better physical condition than others, mechanisms exist so that almost all experience stress. The stronger trainees may be required to carry an extra 25 pounds of machine gun or radio on a speed march. Trainees doing calisthenics are not allowed to look at one another so that they can locate a group norm; therefore, each trainee may be required to do his own personal maximum of pushups. There are other forms of physical stress—hunger, thirst (in field training), and sleep deprivation. . . .
>
> Psychological stress has a number of sources. Fear of failure and the companion fear of being recycled (repeating part of basic training in another company) are among the most severe types of psychological stress, especially for marginal soldiers. Psychological stress is also generated intentionally by arbitrary and sometimes conflicting demands. One drill sergeant said in an interview that he would see to it that his platoon, which had been doing very well, "won't be able to do anything right tomorrow."[15(p15)]

Stress can produce beneficial as well as detrimental consequences:

> Stress can in some cases have an energizing effect, causing those who are prepared and able to do so to rise to the occasion of a stressful situation by rendering an exceptional performance. The probability of such a productive response is enhanced by training and experience, and indeed much of a military unit's preparatory efforts are

devoted to developing the capacity to perform well under stress.

. . . .

We must also recognize that there is another kind of stress, one which decreases the effectiveness of leaders and units. . . . Such stress is not the result of a deliberate effort to use it for productive purposes, but rather derives accidentally or collaterally from policies and practices that are otherwise motivated. It serves no useful purpose, but instead undermines individual and unit effectiveness. More importantly, it results from institutional approaches that leaders as practicing managers have some capacity to change. . . . We are talking here of some middle ground between stress which is deliberately created for positive reasons, on the one hand, and stress which is in the nature of things and cannot be avoided on the other.[16(pp176-177)]

While psychiatric reactions to combat stress have long been recognized as a significant source of lost troop strength, reactions to chronic occupational stress in the peacetime military have received relatively little attention. However, chronic occupational stress in the military poses a threat to military performance in noncombat as well as combat situations and jeopardizes attainment of the peacetime mission of preparing military personnel for combat.

This chapter examines the problem of burnout in the military. The symptoms of burnout are emotional, cognitive, behavioral, and somatic. Burnout may impair combat readiness and decrease resistance to combat stress breakdown through its effects on group cohesion, morale, job performance, and physical and psychological health.

DEFINITION AND DESCRIPTION

While definitions of burnout vary, the commonly accepted view is that burnout is a means of coping with a difficult work situation.[17] One definition is that burnout is a "commonly employed set of maladaptive coping reactions to high and continuing levels of perceived job stress and personal frustration."[18(p7)] An alternative definition[8,19] is that burnout is the experience of occupational tedium or physical, emotional, and mental exhaustion. Most commonly, burnout is defined as a syndrome of emotional exhaustion, depersonalization, and a lack of a sense of personal accomplishment that occurs in response to chronic exposure to occupational stressors.[20]

Individuals who are burned out feel psychologically drained or emotionally exhausted. They feel that their coping resources are being severely taxed by their work, and they feel incapable of dealing with any additional stress. They feel "at the end of their rope." Often they suffer from "professional depression," that is, they feel sad or unhappy about their work and have little enthusiasm or energy for their work.[21] In addition, they feel that they have little emotional energy left for involvement with other people. Human service professionals who are burned out are less involved in the problems of their patients or clients and may even view friends and family members as a further drain on their limited coping resources.[19]

Another sign of burnout is decreased interpersonal sensitivity, also referred to as depersonalization. Burned-out individuals often develop negative, callous, dehumanizing attitudes toward patients or coworkers.[8,20] This suggests that burnout poses a threat to unit cohesion, which is vital to effective military performance[22] and to prevention of psychiatric breakdown in combat.[23]

People experiencing depersonalization become distrustful of the people with whom they work. They tend to view patients or clients as deserving of their own problems. They distance themselves from people at work in a variety of ways. They may come to treat other people not as individuals but rather as members of some category—for example, as members of a particular rank group or type of unit. Human service providers who are burned out may react to patients or clients in a strictly intellectual manner. They may view patients or clients only in terms of their problems; the familiar example is when a healthcare provider refers to a patient not by name but as "the gall bladder in Room 41."

Medical personnel who are burned out limit their interactions with patients. For example, physicians who are high in emotional exhaustion report that they cope by doing work that does not involve interacting with people, such as paperwork.[20] Nurses who are burned out spend less time with patients.[24]

Burned-out medical personnel may also reduce their emotional involvement with patients by delivering mechanical medical care. Glass[25] observed this happening in psychiatrists who served in combat theaters during World War II. As Glass suggests, burnout can have deleterious effects on the quality of medical care provided:

> The psychiatrist himself is likely to become weary and emotionally exhausted in combat. . . . Under these conditions the psychiatrist may at times lose his diagnostic sense and emotional balance. All patients then begin to look alike to him, and he may identify himself with his patients and see them as all equally deserving of evacuation; or seeing them all as volitionally motivated, he may adopt a harsh policy, assume a severe and caustic manner, and return to duty soldiers who are completely unfit for combat.[25(pp61-62)]

In addition to emotional exhaustion and depersonalization, people experiencing burnout believe that they are not accomplishing anything worthwhile at work. They feel that their accomplishments are falling far below the expectations held by themselves and others. In fact, their perceptions that their productivity has decreased are likely to be accurate. Burned-out workers take more frequent work breaks and are absent more often than their colleagues.[26]

Another symptom associated with burnout is a desire to avoid decisions, problems, or changes at work. This avoidance is especially likely in individuals who are dissatisfied with their accomplishments at work.[27] This finding suggests that burnout, by stifling initiative and impairing performance, jeopardizes attainment of the military mission.

Burnout is also associated with a greater tendency to report somatic complaints,[28] health problems,[19,29] and difficulty sleeping.[19] Chronic occupational stress has been associated with increased risk of developing cardiovascular disease.[30,31] Stress alters immune functioning, increasing susceptibility to infections,[32,33] and influences cancer progression.[34]

Chronic occupational stress may also increase health-impairing behaviors. Burnout is associated with increased use of drugs to cope with work-related stress,[19,35] including the use of prescription drugs to calm down.[24] In drug addicts trying to overcome their habit, stress makes relapse more likely. Individuals often consume more nicotine and alcohol when under stress, and their eating habits may change.[36]

The pervasive nature of burnout is suggested by the dissatisfaction individuals suffering from burnout report with their careers, their lives, and their marriages.[5] Because burnout is associated with a greater desire to change jobs[8,20,35,37] and with actual job turnover,[21,37] burnout may hinder the retention of trained military personnel.

Recruitment and retention of nurses are tremendous problems for the military, which currently faces a shortage of both registered nurses and licensed practical nurses.[38] Nurses who are burned out are more likely to change jobs than their colleagues who are not burned out, suggesting that alleviating burnout may facilitate retention of military nursing personnel.[21]

While burnout is associated with decreased job satisfaction, the correlations are not so high as to suggest that burnout is synonymous with job dissatisfaction.[26,37,38,39,40,41] Individuals suffering from burnout may be satisfied with their job but dissatisfied with their work performance.

Organizational consequences of burnout include decreased productivity, increased healthcare costs, increased absenteeism,[21] increased tardiness,[19] and unauthorized extension of work breaks.[42] Burnout may impair not only the quantity but also the quality of the "product" rendered by the organization. In human service organizations, staff burnout may lead to deterioration of the quality of services rendered to clients, even though the organization's statistical reports may remain stable or even improve.[43] While this obviously has implications for human service providers in the military, its implications for other types of military personnel are less obvious. In combat troops, for example, burnout may be prevalent when, despite a unit's improvement on objective indicators, its mission readiness is deteriorating.

In fact, burnout may be a useful description of "the shift in emphasis from *being good* to *looking good*"[44(p28)] that followed the initial success of the Unit Manning System (COHORT [cohesion, operational readiness, and training]) experiment. The purpose of the COHORT program was to develop highly cohesive, high-performance units through personnel stabilization and special training efforts. The demanding training pace was coupled with expectations that the units would perform flawlessly under high-visibility conditions. Eventually, the intense pressure led to impaired performance; decreased cohesion; reduced motivation; and authoritarian, centralized leadership, symptoms that arguably could be attributed to burnout.

Burnout vs Other Military Stress Reactions

This book discusses various psychiatric syndromes that occur in response to military occupational stressors. These syndromes are distinguishable according to the chronic or acute nature of the stressor, the chronic or acute nature of the response, and the intensity of the stressor. For example, combat stress reaction (also still called "battle fatigue") may occur as a reaction to acute or chronic combat stress. Acute combat stress reaction is a readily reversible condition accompanied by heightened physiological arousal.[45] In contrast, chronic combat stress reaction is recalcitrant to treatment and is accompanied by physiological hypoarousal. Posttraumatic stress disorder (PTSD) is a chronic reaction to an acute stressor, which may be combat or another traumatic event. Individuals experiencing PTSD show signs of heightened physiological arousal.

Burnout is similar to chronic combat stress reaction in that it is a state of hypoarousal that occurs as a result of chronic exposure to stressors.[45] The signs and symptoms of the two syndromes are similar. Manifestations of chronic combat reaction include depression, paranoia, decreased tolerance for frustration, excessive complaining, withdrawal from social interaction, sleep disturbances, weight loss, and abuse of alcohol and drugs. The differences between burnout and chronic combat stress reaction may be more quantitative than qualitative, the two conditions differing in intensity of the stressor (combat versus more mundane peacetime occupational stressors) and intensity of the response.

The Process of Burning Out

Many theories have been offered to explain how burnout develops. One theory[46] is that burnout begins when an individual who is extremely committed to an unsatisfying job increases the number of hours worked in order to attain high expectations held by others or, more likely, by the individual. As the number of hours worked increases, exposure to workplace stressors increases, draining the person's "finite store of 'adaptation energy.'"[46(p43)] Consequently, the person's efficiency decreases. The person's response to feeling unproductive is to work more, which further increases exposure to workplace stressors and depletes the person's energy level. This self-perpetuating cycle is likely to result in burnout unless the individual takes time away from normal work duties to recover.

This theory is consistent with Selye's[47] description of the stress response, which he called the General Adaptation Syndrome. According to Selye, initial exposure to a stressor is associated with increased resistance as the person tries to overcome the threat associated with the stressor. Prolonged exposure to the stressor eventually leads to the depletion of adaptive resources, to the breakdown of resistance, and finally to a state of exhaustion.

The progressive erosion of coping resources is apparent in the following description of soldiers suffering from old sergeant syndrome:

> With self-esteem as the mainstay of their personalities, they were able to resist the terrific onslaught of the combat environment. During their early combat careers they proved themselves able to "take it," but once a break in efficiency occurred, self-confidence became progressively weakened. Yet responsibility was not slackened but often was increased. Forced to carry the same or a heavier load in the face of death and destruction, a cycle between increased responsibility and hesitancy to accept it was set up. This conflict was productive of a progressive and insidious type of anxiety.[1(p320)]

The development of a decreased sense of personal accomplishment has been explained from the perspective of attribution theory.[20,48] This viewpoint suggests that when helping professionals note that they have become less responsive to the needs of the people they are supposed to help they blame themselves and view themselves as inadequate. Because exposure to workplace stressors has been relatively constant, it is difficult for individuals to identify a situational cause for their increasingly negative attitudes toward others.

When burnout develops, it is usually not because exposure to workplace stressors has suddenly increased, but rather because an individual's ability to cope with chronic occupational stressors has eroded over time. The result is a dispositional attribution to self or to the people with whom one works. A dispositional attribution to self is especially likely for individuals who do not discuss personal feelings with colleagues and therefore feel that their experiences are unique. Sharing a sense of depersonalization with colleagues would help individuals identify the situational causes of their own behavior.

When a dispositional attribution to the people with whom one works is made to explain workers' decreased sense of personal accomplishment, helping professionals may develop negative, dehumanizing views toward clients or patients. When helping professionals sense that their efforts are not producing positive changes in recipients' lives, they may blame recipients for their own problems. This attitude is consistent with the "just world hypothesis," the tendency to blame victims for their own misfortune. Viewing recipients as too lazy, stupid, bad, or weak to change their own life circumstances allows providers to avoid feeling ineffective.[48]

A lack of feelings of personal accomplishment can produce depersonalization not only in those who provide health and social services to military personnel and family members, but also in leaders who are frustrated with the progress of the soldiers they are expected to lead. Trying to fulfill the peacetime training mission can be frustrating for leaders when competing missions and lack of facilities, equipment, or other resources make it difficult to produce the desired change in trainees.

This process occurred following the Vietnam conflict when the Army was plagued with indiscipline, drug abuse, and racial incidents.[49] In response to these problems, NCOs developed an authoritarian leadership style. They emphasized strict discipline, believing that yelling at soldiers and remaining aloof from them was the best way to motivate them. Socializing with subordinates was viewed as unprofessional, as fraternization. The lesson that caring for the troops produces better soldiers was forgotten. While the appropriateness of the term *burnout* to describe this process is debatable, the process seems parallel to that described in healthcare workers.

Some writers[50] have argued that organizations as well as individuals can burn out, implying that burnout is contagious among members of a work group. This contention makes intuitive sense. When a work environment is stressful, burnout is likely to be common. When employees become burned out, they become more difficult to get along with and less productive. This situation increases the emotional strain as well as the workload of the other employees, thus increasing the likelihood that they too will burn out.

Some investigators have argued that there are stages of burnout. For example, one model[12] postulates eight phases of burnout, with depersonalization and a lack of a sense of personal accomplishment occurring in the early stages, and emotional exhaustion developing in the later stages. Evidence for such a stage model is weak at best.

OCCUPATIONAL FACTORS ASSOCIATED WITH BURNOUT

Researchers have tried to determine why burnout is more likely in some work environments than in others. Occupational characteristics examined in relation to burnout include overload, role ambiguity, role conflict, lack of control, lack of positive feedback, and stressful interpersonal duties.

Overload

The common-sense notion of burnout is that it is caused by the stress of working too hard for too long. There is evidence to support this belief. For example, studies of teachers[51,52] show that those who have larger numbers of students have higher levels of burnout in general and of emotional exhaustion in particular. The comments of a staff officer involved in the Unit Manning System echo reports of a relationship between overload and emotional exhaustion: "Doesn't anyone have the guts to set priorities? Everything is number one priority, and we're just using up the troops."[44(p28)] The effects of overload extend beyond emotional exhaustion. In a study[8] of social service providers, caseload was positively correlated with occupational tedium, with the development of negative attitudes toward clients, and with the desire to change jobs. It was negatively correlated with liking the job, liking the agency, and being satisfied with the job.

A study[14] of Army personnel assigned to rapid deployment force units found that the relationship between hours worked and burnout was different for junior enlisted personnel and NCOs. Among junior enlisted personnel, the more hours worked per day, the greater the emotional exhaustion. Among NCOs, those who reported working a greater number of hours per day also reported *more* of a sense of personal accomplishment. Nevertheless, NCOs who indicated that their time off was insufficient to allow them to take care of personal business reported greater emotional exhaustion.

The difference in relationship between hours worked and burnout for NCOs and junior enlisted personnel can be easily explained. NCOs spend a lot of time on tasks that they perceive as meaningful but trainees perceive as meaningless. Because it is difficult to measure the performance of soldiers serving in the combat arms in peacetime, military leaders often view the number of hours spent training for combat as an indicator of the effectiveness of training. By definition, 8 hours of training is viewed as better than 4 hours, and 12 hours is even better. Long hours in the field may produce burnout if those hours are viewed as unnecessary and meaningless by trainees. NCOs have more control than junior enlisted personnel over how they spend their work time and, therefore, are less likely to spend long hours on tasks they perceive as meaningless.

When superiors do not properly manage subordinates' time, working long hours can be especially frustrating for subordinates:

> One day we hung around the motor pool til 1630 doing nothing, then suddenly we got word that we had to prepare twelve vehicles to be turned in for scrapping, and they had to be ready by 0730 the next day. So we work all night on trucks that are to be junked. Is this the mission?[44(p21)]

This kind of inadequate planning can weaken morale, reduce confidence in leaders, and produce burnout. Leaders' expectations that subordinates work unnecessarily long hours can ultimately be counterproductive.

Maslach suggests that longer work hours promote greater burnout only to the extent that those hours involve "continuous direct contact with patients or clients,"[48(p37)] especially with patients or clients who are in some way difficult to deal with. It may not be the amount of time spent in direct contact with clients per se, but dissatisfaction with the nature of that contact that best predicts burnout.[8]

A widely accepted assertion of military leaders is that they spend 90% of their time dealing with 10% of their soldiers. In other words, they spend a grossly disproportionate amount of time with the worst soldiers—that is, those who have gone absent without leave (AWOL), bounced checks, or have other disciplinary problems. Because soldiers who are doing well are less likely to come to the attention of NCOs, spending time with "problem" soldiers contributes to a lack of a sense of personal accomplishment among NCOs. Most NCOs do not mind spending long hours working but do mind spending them needlessly. For example, NCOs see helping soldiers with their personal finances as a distraction from mission-related work.

Overload involving responsibility for the well-being of other people is especially likely to result in stress and adverse health effects (eg, among air traffic controllers).[53] This finding suggests that in addition to direct contact with patients or clients, responsibility for those patients or clients may independently contribute to burnout. Consistent with this finding is Sobel's[54] observation that the soldiers who were most prone to develop old sergeant syndrome were those who had before breakdown a great deal of responsibility for other soldiers. For NCOs and officers, who are legally charged with looking after the welfare of the troops in their command, responsibility for subordinates may contribute to burnout.

The relationship between burnout and workload is complex. Long hours coupled with perceptions that the time is not well spent are likely to lead to burnout. Overload can contribute to burnout, but it is only one of a number of factors implicated in burnout.

Role Ambiguity

Role ambiguity occurs when a person is uncertain about role expectations in a job.[11] The person is confused about the responsibilities and rights associated with the job, about how best to perform the job, and about the criteria used to evaluate job performance. Role ambiguity is positively correlated with depersonalization, emotional exhaustion, and lack of a sense of personal accomplishment.[11] Role ambiguity is also associated with job dissatisfaction, physical symptoms of stress, job turnover, and impaired job performance.[27] Burnout is lessened when organizational rules and policies are clearly communicated and workers know what to expect from their jobs.[7]

In the military, "other duties as assigned" is part of every service member's job description; this may produce role ambiguity. The mission is often defined on an ad hoc basis and redefined daily: Painting the barracks may be defined as the mission one day, and conducting field training exercises may be the mission the next. Inconsistent application of the criteria used in making retention and promotion decisions may also promote role ambiguity.

Role Conflict

Role conflict occurs when a person cannot reconcile the inconsistency between two or more sets of expected role behaviors. Role conflict increases the likelihood of burnout.[11,55] In a study of enterostomal therapists, role conflict was cited as the most common cause of burnout.[56]

Military leaders are charged with fulfilling the mission and looking after the welfare of the troops. These responsibilities may conflict; an example is when impossible or stupid missions are called for by superiors even though they may demoralize, frustrate, or simply waste the time of subordinates.

Role conflict may be especially high in so-called "boundary positions,"[53(p62)] that is, positions that involve interacting with people both inside and outside an organization or work group. This assertion is supported by findings of higher role conflict in middle managers than in blue-collar employees.[57] Military personnel occupying boundary positions include company-level and platoon-level senior NCOs as well as lieutenants in charge of a platoon. Individuals in the military with more than one professional identity—for example, military officers who are also nurses—also occupy boundary positions and may be especially likely to experience role conflict.

Military medical personnel may experience conflict between their roles as healthcare providers acting on behalf of individual patients and their roles as military personnel serving the military mission. The duty of the military physician is to maximize combat strength. In the civilian community, those who are most severely injured or most seriously ill are generally treated first. In a combat situation, individuals who are most salvageable may be at highest priority for treatment; the worst injured may be treated last. Effective treatment as well as ineffective treatment may pose a threat to the patient's life because treatment may lead to return of the successfully treated service member to combat.

Role conflict is also likely when an employee is expected to do more than is possible given the constraints of time and resources. The army's philosophy of "do more with less" may promote burnout. Lack of administrative support, as manifested in insufficient funds or equipment to accomplish all of several competing organizational goals, may produce role conflict. A senior officer commented on the chronicity of this problem:

> Throughout my service the demands on the army and organizations in it have often been out of proportion to the people and resources available. The army seldom adjusted goals that had been established prior to reductions in force and budget cuts. Too many "can do" commanders at brigade level and above tried to do them all. . . . The troops and the army as an organization paid the price.[58(p39)]

Sometimes an organization makes incompatible demands, producing role conflict. An emphasis on short-term results may compromise the longer term interests of the organization. For example, during the Unit Manning System experiment, pressure for quick results produced an emphasis on looking good that occurred at the expense of being good.[44] The short-sighted "zero defects" approach creates an atmosphere in which a leader will ask a unit member who is particularly adept at a particular task to always perform that task for the unit. As a result, other unit members will not learn how to perform the task, thereby decreasing the unit's preparedness for combat.

Another source of role conflict is an incompatibility between demands and abilities, as occurs when an individual is assigned a task but lacks the adequate training to perform that task.[56] Individuals whose education and training did not provide them with the necessary skills and knowledge to perform the tasks expected of them may be especially prone to burnout.[43] A study[20] of public contact employees revealed that employees who felt that their job training had been inadequate scored higher on all burnout measures.

Role conflict may also stem from an incompatibility between work and home responsibilities. Civilian healthcare workers complain that the demanding nature of their work interferes with their family responsibilities.[59] For military medical personnel, changes of assignment and temporary duty create additional friction between work and family responsibilities. This friction may explain why burnout is reportedly higher among military nurses than among civilian nurses,[3] even among those who work at the same hospital. Whether resulting from competing work demands or from conflicting work and home responsibilities, role conflict has been associated with increased burnout.[41]

Lack of Job Control

Being unable to control or predict events can be stressful.[60] The military organization exerts greater control over its personnel than most civilian organizations, for example, by restricting where they live and what they wear. Furthermore, soldiers complain that being unable to predict the length of the duty day wreaks havoc on their personal lives.[44] This lack of control has pervasive effects on soldiers and their families, as indicated by the wife of an active duty member:

> I've just given up planning anything! Meals, movies, vacations. To hell with it! We plan it, and get it all set up, and they send him off. I don't trust his commander. He just wants to look good, and he'll volunteer Jack for anything that comes along.[44(p38)]

Military personnel may also view the decisions of a promotion or retention board as uncontrollable and unpredictable. In the U.S. Army, these decisions are made by a group of individuals unknown to the person being evaluated. The priorities of the individuals making the decisions are to some extent unknown and may conflict with those of the service member's raters.

Healthcare professionals, especially physicians, have a great deal of job autonomy; however, they have limited control over the outcomes of their work. Sometimes patients misunderstand the treatment regimen or do not comply with it for other reasons. Sometimes patients simply cannot be helped given the constraints of current medical knowledge.

Exposure to uncontrollable or unpredictable stressors or both can lead to increased stress, impaired job performance, and increased insensitivity toward other people. These effects may persist even after exposure to the uncontrollable or unpredictable situation has ended.[60,61]

Individuals who perceive that they have control over various aspects of their work report less burnout.[62,63] When employees are allowed to work independently and have input into decision making, burnout is less likely.[7,56] Junior enlisted personnel tend to have little autonomy in their jobs, and this lack may explain why they are more likely than officers or NCOs to develop burnout.[14]

Responsibility without appropriate decision-making input may be especially stressful. This predicament is illustrated by the comments of a squad leader who stated: "I'm responsible for training my squad, but I have no input to the training schedule. I know what my men need to practice, but I get no training time."[44(p26)] Decisions are made at higher levels in organizations with high burnout levels,[37] suggesting that micromanagement contributes to burnout:

> A number of company commanders said that their bosses constrained their autonomy, punished independence, and compromised their credibility. . . . One platoon leader complained that after positioning a machine gun in a defensive maneuver he was required to change its location three times after successive visits from the company, battalion, and brigade commanders. The lieutenant, noting that the weapon ended up in about the same position where he had first placed it, lamented, "You'd think after two years they'd realize I know where to put the damned thing."[44(pp26-27)]

Despite the generally positive effects of having control, a caveat about control must be presented here: The effects of control over a stressful situation depend on the individual and the context.[64,65] Having control is not always beneficial. For example, a person who is given control over a task but does not have the requisite training is likely to experience stress. Thus, giving subordinates as much control as possible over their work will minimize burnout only to the extent that this control is appropriate given their level of training and experience.

Lack of Positive Feedback

If an employee does not receive sufficient information about the effectiveness of his work, burnout is more likely.[8,26] In human service occupations, feedback about the success of one's work comes from clients or patients as well as from supervisors and colleagues. For example, medical personnel often do not receive adequate feedback about the effectiveness of their work. If a patient does not return for a follow-up visit, the provider usually does not know whether the patient has improved to the point of no longer needing treatment, has sought treatment elsewhere, or has dropped out of the healthcare system in frustration. When medical personnel do receive feedback it is more likely to be bad than good; it has been said that the successes go away and the failures keep coming back.[20] Providers get a distortedly negative view of their own effectiveness because the patients for whom treatment has failed are more likely to return than those who have been successfully treated.

Stressful Interpersonal Duties

Medical personnel engage in emotionally taxing interactions with people who are sick, in pain, anxious about their health and their future, and possibly dying. In the military, this is especially true because medical personnel in wartime treat patients whose wounds were inflicted by weapons systems whose destructiveness and lethality are unmatched in the civilian community. Added to this burden is the difficult job of informing patients and their loved ones about a grim prognosis or about a diagnosis with tremendous emotional impact such as breast cancer or acquired immunodeficiency syndrome.

Superimposed on the difficulty of interacting with people who are suffering is the unpleasant nature of some of the treatments provided by medical personnel. Patients who are asymptomatic on arrival at the dentist's office often leave in considerable pain as a result of dental procedures. As a result, dentists find that patients are often fearful or hostile toward them. Similarly, nurses who work in burn units inflict agonizing pain on their patients through the dressing changes and debridement necessary to treat burn wounds. Because the nursing profession is oriented to relieving suffering, it can be extremely stressful for nurses when a patient's response to treatment is not the gratitude nurses expect but rather hostility and uncooperativeness.[66]

Medical personnel report that having a great deal of responsibility for the well-being of their patients is stressful.[59] When a patient dies or fails to improve, healthcare providers sometimes blame themselves. In a study[56] of enterostomal therapists, respondents identified working with clients whose prognosis was poor as a stressor that contributed to burnout. Another study[67] reported that physicians' ratings of the stressfulness of various patient scenarios varied according to the degree of threat to the patient's life and the extent to which the best course of action was unclear. Patient scenarios involving both threat to the patient's life and decision-making uncertainty were rated as more stressful than those involving only one or the other factor. Events requiring fast action on the part of the physician were rated as highly stressful. In combat or in a peacetime emergency situation, any or all of these factors may be operating.

In addition to medical personnel, people in other military occupational groups may regularly experience emotionally draining interpersonal interactions. Supervisors often must help subordinates deal with both personal and work-related problems that interfere with employees' job performance, and this may increase their susceptibility to burnout.[68,69] Social workers, family assistance workers, rescue workers, and military police also perform difficult interpersonal duties and may therefore be especially susceptible to burnout.

The types of jobs that are likely to promote burnout are those that require continuous, direct contact with other people in emotionally taxing situations; those that require long hours of work performing tasks of questionable utility; those that are unclear as to workers' rights, duties, and responsibilities; and those that do not give workers adequate control over their work.

THE INFLUENCE OF INTRAPERSONAL AND SOCIAL FACTORS

Individual Characteristics

This chapter views burnout as a subcategory of occupational stress.[70] The transactional model of stress proposes that, for a stress response to occur, an individual must appraise a stimulus or event as harmful, threatening, or challenging.[71] This model suggests that individual differences in the appraisal of events explain why some people burn out while others in the same situation do not. Some people thrive under workplace conditions that others find extremely aversive. The concept of Person–Environment Fit[72] highlights the importance of matching the individual worker's preferences regarding job characteristics with the demands of the job itself; this perspective suggests that burnout is more likely when there is a misfit between the individual worker and the work environment.[70]

Few studies have examined personality traits as they pertain to burnout; however, one study[5] investigated this issue in physicians. Physicians who had low self-esteem, low self-confidence, proneness to dysphoria and obsessive worry, social anxiety, passivity, or withdrawal from others when assessed just before entering medical school had higher levels of burnout when reassessed an average of 25 years later. Physicians who had indicated greater adherence to religious and moral rules and who had expressed interest in poetry, dramatics, and science were less likely to burn out.

The manner in which a person expresses anger may be related to the type of burnout response that develops. In a study[27] of nurses, those who tended to direct anger toward other people were more likely to report depersonalization, while those who tended to direct anger toward themselves were more likely to experience a burnout response that included an avoidance of decisions or problems.

Military service members who have problems at home or in other aspects of their personal life may be at increased risk for developing burnout.[43,70] Burnout is more likely among individuals who are unhappily married than among those who are happily married.[5] Military assistance programs designed to help troubled families may augment the service member's resources for dealing with stress at work.

Morale

Morale is "the enthusiasm and persistence with which a member of a group engages in the prescribed activities of that group."[73(p454)] The military concept of morale is similar to the concept of organizational commitment in the civilian literature. Individuals who are committed to a particular organization are willing to invest a great deal of time, effort, and emotional energy for the organization's benefit. They have a strong desire to continue their association with the organization and believe in the organization's values and goals.

Several writers[2,17] claim that the most dedicated and committed workers are at greatest risk for burnout. Others[46] invoke a "workaholic personality type" to describe those who are most likely to burn out. Sobel[1] noted that the soldiers who suffered from old sergeant syndrome were those who, in the past, handled responsibility well, were excellent leaders, and related well to other people. In fact, many of them had received citations, awards, and medals for their outstanding performance.[54] These observations suggest that military personnel who strongly believe in the military and are willing to work hard to further its goals—those who, in the absence of burnout, would be most valuable to the military—are most vulnerable to burnout.

Commitment may be viewed as the extent to which a person has stakes in a given situation.[71] A worker is more likely to appraise a situation as harmful, threatening, or challenging when the situation involves something that is personally significant. Workers who have put little time, effort, or emotional energy into their work would be less likely to appraise work-related events as stressful and less likely to burn out. Sobel describes the case of a 29-year-old first sergeant of excellent capabilities who was evacuated for exhaustion:

> Subsequently it was discovered that he had carelessly left his company records strewn about a command post and that they had been picked up by a British patrol. This sergeant had been extremely careful with secret information and papers. Despite the diminution in efficiency, as shown by this case, there was no loss of motivation, and these men continued, sometimes desperately, in a job they had become incapable of handling. This led to severe conflict and guilt feelings with the result that their anxiety increased progressively to the point where evacuation became imperative. Guilt over letting their buddies down was a constant feature and was directly proportionate to the state of morale in the unit, as is the incidence of the entire syndrome.[1(p317)]

Despite claims that the most committed workers are at greatest risk for burnout, the dominant view of commitment as a risk factor for burnout is incomplete. In fact, commitment can help mitigate burnout. Research suggests that commitment enhances the ability to cope with a stressful work environment[74] and moderates the adverse effects of occupational stress on job performance.[57] Commitment to army values may protect personnel of all ranks from the development of burnout.[14] Taken together, the results suggest that there may be some optimal level of commitment, and deviations in either direction from the optimum increase an individual's susceptibility to burnout.

Causal relationships between burnout, on the one hand, and morale and commitment, on the other, are unclear. The most likely scenario is that morale and commitment influence susceptibility to burnout[2,17,74] and that burnout in turn has negative effects on morale and commitment.[75,76] Conditions that foster low morale are likely to encourage the development of burnout. While commitment and morale are important, they may not be sufficient to prevent burnout in an nonsupportive work environment. In the long run, commitment to a job that does not provide adequate support and rewards for hard work is likely to be harmful to the worker although initially a committed worker can maintain superior performance and high morale despite an indifferent or frustrating work environment.

Cohesion

"Loosely defined, cohesion represents feelings of belonging, of solidarity with a specifiable set of others who constitute a 'we' as opposed to 'them.'"[77(p6)] Cohesive units provide better social support to their members than noncohesive units. The social support provided by coworkers can take the form of instrumental, informational, or emotional aid. Coworkers can provide information that directly aids in the performance of job duties—for example, by providing instructions regarding how to perform a particular task. Coworkers can help reduce overload by directly assisting with job duties. They can provide information that reduces role ambiguity and can provide feedback regarding one's job performance. In addition, coworkers can provide emotional support for a colleague suffering from occupational stress, either directly or by increasing awareness of the situational causes of a stressful job situation.

Research[69,78,79] supports an association between social support and increased resistance to burnout. Burnout is inversely related to the perceived friendliness and support of coworkers,[7] to satisfaction with coworkers,[35] and to having coworkers with whom one feels comfortable discussing difficult clients and sharing work responsibilities.[8] Receiving feedback and support from colleagues and supervisors is negatively related to burnout.[8] Supervisor support may be particularly important in minimizing burnout.[52,69] Perceived impatience or defensiveness of supervisors predicts extended absence from work.[21] A study[14] of U.S. Army personnel assigned to rapid deployment force units found that measures of cohesion were more important than objective stressors or characteristics of the individual in predicting burnout.

Sobel[1,54] described the loss of group cohesion in soldiers suffering from old sergeant syndrome. These soldiers had been either original members of their divisions or had been with their divisions for an extended period. These soldiers were survivors in that they were among the few remaining long-term members of their unit. They had close bonds with the few remaining unit old-timers and spent a great deal of time with them relating battle experiences. These discussions made them feel less vulnerable by reminding them that they had survived so many battles. However, as attrition of the long-term unit veterans occurred, these soldiers failed to form strong bonds to new soldiers. This failure contributed to the erosion of self-confidence, to weakened defenses against anxiety, and to other manifestations of a severe battle reaction. Sobel noted that "loyalty to the group" was the final defense against anxiety that was weakened before breakdown.

Leadership Qualities

Caring leadership that relies on competence rather than rank for its power to motivate troops can prevent burnout. Authoritarian leadership, that is, the use of rules and pressure to keep workers under control, is associated with greater likelihood of burnout.[7] Leaders who rigidly control the work environment and do not seem to care about their subordinates create an atmosphere of poor morale and disappointing productivity, as illustrated by the following anecdote:

> One athletically gifted private, capable of earning maximum points on the army physical readiness test, said that he had purposely achieved only barely passing scores on the test to reduce the chances that his company would receive a physical training gold streamer: "The captain doesn't deserve a gold streamer. He does nothing for us; he just uses us." Fellow COHORT soldiers applauded this act of subtle insubordination because they, too, felt the commander did not merit receiving the award.[44(p51)]

The captain probably was low in consideration and high in structure. Leaders who are high in consideration emphasize the well-being of group members and create an atmosphere of trust, respect, and two-way communication. Those who are high in structure emphasize organizing group activities to achieve organizational goals. These two leadership qualities were examined in a study[40] that assessed the relationship between the leadership style of the head nurse and burnout among staff nurses. The higher the head nurse was in consideration, the lower the staff nurse burnout. Head nurse structure by itself did not relate to burnout, although it did interact with consideration. Specifically, staff nurse burnout was highest if the head nurse was low in consideration *and* high in structure. If the head nurse was high in consideration, the amount of structure had little influence on burnout scores. The combination of low consideration and low structure also produced relatively low burnout scores.

Supervisors who are high in consideration may reduce burnout by appearing more approachable to subordinates who need to discuss their work-related problems. A study of civilian nurses[35] revealed that those who indicated a greater use of talking with the supervisor to cope with occupational stress had relatively low burnout levels. Similarly, nurses at a military medical facility were less likely to develop emotional exhaustion when faced with workplace stressors if their supervisor was supportive.[80] These results suggest that good communication between supervisors and subordinates may help subordinates cope with a stressful workplace, thus minimizing the likelihood of burnout in subordinates.

Individuals who are experiencing burnout report less satisfaction with their supervisors.[35] When workers perceive supervisors as nonsupportive or inept, burnout is more likely.[56] In military populations, confidence in senior leaders and perceptions that leaders care about the well-being of their subordinates are negatively associated with burnout.[14] Therefore, it is important that leaders be viewed as competent and caring by the troops if burnout is to be kept to a minimum.

RECOGNITION AND REDUCTION OF BURNOUT

Recognizing Burnout in Self and Others

The best line of defense against burnout is to ensure that all military personnel know what burnout is and what its symptoms are. Although awareness of burnout is a prerequisite for its prevention and treatment, the potential pitfall of increased awareness is the development of "medical students syndrome," whereby learning about burnout leads to a self-fulfilling prophecy.[18]

Individuals can accurately perceive the extent to which a coworker is experiencing burnout.[19] Because military leaders are responsible for the job performance and well-being of subordinates, it is important that leaders be able to recognize burnout. In addition, unit members should be able to recognize burnout in their peers.

Several psychometric instruments have been devised for assessing burnout; the Maslach Burnout Inventory (MBI)[81] is the most widely used. The MBI consists of 25 items that yield frequency scores for each of three subscales, specifically emotional exhaustion, depersonalization, and personal accomplishment. The reliability and validity of the MBI are well established.[26,81] The three subscales tap relatively independent dimensions of burnout; therefore, subscale scores rather than total burnout scores are typically used.

Because the authors of the MBI view burnout as a phenomenon afflicting human service providers, validation efforts have focused almost exclusively on this occupational group. A modified version of the MBI was developed for use in a commercial setting and is appropriate for use with a wider range of populations than the original version.[12] Because ratings of the intensity and frequency of experienced burnout symptoms are moderately to highly correlated,[7,26] the modified version of the MBI requires only that respondents rate the extent to which each item is descriptive of themselves. Factor analysis of responses to the modified MBI supports the validity of the three subscales—emotional exhaustion, depersonalization, and lack of a sense of personal accomplishment for assessing a military population.[14]

Another questionnaire used to assess burnout is the Tedium Scale,[19] which consists of 21 items designed to assess physical exhaustion (feeling tired and weak), emotional exhaustion (feeling depressed or trapped), and mental exhaustion (feeling worthless and disillusioned). Unlike the MBI, the Tedium Scale yields a total burnout score. The reliability of the Tedium Scale is satisfactory.[19] The Tedium Scale is easier to administer, score, and interpret than the MBI but provides less specific information about the manifestations of burnout.

Reducing Burnout

Burnout results from an interaction between a person whose coping abilities are wearing thin and an unpleasant work environment. This interaction suggests that efforts to minimize burnout should focus both on enhancing individuals' coping resources and on reducing workplace stressors.

An individual's resistance to stress is a product of many different factors, including the person's physical health, mental health, and social support. The adoption or maintenance of health-promoting behaviors, such as physical exercise, proper diet, adequate rest, and restraint from excessive consumption of alcohol and caffeine, should be encouraged. Because it can be extremely difficult to change habits when under stress, it is important that health-promoting behaviors become habitual before the person becomes burned out.

Because an individual's appraisal of a situation determines whether a stress response will occur,[71] informing workers about the benefits they can expect from undertaking potentially stressful assignments may help reduce burnout. For example, it may be possible to emphasize the career or growth opportunities in an overseas assignment so that the service member does not dwell on the negative aspects, such as the inconvenience of a household move or the separation from family that occurs during an unaccompanied tour. Leaders should ensure that subordinates understand how the successful completion of a particularly stressful or challenging task will contribute to the military mission. This will enable individuals who adopt the ideology or philosophy of the military to put potentially stressful events into a meaningful context and thereby minimize potentially adverse effects.[74]

Burnout can be minimized through realistic training in which soldiers are taught how to deal with workplace stressors. The importance of training is revealed by a study[67] that found that physicians with more training rated a number of patient scenarios as less stressful than their colleagues with less training. Similarly, a study of nursing assistants found lower levels of burnout among those who received training for work with the cognitively impaired.[79] Military training exercises are designed to simulate combat conditions; however, soldiers may not be adequately prepared to deal with peacetime occupational stressors. Increased training in how to resolve conflicts with coworkers, superiors, and subordinates; how to make difficult decisions; and how to improve communication between superiors and subordinates might better prepare soldiers for military service in peacetime.

Military training not only fails to prepare military personnel for some of the stressors they will encounter in peacetime, it may actually hamper their ability to cope with some types of missions. For example, U.S. Army paratroopers deployed to multinational peacekeeping operations in the Sinai in 1981 reported boredom and monotony.[82] The values inculcated through their training, that is, an emphasis on fighting to achieve military objectives, may have conflicted with the orientation needed to conduct peacekeeping operations.[82] Training that encourages combat troops to view this type of operation as a meaningful and appropriate use of their efforts and skills would help prevent adverse psychological reactions.

Training and experience can mitigate the stressfulness of some events but other events are so inherently stressful that increased knowledge and experience cannot mitigate their impact. In the study of physicians previously mentioned,[67] training reduced the stressfulness of events previously designated as medium or low stress but did not reduce the stressfulness of events previously designated as high stress. A supportive work environment can mitigate the effects of highly stressful events.

Military leaders can do much to ameliorate burnout by establishing conditions that foster the development of morale and cohesion. (See Chapter 1, "Morale and Cohesion in Military Psychiatry.") Good communication between and among soldiers and leaders is crucial to preventing burnout. Military leaders can reduce role conflict and role ambiguity by developing clear job descriptions and involving subordinates in the development of meaningful and achievable personal and unit goals.[11] They can minimize burnout by ensuring that organizational goals and regulations are unambiguously communicated to subordinates. Improved communication between leaders and subordinates can help ensure that sacrifices made for the sake of the mission are perceived as necessary and meaningful. Increased awareness of how peers are reacting to the work environment may help service members realize that their own reactions are a normal response to a stressful environment.

Mission requirements sometimes mandate increased work hours; however, military personnel should receive time off to recover when mission requirements abate. Extra duty should be kept to a minimum. These measures are likely to provide the added benefit of increasing subordinates' perceptions that leaders care about them. Individuals who have control over the amount of time they devote to their work should be taught that while working long hours is at times necessary to achieve military objectives, working harder and longer does not guarantee enhanced productivity. Military personnel must learn to pace themselves so that they can sustain an optimal level of functioning, reserving some energy for dealing with stressful situations should they arise.[45]

In jobs that involve dealing with patients or clients, burnout can be alleviated by reducing the number of hours of stressful patient contact.[53] This reduction can be accomplished by interspersing patient contact with administrative tasks or other types of work, by encouraging attendance at professional meetings, and by encouraging participation in job-relevant courses.

Medical personnel whose work involves emotionally demanding interactions with patients may benefit from caregiver support groups[11] or from consultation with mental health professionals. In one hospital, a liaison psychiatrist helped the staff of a burn unit improve their work environment.[83] Using the Work Environment Scale,[84] the psychiatrist assessed staff members' perceptions of the work environment as well as their preferences for an ideal work environment. Through a series of biweekly meetings, the psychiatrist sought to reduce the discrepancy between the actual and preferred environments by discussing staff members' perceptions of the work environment and by helping them plan and implement changes in their workplace. The effectiveness of the intervention was demonstrated by reduced discrepancies between staff members' actual and preferred work environments.

Another way to minimize burnout in healthcare providers is to ensure that they receive feedback about the positive outcomes of their work. One way to provide this feedback in high-stress healthcare occupations is for providers to invite former patients and their families to an informal social gathering.[85] At these "alumni parties," care providers have an opportunity to see that patients formerly under their care have improved as a result of the care provided. This reinforces providers' perceptions that the work they perform is meaningful and appreciated. Interacting with patients outside of the healthcare setting would provide the added benefit of countering the development of depersonalization.

Because the presence of negative conditions and the absence of positive conditions in the workplace are independent of each other,[4] efforts to reduce burnout should not only try to reduce negative job-related experiences but also to enhance positive experiences. This approach suggests the importance of formally recognizing outstanding job performance both informally on a personal level and more formally through the use of awards and medals. Employees who perceive their work as higher in incentives and rewards are less likely to develop burnout.[79]

SUMMARY AND CONCLUSION

Chronic occupational stress can lead to burnout. Symptoms of burnout include feeling emotionally exhausted, being less sensitive to people at work, and being disappointed with one's accomplishments at work. Burnout in military personnel has received little attention; however, this chapter contends that burnout poses a threat to the military mission in peacetime *and* in wartime. Burnout may adversely affect the performance, commitment, retention, cohesion, morale, and physical health of military personnel. Military leaders can do much to prevent or ameliorate burnout. By fostering the development of horizontal and vertical cohesion, by providing realistic training that prepares service members for the types of stressors they are likely to encounter in peacetime military service, by making sure that the sacrifices expected of subordinates are necessary and meaningful, and by increasing awareness of organizational goals and giving workers as much autonomy as practicable in achieving them, burnout can be minimized.

REFERENCES

1. Sobel R. The "old sergeant" syndrome. *Psychiatry.* 1947;10:315–321.
2. Freudenberger HJ. Staff burnout. *J Soc Issues.* 1974;30:159–165.
3. Bartz C, Maloney JP. Burnout among intensive care nurses. *Res Nurs Health.* 1986;9:147–153.
4. Pines AM, Kanner AD. Nurses' burnout: Lack of positive conditions and presence of negative conditions as two independent sources of stress. *J Psychosoc Nurs Ment Health Serv.* 1982;20(8):30–35.
5. McCranie EW, Brandsma JM. Personality antecedents of burnout among middle-aged physicians. *Behav Med.* 1988;14(1):30–36.
6. Neale AV. Work stress in emergency medical technicians. *J Occup Med.* 1991;33(9):991–997.
7. Savicki V, Cooley A. The relationship of work environment and client contact to burnout in mental health professionals. *J Counsel Dev.* 1987;65(5):249–252.
8. Pines A, Kafry D. Occupational tedium in the social services. *Social Work.* 1978;23:499–507.
9. Matthews DB. A comparison of burnout in selected occupational fields. *Career Dev Q.* 1990;38:230–239.
10. Jackson SE, Maslach C. After-effects of job-related stress: Families as victims. *J Occup Behav.* 1982;3:63–77.

11. Schwab RL, Iwanicki EF. Perceived role conflict, role ambiguity, and teacher burnout. *Educa Admin Q.* 1982;18(1):60–74.

12. Golembiewski RT, Munzenrider R, Carter D. Phases of progressive burnout and their work site covariants: Critical issues in OD research and praxis. *J Appl Behav Sci.* 1983;19(4):461–481.

13. Shelley JJ, Wong M. Prevalence of burnout among military dentists. *Milit Med.* 1991;156:113–118.

14. Wilcox VL, Garrigan J, Manning FJ. Levels and predictors of burnout in Army personnel. 1992. Unpublished manuscript.

15. Faris JH. The impact of basic combat training: The role of the drill sergeant. In: Goldman NL, Segal, DR, eds. *The Social Psychology of Military Service.* Beverly Hills, Calif: Sage; 1976: 11–24.

16. Sorley L. The leader as practicing manager. In: Buck JH, Korb LJ, eds. *Military Leadership.* Beverly Hills, Calif: Sage; 1981: 167–193.

17. Kamis E. An epidemiological approach to staff burnout. In: Jones JW, ed. *The Burnout Syndrome—Current Research, Theory, Interventions.* Park Ridge, Ill: London House; 1982: 54–67.

18. Paine WS. The burnout syndrome in context. In: Jones JW, ed. *The Burnout Syndrome—Current Research, Theory, Interventions.* Park Ridge, Ill: London House; 1982: 1–29.

19. Pines AM, Aronson E, Kafry D. *Burnout: From Tedium to Personal Growth.* New York: The Free Press; 1981.

20. Maslach C, Jackson SE. Burnout in health professions: A social psychological analysis. In: Sanders GS, Suls J, eds. *Social Psychology of Health and Illness.* Hillsdale, NJ: Erlbaum; 1982: 227–254.

21. Firth H, Britton P. "Burnout," absence and turnover among British nursing staff. *J Occup Psychol.* 1989;62:55–59.

22. Manning FJ, Ingraham LH. An investigation into the value of unit cohesion in peacetime. In: Belenky G, ed. *Contemporary Studies in Combat Psychiatry.* Westport, Conn: Greenwood; 1987: 47–67.

23. Steiner M, Neumann M. Traumatic neurosis and social support in the Yom Kippur War returnees. *Milit Med.* 1978;143:866–868.

24. Cronin-Stubbs D, Brophy EB. Burnout: Can social support save the psych nurse? *J Psychosoc Nurs Mental Health Serv.* 1985;23(7):8–13.

25. Glass AJ. Psychiatry at the division level. In: Hanson FR, ed. *Combat Psychiatry: Experiences in the North African and Mediterranean Theaters of Operation, American Ground Forces. World War II.* Washington, DC: GPO; 1949: 45–73.

26. Maslach C, Jackson SE. The measurement of experienced burnout. *J Occup Behav.* 1981;2:99–113.

27. Firth H, McKeown P, McIntee A, Britton P. Professional depression, "burnout" and personality in longstay nursing. *Int J Nurs Stud.* 1987;24(3):227–237.

28. Belcastro PA. Burnout and its relationship to teachers' somatic complaints and illnesses. *Psychol Rep.* 1982;50:1045–1046.

29. Stout JK, Williams JM. Comparison of two measures of burnout. *Psychol Rep.* 1983;53:283–289.

30. Haynes SG, Feinleib M. Women, work and coronary heart disease: Prospective findings from the Framingham Heart Study. *Am J Public Health.* 1980;70(2):133–141.

31. Karasek R, Baker D, Marxer F, Ahlbom A, Theorell T. Job decision latitude, job demands, and cardiovascular disease: A prospective study of Swedish men. *Am J Public Health.* 1981;71(7):694–705.

32. Jemmott JB, Locke SE. Psychosocial factors, immunologic mediation, and human susceptibility to infectious diseases: How much do we know? *Psychol Bull.* 1984;95(1):78–108.

33. Ader R, Felton D, Cohen N. *Psychoimmunology.* San Diego, Calif: Academic Press; 1991.

34. Sklar LS, Anisman H. Stress and cancer. *Psychol Bull.* 1981;89(3):369–406.

35. Albrecht TL. What job stress means for the staff nurse. *Nurs Admin Q.* 1982;7:1–11.

36. Grunberg NE, Baum A. Biological commonalities of stress and substance abuse. In: Shiffman S, Wills TA, eds. *Coping and Substance Use.* New York: Academic Press; 1985: 25–62.

37. Weinberg S, Edwards G, Garove WE. Burnout among employees of state residential facilities serving developmentally disabled persons. *Children Youth Serv Rev.* 1983;5:239–253.

38. Secretary's Commission on Nursing. Military nurses task force report on the military nursing shortage. In: *Support Studies and Background Information.* Vol 2. 1988; VI–A–1—VI–C–1.

39. Leiter MP. Burnout as a function of communication patterns. *Group Org Studies.* 1988;13(1):111–128.

40. Duxbury ML, Armstrong GD, Drew DJ, Henly SJ. Head nurse leadership style with staff nurse burnout and job satisfaction in neonatal intensive care units. *Nurs Res.* 1984;33(2):97–101.

41. Bacharach SB, Bamberger P, Conley S. Work-home conflict among nurses and engineers: Mediating the impact of role stress on burnout and satisfaction at work. *J Organ Behav.* 1991;12:39–53.

42. Jones JW. Dishonesty, burnout, and unauthorized work break extensions. *Personality Social Psychol Bull.* 1981;7(3):406–409.

43. Carroll JFX. Staff burnout as a form of ecological dysfunction. *Contemp Drug Problems.* 1979;(Summer):207–225.

44. Marlowe DH. *Unit Manning System Field Evaluation.* Washington, DC: US Department of the Army, Walter Reed Army Institute of Research; 1987. Technical Report No. 5.

45. Rahe RH. Acute versus chronic psychological reactions to combat. *Milit Med.* 1988;153(7):365–372.

46. Homer JB. Worker burnout: A dynamic model with implications for prevention and control. *System Dynamics Rev.* 1985;1(1):42–62.

47. Selye H. The General Adaptation Syndrome and the diseases of adaptation. *J Clin Endocrinol Metab.* 1946;6(2):117–230.

48. Maslach C. Burnout: A social psychological analysis. In: Jones JW, ed. *The Burnout Syndrome—Current Research, Theory, Interventions.* Park Ridge, Ill: London House; 1982: 30–53.

49. Ingraham L. *Fear and Loathing in the Motor Pool.* Washington, DC: Walter Reed Army Institute of Research; 1987. Report WRAIR NP–86–9.

50. Rountree BH. Psychological burnout in task groups: Examining the proposition that some task groups of workers have an affinity for burnout, while others do not. *J Health Human Resources Admin.* 1984;7:235–248.

51. DePaepe J, French R, Lavay B. Burnout symptoms experienced among special physical educators: A descriptive longitudinal study. *Adapted Physical Activity Q.* 1985;2:189–196.

52. Russell DW, Altmaier E, Van Velzen D. Job-related stress, social support, and burnout among classroom teachers. *J Appl Psychol.* 1987;72(2):269–274.

53. Kahn R. Job burnout: Prevention and remedies. *Public Welfare*. 1978;36(2):61–63.

54. Sobel R. Anxiety-depressive reactions after prolonged combat experience—the "old sergeant syndrome." *Bull US Army Med Dept*. 1949;9(Suppl *Combat Psychiatry*):137–146.

55. Jackson SE, Schwab RL, Schuler RS. Toward an understanding of the burnout phenomenon. *J Appl Psychol*. 1986;71(4):630–640.

56. Cronin-Stubbs D. Professional burnout part two: A survey of enterostomal therapists. *J Enterostomal Therapy*. 1982;9(4):14–16.

57. Jamal M. Relationship of job stress to job performance: A study of managers and blue-collar workers. *Human Relations*. 1985;38(5):409–424.

58. Collins AS. *Common Sense Training: A Working Philosophy for Leaders*. San Rafael, Calif: Presidio; 1978.

59. Wolfgang AP. Job stress in the health professions: A study of physicians, nurses, and pharmacists. *Behav Med*. 1988;14(1):43–47.

60. Glass DC, Singer JE. *Urban Stress: Experiments on Noise and Social Stressors*. New York: Academic Press; 1972.

61. Cohen S. Aftereffects of stress on human performance and social behavior: A review of research and theory. *Psychol Bull*. 1980;88(1):82–108.

62. McDermott D. Professional burnout and its relation to job characteristics, satisfaction, and control. *J Human Stress*. 1984;10:79–85.

63. Arches J. Social structure, burnout, and job satisfaction. *Social Work*. 1991;36(3):202–206.

64. Averill JR. Personal control over aversive stimuli and its relationship to stress. *Psychol Bull*. 1973;80(4):286–303.

65. Thompson SC. Will it hurt less if I can control it? A complex answer to a simple question. *Psychol Bull*. 1981;90(1):89–101.

66. Quinby S, Bernstein NR. Identity problems and the adaptation of nurses to severely burned children. *Am J Psychiatry*. 1971;128(1):58–63.

67. Herrera H. Work stress perceived by physicians. Presented at the North Atlantic Treaty Organization (NATO) Advanced Study Institute on Environmental Stress, Life Crises, and Social Adaptation; 18 August 1978; Cambridge, England.

68. Jackson SE. Organizational practices for preventing burnout. In: Amarjit S, Schuler RS, eds. *Handbook of Organizational Stress Coping Strategies*. Cambridge, Mass: Ballinger; 1984: 89–111.

69. Ross RR, Altmaier EM, Russell DW. Job stress, social support, and burnout among counseling center staff. *J Counsel Psychol*. 1989;36(4):464–470.

70. MacNeill DH. The relationship of occupational stress to burnout. In: Jones JW, ed. *The Burnout Syndrome—Current Research, Theory, Interventions*. Park Ridge, Ill: London House; 1982: 68–88.

71. Lazarus RS, Folkman S. Coping and adaptation. In: Gentry WD, ed. *Handbook of Behavioral Medicine*. New York: Guilford; 1984: 282-325.

72. Loftquist LH, Dawis RV. *Adjustment of Work*. New York: Appleton-Century-Crofts; 1969.

73. Manning FJ. Morale, cohesion, esprit. In: Mangelsdorff AD, Gal R, eds. *Handbook of Military Psychology*. New York: Wiley; 1991: 453–470.

74. Cherniss C, Krantz DL. The ideological community as an antidote to burnout in the human services. In: Farber BA, ed. *Stress and Burnout in the Human Service Professions*. New York: Pergamon; 1983.

75. Miller KI, Ellis BH, Zook EG, Lyles JS. An integrated model of communication, stress, and burnout in the workplace. *Communication Res*. 1990;17(3):300–326.

76. Leiter MP, Maslach C. The impact of interpersonal environment on burnout and organizational commitment. *J Organ Behav*. 1988;9:297–308.

77. Ingraham LH, Manning FJ. Cohesion: Who needs it, what is it, and how do we get it to them? *Milit Rev*. 1981;61(6):2–12.

78. Koeske GF, Koeske RD. Work load and burnout: Can social support and perceived accomplishment help? *Social Work*. 1989;(May):243–248.

79. Chappel NL, Novack M. The role of support in alleviating stress among nursing assistants. *Gerontologist*. 1992;32(3):351–359.

80. Constable JF, Russell DW. The effect of social support and the work environment upon burnout among nurses. *J Human Stress*. 1986;12:20–26.

81. Maslach C, Jackson SE. *Maslach Burnout Inventory Manual*. Research edition. Palo Alto, Calif: Consulting Psychologists Press; 1981.

82. Segal DR, Harris JJ, Rothberg JM, Marlowe DH. Paratroopers as peacekeepers. *Armed Forces Society*. 1984;10(4):487–506.

83. Koran LM, Moos RH, Moos B, Zasslow M. Changing hospital work environments: An example of a burn unit. *Gen Hosp Psychiatry*. 1983;5:7–13.

84. Moos R. *Work Environment Scale Manual*. Palo Alto, Calif: Consulting Psychologists Press; 1981.

85. Sande D. Preventing burnout in intensive care nurseries. *Pediatr Nurs*. 1983;9:364–366, 394.

Chapter 4

PSYCHIATRIC ASPECTS OF DISEASES IN MILITARY PERSONNEL

JOSEPH M. ROTHBERG, Ph.D.*

*Research Mathematician, Department of Military Psychiatry, Walter Reed Army Institute of Research, Washington, D.C. 20307–5100

INTRODUCTION

The intent of this chapter is to describe some of the ways that the behavior of soldiers and their leaders can modulate the occurrence of manpower loss due to disease. The actions (and inactions) of soldiers that remove troops from fighting status may be a form of "voluntary casualty" whose prevention is a command issue. For example, preventing the ineffectiveness that arises from malaria is more likely to be successful in the short run if viewed as a behavioral problem (how to ensure that the soldiers take the prophylactic pill) than as a medical problem (how to develop a longer lasting prophylaxis).

The U.S. Army has long recognized that it is engaged in a continuous battle to resist the attacks of what Heggers calls "natural biological warfare."[1] Because past wars have seen more soldiers removed from combat because of disease than from battle injuries, improvements in the health of soldiers can potentially restore more troops to combat status than eliminating all battle casualties. A remarkable description of the impact of infectious diseases and the stress of continuous jungle combat on the fighting strength of Merrill's Marauders, a World War II fighting unit in the China-Burma-India theater, is found in the compilation of the original reports by Stone[2] and the reprint of the 1945 Historical Division report.[3]

> McGee's forces were attacked. The Japanese were not present in great strength, but the 2d Battalion was so wasted by fatigue, dysentery, malaria, and malnutrition that the unit was not effective for combat. During the engagement, several men went to sleep from exhaustion. Colonel McGee himself lost consciousness three times and between relapses directed the Battalion from an aid station."[3(p113)]

The debilitating effects of the medical problems far exceeded the losses from hostile fire and led to the dissolution of the unit.

The focus of this chapter is on the statistics of major infectious diseases armywide and theaterwide and is intended to alert the reader to some major causes of noneffectiveness in prior wars. Although the behavioral, biological, and social components of every disease can be influenced by command policies, this chapter focuses on four diseases that were significant in World War II and the ways that they were manifest in the Korean and Vietnam conflicts. The emphasis of the disease descriptions is on their social and psychological aspects.

A GENERAL FRAMEWORK OF DISEASE COMMUNICATION

The loss of manpower because of combat stress can be thought of as a specific instance of the general process of disease-related loss of manpower. The author adopts a broad view of disease to include those behavioral and psychological processes that remove soldiers from combat for varying periods.

The framework for considering disease-related manpower-loss is an epidemiological agent–vector–host disease model (where the agent is the "germ" or pathological entity, the vector is the intermediate vehicle of transmission, and the host is the soldier). The author considers the end product (a noneffective soldier due to disease) to depend on a sequence of events (where each event in the sequence can be analyzed separately). Such a framework expands the options for informing command policies in ways that can be applied to reduce the loss of manpower. The functional relations defining the model are that a pathogen causes a disease if there are enough vectors and if the probability of sequential transmission is high enough. This transmission is composed of four significant events: (1) the host becomes diseased after exposure to the pathogen (an event that occurs with probability, P_1), (2) the pathogen is introduced by contact with the infected vector (with probability, P_2), (3) the vector makes contact with the host (with probability, P_3), and (4) the vector has acquired the pathogen from the reservoir (with probability, P_4). As a sequential chain terminating with a noneffective soldier (seen in the following diagram), the probabili-

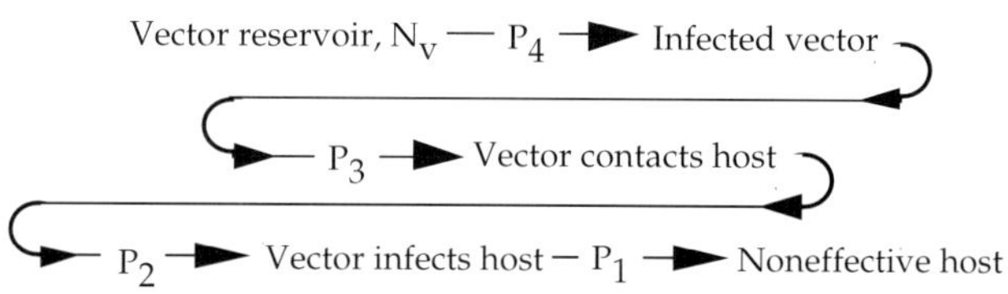

ties are combined by multiplication corresponding to the observation that reducing any one necessary step serves to limit the overall value of the chain to that value or less.

In statistical terms, the probability chain is multiplicative and conditional on the number of vectors (N_v). Disease results when the product of that number of vectors and the probabilities of the events of the chain exceed some critical threshold. In addition, P_1, the probability of becoming diseased, given exposure, can be subdivided into categories (defined by the length of time that the disease state renders the soldier noneffective) to reflect disease severity. For completeness, P_1 can also be expanded to reflect the individual's prior history of exposure.

The various strategies that have been used by the military medical services in previous wars to reduce the impact of disease may all be interpreted in terms of their contribution to modifying this chain of probabilities, the number of vectors, or the average duration of noneffectiveness.

In the following discussion will be found armywide data on the rates of occurrence of four selected disorders that were frequent or exceptional problems in World War II, some discussion of both the precipitants and consequences of those diseases, and consideration of some of the public health issues (screening, ambulatory care, vectors, and hygiene) related to the control of these disorders. Those diseases are also considered during the Korean and Vietnam conflicts. The data are drawn from the published medical records. The reader with a continuing interest in this area is referred to the American Public Health Association's *Control of Communicable Diseases in Man*[4] for a brief description of the history of the various communicable diseases and information on how to recognize a specific disease, to recognize the modes of disease transmission, and to manage the patient so that the disease does not spread.

MAJOR WORLD WAR II DISEASES: THE BIG FOUR

During World War II, Reister[5] reports that there were about 3 million admissions for infectious and parasitic diseases among U.S. Army personnel. These admissions amounted to an annual rate of 117 per 1,000 strength and, as a major diagnostic category, were second only to diseases of the respiratory system (an annual rate of 177 per 1,000), which were handled separately. The grand total for diseases was 15 million admissions, with an additional 2 million nonbattle injuries. The category of infectious and parasitic diseases accounted for 18% of the 339 million soldier-days lost due to hospitalization (noneffectiveness) for a disease or nonbattle injury. Because of the differences in the average number of days per admission, the more frequent respiratory diseases hospitalizations accounted for only 12% of the lost days. Among the medical conditions that were of concern during that time, there are four that will be discussed below: tuberculosis (TB), venereal diseases (VDs), malaria, and hepatitis. The annual rates for these conditions during World War II and the Korean and Vietnam conflicts are presented in Table 4–1. Comparisons with World War I data are made in the text. These four diseases were selected because they occurred frequently in the military or civilian communities and thus represented sig-

TABLE 4–1

ANNUAL ADMISSION RATES PER 1,000* OF SELECTED DISEASES BY YEAR AND AREA

	Tuberculosis	Venereal Disease	Malaria	Hepatitis
World War II worldwide				
1942	1.7	40.4	6.8	15.2
1943	1.2	41.4	22.3	4.2
1944	0.8	44.6	19.0	3.6
1945	1.2	65.6	10.8	10.1
Korea				
1950	0.9	44.7	11.0	19.0
1951	1.0	150.5	10.0	16.8
1952	0.8	192.9	12.5	5.8
Vietnam				
1965	0.2	277.4	48.5	5.7
1966	0.1	281.5	39.0	4.0
1967	0.1	240.5	30.7	7.0
1968	0.1	195.8	24.7	8.6
1969	0.1	189.7	20.8	6.4
1970	0.1	223.0	23.1	7.6
1971	0.0	326.4	16.5	9.6
1972	0.2	698.9	5.0	10.0

* Includes carded for record only.

nificant medical noneffectiveness, or had the potential to do so.

Tuberculosis

TB was the leading cause of civilian disease death in the military age group during the World War II years as reported by Long.[6] Because the annual case rate in the military was only slightly more than 1 per 1,000, TB was not a major cause of noneffectiveness during the war despite the fact that an average case extended for 113 days. The TB rate was reduced to one-ninth of the value of World War I by the policy of rejecting entry into the army of both active and arrested cases of TB. The screening program was a considerable success for the army and had the overall public health benefit of detecting and identifying cases of TB in the civilian population.

The agent–vector–host chain for TB begins with the observation that the agent, the tuberculosis bacterium, is commonly found in the environment. The vector may be bacteria-containing droplets exhaled by other diseased individuals or other respiratory carriers (P_4 is large). When in an area where TB is endemic, every sneeze must be assumed to be contaminated and to provide exposure (P_3 is high). Based on the observations that a large fraction of soldiers are positive reactors to the test for prior exposure to TB (P_2 is high) but that there are a small number of TB cases, current soldiers appear to be relatively resistant to TB (P_1 is small). The TB screening of soldiers before enlistment keeps out those with preexisting disease. The aggressive handling of those with compromised immune systems (for whom P_1 is large so that they are more likely to contract TB) has minimized that source of cases.

Venereal Diseases

The VDs amounted to over one-third of all infectious and parasitic disease cases during World War II.[5] The noneffectiveness rate is calculated using only the inpatient cases, and the rate was relatively low because the largest proportion of cases did not interfere with duty and were treated on an outpatient basis where they appear as carded for record only (CRO). The rate for VD in World War II was only about one-half of the rate observed during World War I (49 per 1,000 versus 87 per 1,000)[5] although Table 4–1 shows increasing values in successive wars. The cluster of VD differs from the other three disease categories because VD is not a single disease and there are few if any outpatient cases for the other diseases. The introduction of penicillin in 1944 did not result in a significant reduction in the recorded VD rate during World War II or subsequent wars.

For these diseases, prevention efforts have historically been concerned with condom use (which reduces P_2), reduced frequency of sexual intercourse (which reduces P_3), and health inspection of prostitutes (which reduces P_4).

Malaria

With a rate of 16 per 1,000 for the entire war, malaria was not a worldwide problem. Within various theaters, however, the malaria rates were not benign and, at the extreme, reached an annualized equivalent rate of 4,000 per 1,000 at Milne Bay in late 1942[7] and 210 per 1,000 in 1943 in the southwest Pacific.[5] There were parallel differences in the noneffectiveness rate, which reached its peak of 14 excused from duty per day per 1,000, in the same theater in 1943. There was a large, but unquantified, performance loss in soldiers who were symptomatic but still deployed and not hospitalized.

The agent–vector–host chain for malaria is well defined with the agent being a parasitic protozoan, *Plasmodium* sp., and the vector being a mosquito, *Anopheles* sp. The probabilities are interpretable as P_4 being the probability that the average anopheles has previously bitten a malaria-infected human, P_3 is the probability of being bitten, P_2 is the probability that the bite transfers the parasite, and P_1 is the probability that the transferred parasite causes the disease. Field malaria discipline consists of administering prophylactic drugs (to keep P_1 low), using physical barriers and repellents (to keep P_3 low), avoiding malaria-endemic areas (to keep P_4 low), and employing mosquito eradication programs (to reduce N_v).

Although malaria was included in the "Big Four" because of the disease's well-defined natural transmission by the mosquito vector, it has an interesting psychiatric sidelight. The prevention and treatment of malaria with quinacrine hydrochloride (Atabrine) during World War II in the India-Burma theater was associated with a number of cases of psychosis. A review of the evidence by Mays[8] concluded that a toxic psychosis occurred in 0.12% of the malaria cases treated with Atabrine, and that Atabrine was indeed responsible for the psychosis. The limitation of the geographic distribution to the India-Burma theater suggested to Glass[9] that the effect is not entirely pharmacologic in nature: "Experiences of other theaters in World War II indicate that Atabrine alone without situational stress and primitive conditions of tropical living does not produce psychotic reactions."[9(p1021)]

Hepatitis

Hepatitis occurred at an annual rate of 8 per 1,000 troops armywide. The highest regional rate occurred in the southwest Pacific with a rate of 26 per 1,000.[5] Before World War II, hepatitis was not considered to be a military disease although many cases of jaundice (many of which were due to hepatitis) occurred during the Civil War. During the process of immunizing soldiers against yellow fever, a contaminated vaccine caused an epidemic of close to 50,000 cases in 1942 as described by Havens[10], and those cases probably represented one-quarter of all of the hepatitis cases that occurred during all of World War II.

The recent availability of hepatitis vaccines has shifted the preventive focus to host resistance (P_1) from the attempts to lower environmental contamination (P_3). The requirements for good sanitation are not relaxed, however, because hepatitis is not the only disease capable of fecal-oral transmission and vaccines are not available for every such disease.

In addition to hygienic issues illustrated by Paul and Gardner[11] in the correlation of hepatitis with the diarrheal and dysentery diseases of poor sanitation, the natural history of hepatitis is a directly psychiatric issue. The disease presentation may include malaise, fatigue, nausea, or other symptoms that can be initially perceived as psychosomatic. A delayed recovery syndrome, referred to as the posthepatitis syndrome and characterized by fatigue and gastro-intestinal disorders after the objective signs disappear, was reported[10] in a small percentage of patients. Havens[10] infers that the syndrome was caused by the interaction of the hepatitis with a preexisting neurosis (neurotic predisposition) because the syndrome responded to adequate diet, physical reconditioning, and indoctrination.

This kind of interaction between individual psychological needs and the sequelae or symptoms of a disease was outlined by Glass[12] in his description of two ways through which soldiers manifest their inability to deal with the combat environment. The first is through overt combat fatigue, which legitimizes withdrawal from combat. The second is one of the following three psychosomatic states that legitimizes delayed return to combat: (1) persistent symptoms with negative somatic findings, (2) persistent symptoms with minor objective findings, or (3) delayed convalescence. Glass[12] makes a strong case for viewing the health behavior of soldiers as multidetermined by physiologic, psychologic, and sociologic forces.

OTHER INFECTIOUS AND PARASITIC DISEASES IN WORLD WAR II

The four diseases mentioned above amounted to 64% of the admissions for infectious and parasitic diseases during World War II. The remaining admissions were divided into viral diseases (21%), with influenza (6%) as the most frequent single disease; bacterial diseases (6%); arthropod infestation (4%); protozoan and helminth infections (3%); rickettsial and fungal diseases (1%); and an unclassified remainder (3%).[5]

THE BIG FOUR IN KOREA

The Korean conflict data arrayed by Reister[13] show that, overall, cases of infective and parasitic diseases were admitted at an annual rate of 48 per 1,000 strength, which was 40% of the value for World War II. The VD CRO cases were tabulated separately and occurred at an annual rate of 57 per 1,000 strength in divisions and regimental combat teams (combat troops), which was a higher annual rate than that recorded for all types of cases (CRO and admissions) during World War II. The VD rate (including CRO) for all troops in Korea was 146 per 1,000. Disposition rates for hepatitis, malaria, or TB are not available for the Korean conflict although the provisional admission data give annual rates of 16 per 1,000 for hepatitis, 11 per 1,000 for malaria, and 1 per 1,000 for TB. The definitive clinical trials of the effect of diet and exercise on the course of hepatitis in over 400 soldiers were done at this time by Chalmers et al.[14] The report of the trials makes no mention of a posthepatitis syndrome, which was present in World War II reports, although a careful reading of the description of their population suggests that the number of their psychotic cases was more than would be expected by chance.

THE BIG FOUR IN VIETNAM

The Vietnam conflict medical data are available as provisional admission data from Neel[15] for 1965 through 1970 and disposition data for selected conditions from Ognibene and Barrett[16] for 1965 through 1972. The overall infectious and parasitic disease rate is not yet available. The average annual VD rate from January 1964 through June 1972 was 325 per 1,000. The rate was not constant and ranged from a low of 190 per 1,000 in 1969 to a high of 699 per 1,000 in the first 6 months of 1972. The average annual rate during 1965 through 1970 for malaria admissions was 31 per 1,000, with a decreasing trend from 48 per 1,000 in 1965, to 22 per 1,000 in 1970.[15] As with World War II, during the Vietnam conflict, small area rates were sometimes very high, and Neel[15] reports that there were at least two maneuver battalions that were rendered ineffective by malaria. Hepatitis was reported at an average annual rate of 6 per 1,000. TB was almost nonexistent, with a reported rate of 0.09 per 1,000 in the 1965 through 1970 period, despite a high endemic rate in the area and intimate contact with the local population as seen in the VD rate.[15]

PUBLIC HEALTH ASPECTS OF THE BIG FOUR

Tuberculosis and Screening

TB is a chronic debilitating disease whose symptoms of depression and fatigue may mimic mental disorders. Screening has been effective in keeping the TB rate low within the military. TB is a disease that had for a time after World War II all but disappeared in both the civilian and military sectors. It has been included here to illustrate screening rather than as a current military medical problem. The appropriate extension of the concept of screening of individuals to prevent their entry into the army for clinical entities other than TB depends on multiple factors. A detection method of adequate sensitivity (cases are identified as cases) and specificity (noncases are identified as noncases) is needed. Screening is not economical for a relatively rare condition when the screening method has inadequate sensitivity because the cost of the screening program may exceed the cost of allowing the cases to appear and be treated within the army. Nor should screening be done with inadequate specificity unless there are an excess of civilians available for service. Because low-specificity screening will incorrectly identify some large fraction of the normals as cases, the rejection of those cases may make it impossible to reach recruiting goals.

Throughout this discussion of screening, the tacit assumptions have been that the underlying condition is truly chronic without remission, that expression of its signs and symptoms interferes with the performance of a soldier's duties, that there is a significant load on the medical system associated with each case, and that there are no overriding external (political) considerations preventing the use of a screening program or following the screening with actions based on the results of the program. TB is a condition that fits the assumptions listed above.

During World War II, screening was an administrative rather than a medical responsibility. It was initially used to reject registrants with any form of VD or with mental disorders or psychoneurotic traits, as well as to reject TB cases. The deferment due to VD was terminated in early 1943 in response to public pressure and therapeutic advances. A psychiatric history was not initially used as a rejection criterion, but that liberal policy was modified in response to complaints from army combat officers to be more restrictive so that even suggestive evidence of emotional instability was cause for rejection. The acute need for soldiers in 1944 led to a reversal of this blanket deferment policy and the introduction of a brief written test to select those who required further psychiatric evaluation before induction into the military.

Venereal Diseases and Ambulatory Treatment

For an acute condition such as VD that can be effectively treated in an outpatient setting, there is a low reported noneffectiveness despite a large number of cases. Realistically, however, that large number of cases represents a considerable number of lost soldier-years, albeit a few hours at a time. The viral VDs and the recently detected types of VD that are resistant to conventional drug treatment suggest that future cases may require more vigorous and repeated outpatient or even inpatient treatment.

The knowledge gained from World War II regarding medical noneffectiveness associated with inpatient hospitalization continues to be applicable today. As summarized by Glass,[17] an almost universal experience of medical officers in World War II concerned the deleterious effect of hospitalization. In a significant number of military personnel, hospitalization seemed to fixate symptoms, retard expected clinical improvement, and negatively influence motivations for return to duty. "During these early years, it became apparent to many wartime psychiatrists and other medical officers that hospitalization in itself created or perpetuated illness and disability."[17(p748)]

In addition to illustrating the desirability and necessity of ambulatory care, VD also serves to illustrate the social aspects of disease processes. VD is sometimes viewed as a behavior problem or a voluntary disease because the prerequisite sexual behavior without proper prophylaxis is unequivocally an individual action within a specific social environment. Attention has been focused by Jones[18] on the observation of Reister that the Korean conflict VD rates were inversely related to combat intensity and directly related to the proportion of combat support troops.

The high VD rate in the Vietnam conflict reflects a variety of social and psychological forces that reduced the efficacy of conventional preventive procedures. Starting with World War II, the U.S. Army policy described by Sternberg[19] has been to provide and encourage wholesome recreation to occupy soldiers' free time as a way to reduce VD rates. The author observes from Neel's[15] data on American troops in Vietnam that the VD rate, including carded-for-record-only cases, varied as the inverse of the troop strength. The rates were lowest when the troop strength was highest and highest when the strength was lowest. The author speculates that the high VD rate after 1969 in Vietnam may reflect changes in the combat intensity and troop composition similar to those that led to the high VD rate during the Korean conflict after mid-1951.[13]

Malaria and Vector Transmission

Malaria is a disease that is transmitted by the bite of a specific type of mosquito if that mosquito had previously bitten an infected human. Direct person-to-person transmission through blood transfusions or illicit drug-use needles has not been reported to be a major nonvector transmission mode.[13] In theory, the disease can be prevented by disrupting the chain of transmission with environmental manipulation to reduce the number of mosquitos and antimalarial drug treatment and prophylaxis to reduce the number of infected humans. In practice, malaria remains a problem when troops are relocated because antimalarial discipline may not be implemented in a timely manner. Prophylaxis is not completely effective and has undesired side effects so that avoiding the vector is frequently a more effective strategy than depending on compliance with an unpleasant prophylactic regimen. The case of malaria that develops after the soldier has failed to take the scheduled malaria prophylaxis is a form of voluntary illness. As with dehydration from failure to maintain scheduled water intake, frostbite from failure to change socks, VD from failure to use a condom, or hepatitis from failure to avoid unsanitary local food, these voluntary illnesses represent manpower loss, which potentially can be avoided by appropriate leadership influences.

Hepatitis and Hygiene

Hepatitis is a communicable viral disease that may present with irritability or even psychosis, incapacitates the patient for weeks, renders him debilitated for months, and may have permanent consequences. The practical modes of transmission are the oral ingestion of fecal-contaminated substances and the injection of hepatitis-contaminated substances or use of hepatitis-contaminated needles. The introduction of the single-use disposable needle and the air-gun immunization system have reduced the patient risk of iatrogenic hepatitis. The health care providers who are exposed to blood or blood products are at elevated risk for hepatitis.[20] The reuse of needles for illicit drug intake remains a transmission route for hepatitis, both type A and type B. The breakdown of primary sanitation is the major cause of the spread of hepatitis in wartime. The primary hygienic goals for the control of hepatitis are to keep human excreta out of the food chain and to provide adequate amounts of uncontaminated or purified water.

ADDITIONAL COMMENTS ON HIV AND AIDS

The human immunodeficiency virus (HIV) is a transmissible agent with a long incubation period and is responsible for the fatal acquired immuno-deficiency syndrome (AIDS). Three army areas immediately impacted by the recent emergence of AIDS are the logistical (blood supply), the psychological (cohesion), and the tactical (deployment). These areas are briefly discussed below.

Current U.S. Army expectation includes the concept that each soldier can be available to serve as a "walking blood bank"[21] to provide emergency blood transfusions for a wounded comrade. Continuous introduction of HIV into army personnel will probably occur both from heterosexual VD and through illegal homosexual acts or intravenous drug abuse. Screening for infection is hampered by the long and variable time between infection with HIV and the ability of current tests to detect the presence of the virus. The presence of a positive HIV test makes that soldier's blood untransfusable; the possibility that the soldier may be infectious through exposure too recent to produce a positive test makes many soldiers' blood untransfusable. A reexamination of blood supply doctrine seems indicated in light of the emergence of HIV.

The small-group performance of the army is maintained by cohesive interpersonal relationships. The HIV-infected soldier is a challenge to the group cohesion. The revelation that HIV infection has occurred raises the question that it may have happened through behaviors (homosexuality or illicit drug use) that are not consonant with those of the other members of the group.

The occurrence of HIV infection among the sexually active, overseas population forces reexamination of the consequences of deployment. HIV infection is endemic in central Africa and has been reported among prostitutes worldwide.[22] The VD transmission to soldiers on overseas deployments is proportional to the probability of occurrence of the other VDs.

SUMMARY

The mission of the U.S. Army Medical Department is the conservation of the fighting strength. Because infectious and parasitic diseases have accounted for large amounts of lost time, even fractional reductions in the number of cases or the average length of stay per case can have a significant impact by returning many soldiers to duty. This chapter has presented some of the trends of the significant diseases (TB, VD, malaria, and hepatitis) of soldiers; some of the traditional responses to those diseases (screening, ambulatory care, vector control, and hygiene); some of the sociological, psychological, and psychiatric aspects of those diseases that can be influenced by command policy; and a framework for thinking about the communication of disease. The intention here has been to remind health professionals of the magnitude of wartime illness and to focus their attention on some of the behavioral factors associated with these diseases.

REFERENCES

1. Heggers JP. Microbial invasion—The major ally of war (natural biological warfare). *Milit Med.* 1978;143(6):390–394.

2. Stone JH. *Crisis Fleeting.* Washington, DC: Office of The Surgeon General, US Department of the Army; 1969.

3. Center of Military History. *Merrill's Marauders February–May 1944.* Washington, DC: US Department of the Army; 1990.

4. Benenson AS. ed. *Control of Communicable Diseases in Man.* 15th ed. Washington, DC: American Public Health Association; 1990.

5. Reister FA. *Medical Statistics in World War II.* Washington, DC: Office of The Surgeon General, US Department of the Army; 1975.

6. Long ER. Tuberculosis. In: *Infectious Diseases*. Vol 2. In: Havens WP, Jr., ed. *Internal Medicine in World War II*. Washington, DC: Office of The Surgeon General, US Department of the Army; 1963: 329–407.

7. Russell PF. Introduction. In: *Communicable Diseases, Malaria*. Vol 6. In: Coates JB, Jr., Hoff EC, Hoff PM, eds. *Medical Department, U.S. Army Preventive Medicine in World War II*. Washington, DC: Office of The Surgeon General, US Department of the Army; 1963: 1–10.

8. Mays JRS. Consultant's composite report of toxic psychoses due to atabrine, India-Burma theater. In: *Overseas Theaters*. Vol 2. In: Glass AJ, ed. *Neuropsychiatry in World War II*. Washington, DC: Office of The Surgeon General, US Department of the Army; 1973: 1087–1094.

9. Glass AJ. Lessons learned. In: *Overseas Theaters*. Vol 2. In: Glass AJ, ed. *Neuropsychiatry in World War II*. Washington, DC: Office of The Surgeon General, US Department of the Army; 1973: 989–1027.

10. Havens WP, Jr. Viral hepatitis. In: *Infectious Diseases and General Medicine*. Vol 3. In: Havens WP, Jr., ed. *Internal Medicine in World War II*. Washington, DC: Office of The Surgeon General, US Department of the Army; 1968: 331–384.

11. Paul JR, Gardner HT. Viral hepatitis. In: *Communicable Diseases Transmitted Through Contact or by Unknown Means*. Vol 5. In: Hoff EC, ed. *Preventive Medicine in World War II*. Washington, DC: Office of The Surgeon General, US Department of the Army; 1960: 411–462.

12. Glass AJ. Psychosomatic medicine. In: *Infectious Diseases and General Medicine*. Vol 3. In: Havens WP, Jr., ed. *Internal Medicine in World War II*. Washington, DC: Office of The Surgeon General, US Department of the Army; 1968: 675–712.

13. Reister FA. *Battle Casualties and Medical Statistics: U.S. Army Experience in the Korean War*. Washington, DC: Office of The Surgeon General, US Department of the Army; 1973.

14. Chalmers TC, Lokhardt RD, Reynolds WE, et al. The treatment of acute infectious hepatitis. Controlled studies of the effects of diet, rest, and physical reconditioning on the acute course of the disease and on the incidence of relapse and residual abnormalities. *J Clin Invest*. 1953;34:1163–1245.

15. Neel S. *Medical Support of the U.S. Army in Vietnam 1965–1970*. Washington, DC: US Department of the Army; 1973.

16. Ognibene AJ, Barrett ON, Jr., eds. In: *General Medicine and Infectious Diseases*. Vol 2. *Internal Medicine in Vietnam*. Washington, DC: Office of The Surgeon General and Center for Military History, US Department of the Army; 1982.

17. Glass AJ. Lessons learned. In: *Zone of the Interior*. Vol 1. In: Glass AJ, Bernucci RJ, eds. *Neuropsychiatry in World War II*. Washington, DC: Office of The Surgeon General, US Department of the Army; 1966: 735–759.

18. Jones FD. Reactions to stress: Combat versus combat support troops. Washington, DC: Walter Reed Army Medical Center; 1977. Mimeograph.

19. Sternberg TH, Howard EB, Dewey LA, Padget P. Venereal diseases. In: *Communicable Diseases Transmitted Through Contact or by Unknown Means*. Vol 5. In: Hoff EC, ed. *Preventive Medicine in World War II*. Washington, DC: Office of The Surgeon General, US Department of the Army; 1960: 139–331.

20. Segal HE, Llewellyn CH, Irwin G, Bancroft WH, Boe GP, Balaban DJ. Hepatitis B antigen and antibody in the U.S. Army. Prevalence in health care personnel. *Am J Public Health*. 1976;66:667–671.

21. Withers BG, Kelley PW, McNeil JG, Cowan DN, Brundage JF. A brief review of the epidemiology of HIV in the U.S. Army. *Milit Med*. 1992;157:80–84.

22. Burrelli DF. HIV–1/AIDS and U.S. military manpower policy. In: Stanley J, Blair JD, eds. *Challenges in Military Health Care*. New Brunswick, NJ: Transaction Publishers; 1993.

Chapter 5

ALCOHOL AND DRUG ABUSE AND DEPENDENCE

HENRY K. WATANABE, M.D.,* PAUL T. HARIG, PH.D.,† NICHOLAS L. ROCK, M.D.,‡ AND RONALD J. KOSHES, M.D.§

*Colonel, Medical Corps, U.S. Army; Medical Member Physical Evaluation Board, Walter Reed Army Medical Center; Guest Scientist, Department of Military Psychiatry, Walter Reed Army Institute of Research, Washington, D.C. 20307–5100

†Lieutenant Colonel, Medical Service Corps, U.S. Army; Director, Army Fitness Research Institute, Army War College, Carlisle Barracks, Pennsylvania 17013–5050

‡Colonel (ret), Medical Corps, U.S. Army; Medical Director, The Rock Creek Foundation, Silver Spring, Maryland 20910–4457

§Medical Director, Adult Services Administration, Commission on Mental Health Services, Department of Human Services, District of Columbia, Washington; Guest Scientist, Department of Military Psychiatry, Walter Reed Army Institute of Research, Washington, D.C.; Assistant Clinical Professor of Psychiatry, Uniformed Services University of the Health Sciences, Bethesda, Maryland; President, Society of American Military Psychiatrists

INTRODUCTION

Among the numerous studies[1,2,3] that have attempted to explain why some occupational groups claim a higher level of excessive alcohol consumption, the common threads of stress and boredom are found. It is not surprising that alcohol and substance abuse could become problems in a combat environment because they are expedient pathways to stress management.

The history of past wars demonstrates this. In the late 1960s and early 1970s, thousands of returning soliers who had served in Vietnam and reportedly used narcotics there aroused public anxiety about the existence of a drug epidemic among U.S.troops.[4]

Before the early 1970s, the military dealt with serious substance abuse by administrative and legal means (discharge and punishment) although it did not respond to every instance of substance abuse. The medical concerns were with treating serious medical complications. However, after 1970, Congress mandated a change from punitive measures to treatment and rehabilitation. Since then, improvements have resulted in providing a comprehensive program based on command responsibility with significant medical interface. Currently, the basic policy in the military services is to keep a sustained effort to prevent substance abuse problems from occurring and to eliminate from the service those who cannot effectively be restored within a reasonable period.

Substance abuse is not tolerated not only because of its physiological effects on the abuser that would jeopardize mission requirements, but also because of its psychosocial implications in the unit. While a kind of cohesion can occur around the use of substances,[1] substance abuse is definitely damaging to the good order and morale of the unit and interferes with mission accomplishment.

The command structure has been charged with the responsibility for the alcohol and drug abuse program. The medical services are to offer consultation and technical supervision to individuals who work for the command and to provide specific and direct medical support for those with identified problems. The purpose of this chapter is to assist medical personnel to achieve those command goals and objectives.

The illegal use of drugs in civilian life and in the military began to steadily increase after 1967, and illicit drug usage among military personnel was reported to have doubled every year from 1967 to 1969.[5] The return from Vietnam of thousands of soldiers who had reportedly used heroin raised public anxiety over the possibility of a drug epidemic, and a congressional investigation confirmed that overseas drug use was prevalent among U.S. troops.[4] Indeed, the Vietnam conflict was the first American war in which drug and alcohol dependency overshadowed combat stress reactions as a problem for military psychiatry. The large prevalence of drug abuse among troops in Vietnam had unique political sensitivity for an administration that had campaigned on a strong law and order platform that tied drug use to rising crime rates. It also added fuel to opponents' demands for immediate troop withdrawals, which, in turn, was perceived as a major political threat to the President's Vietnamization program.[6]

In response, the administration created a drug abuse office within the Federal Government, emphasizing the prevention of drug abuse through education and law-enforcement procedures focusing on detection. The day after the President declared a national counteroffensive against drug abuse, the U.S. Army in Vietnam began urine testing for opiates for all soldiers completing their tours. Detoxification, treatment, and rehabilitation were provided to those who were identified as heroin abusers. Army regulations were soon modified to create an amnesty for those who voluntarily turned themselves in for treatment. This amnesty was a big step because it eliminated criminal consequences to treating individuals for problems with narcotics. By November 1971, unannounced testing for amphetamines and barbiturates, as well as opiates, had commenced worldwide, and treatment programs were being phased in throughout the world.[7]

Recently, the epidemic of crack and cocaine use in the civilian population has had parallel consequences in the military. Given the generally poor rate of rehabilitation for these substances using conventional treatments, the appearance of cocaine and crack on the military scene has resulted in significant manpower losses. Koshes and Shanahan[8] tracked the disposition of soldiers who tested positive for cocaine at a U.S. Army training post. All of those who tested positive were dismissed from the service, many of whom were high-ranking enlisted soldiers with many years of service.

HISTORY

Pre-1971

Alcohol problems have existed in most of the armies throughout the world since historical records have been kept. Narcotic addiction occurred during the Civil War, World War I, World War II, the Korean conflict, and the Vietnam conflict, as well as with soldiers stationed in the continental United States and overseas between and after the conflicts. Substance abuse has always been a potential occupational hazard for medical personnel. As Farley has observed, "Addiction to mood altering chemicals ... is also a major problem in the medical profession and particularly in the specialty of anesthesia."[9(p1)] This is in part because anesthesiologists have legal (although controlled) access, in part because of the high stress and responsibilities of the profession, and in part because of a tendency for educated medical professionals to rationalize that they can self-administer dangerous and addictive drugs safely.

The highly addictive properties of controlled medical substances such as the anesthetic fentanyl [10] create unique problems for medical providers. The temptations of access and the dangers of self-administration of these drugs by military medical personnel was evidenced in a near-epidemic of fentanyl abuse among tri-service anesthesiologists and nurse anesthetists in the early 1980s. This abuse led to the special rehabilitation program for military personnel that is dictated by a quality assurance regulation.[11] This regulation linked substance abuse rehabilitation and medical quality assurance. The purposes were to ensure that during rehabilitation, the practice credentials of drug-dependent health professionals were restricted, and that their recovery was carefully monitored by medical authorities. These policies reflected impaired health provider statutes that were enacted by the state regulatory authorities. These statutes encourage rehabilitation and full return to practice but also protect the consumer from possible harm during the provider's recovery.

During the 1800s, intoxication and delirium tremens (DTs) from bromides resulted in many hospital admissions. Barbiturate intoxications were a common problem in the 1900s. The introduction of lysergic acid (LSD) in the 1950s resulted in newer problems related to psychosis. Since then, many more chemical agents have been utilized with resultant problems for the military and civilian communities.[2]

During the Russo-Japanese War (1904–1906), the Russians identified three common types of "mental cases": depressive syndrome, general paresis, and alcohol psychosis.[12] In the U.S. Army, from 1907–1917, admissions for alcohol problems were 16 per 1,000 troops per annum.[13] During World War II, the alcohol admission rate was 1.7 per 1,000 troops per annum, while the drug addiction rate was 0.1 per 1,000 troops per annum. Combined, they made up 4.7% of all psychiatric diagnosis.[14] Since World War II and until 1970, the pattern had remained the same. However, in the 1970s drug abuse problems increased significantly in the armed forces.[2]

Attempts at solving the problems have been historically poor. The Federal Anti-Narcotic Act in 1914, the infamous prohibition act of 1919 to 1933, and the Federal Addiction Rehabilitation Act of 1966 were national attempts focusing mostly on the civilian community.

Post-1971

The subject of alcohol rehabilitation deserves special attention in this chapter because alcohol problems have traditionally been handled somewhat apart from other drugs of abuse, yet treatment policies were closely influenced by the Department of Defense (DoD) drug counteroffensive. Initially, the recognition of the occupational significance of alcoholism and support for its treatment was stimulated by several congressional initiatives, including the passage of important enabling legislation and the establishment of the National Institute on Alcohol Abuse and Alcoholism to coordinate research and public information. The first such law, the Comprehensive Alcohol Abuse and Alcoholism Prevention, Treatment, and Rehabilitation Act,[15] was sponsored by Senator Harold Hughes, a recovering alcoholic, and provided the country's first comprehensive national policy on alcoholism since the repeal of Prohibition. Among its provisions, it mandated treatment and rehabilitation for federal employees, prohibited discrimination against alcoholics by hospitals that received federal funds, safeguarded the confidentiality of treatment records, and encouraged worksite programs to identify and treat drinking problems.

The year 1971 marked a turning point for military alcoholism programs when Senator Hughes introduced a companion law, Public Law 92–129, that directed the Secretary of Defense to "identify, treat and rehabilitate members of the armed forces who are drug or alcohol dependent."[3(p646)] Consequently, military treatment for chronic alcohol problems received increased visibility as it drew energy from incentives to combat the drug crisis that had been festering during Vietnam. This visibility was clearly a mixed blessing because DoD policies on drug abuse had begun to migrate away from the early focus on rehabilitation.

In 1980, a comprehensive policy directive expressed the policy goal as follows: "To be free of the effects of alcohol and drug abuse; of the trafficking in illicit drugs by military and civilian members of the Department of Defense; and of possession, use, sale, or promotion of drug abuse paraphernalia."[16] The policy clearly stated that drug and alcohol abuse were incompatible with the high standards of performance, military discipline, and readiness. The emphasis on prevention and control resulted from the recognition that drug abuse and drug addiction were not synonymous,[17] bolstered by the results of a worldwide survey[18] that found drug use was most prevalent among 18- to 25-year-olds who had not developed the mature lifestyles that preclude abuse. Thereafter, the drug problem was reinterpreted to exist more from a lack of discipline than from addiction. Accordingly, greater emphasis was placed on prevention programs directed at all military personnel and on more punitive policies aimed at drug and alcohol abusers.[19]

The reaction to the crash of a jet aircraft on the USS *Nimitz* in 1981 further emphasized the military's problem with drugs by revealing the high incidence of marijuana use among those sailors who were killed in the crash.[19] A stringent policy of zero tolerance by military authority emerged from this incident, with greater emphasis on random urine testing for drugs and severe disciplinary consequences on users of illicit drugs. Along with the view that drug abuse reflected indiscipline more than addiction came an emphasis on command sponsorship of the treatment system; that is, the alcohol and drug prevention and control programs were regarded as commanders' programs. By placing policy for these programs in line, rather than medical, channels the DoD emphasized that its primary value was for manpower conservation and the benefits were the avoidance of heavy replacement costs of skilled personnel. Thus, criteria for admission to rehabilitation programs came to include a commander's approval and implied latitude to discharge in lieu of treatment.

As the substance abuse policy was implemented and expanded, military and civilian personnel were trained specifically for the Alcohol and Drug Abuse Prevention and Control Program (ADAPCP), and treatment facilities were created, expanded, and evaluated. Total annual DoD outlays for drug and alcohol prevention and control exceeded $228 million in fiscal year 1987 and involved over 4,600 man years of effort.[3] These expenditures included the costs (including personnel) for biochemical testing, education, treatment, training, and evaluation. In fiscal year 1988, for example, more than 47,000 of the 2.1 million active duty military personnel received treatment for drug and alcohol problems. Nearly 39,000 of these individuals were treated as outpatients in 400 nonresidential facilities, while approximately 8,000 were treated as inpatients in 52 residential facilities.[19] This made the DoD a major provider of inpatient alcoholism treatment and one of the world's largest integrated occupational health programs targeted on substance abuse and chemical dependency.

In 1986, DoD policies on drug and alcohol abuse were placed in a broader context of health promotion that emphasized the value of healthy lifestyle on personal readiness.[16] By implication, alcohol abuse and drug abuse were characterized as unhealthy behaviors that are incompatible with military service. Concurrently, an emphasis on deterrence through routine urine drug screening and stringent zero tolerance policies for those detected for drug use or convicted of drunk driving has achieved significant reductions in drug abuse in the military.[19] From 1982 to the present time, worldwide surveys[19] have confirmed the substantial reduction in the use of illicit drugs and related medical and disciplinary problems.

Changing Trends, Unchanging Risks

Progress in reducing alcohol abuse and alcoholism among those in higher military ranks has not, however, been as pronounced as the counter-drug program results. Bray and colleagues[19] reported standardized comparisons of prevalence of alcohol and drug use among military personnel and civilians with 1985 data. These analyses, which controlled for demographic differences, indicate that drug use was significantly lower among military personnel than for civilians, while heavy drinking was significantly higher. The analyses concluded that the zero tolerance policies for drug use in the military had been effective, but military life may be conducive to a greater likelihood of abusive levels of alcohol use among military personnel than among civilians in general.

Why the difference? Although there is a substantial research literature[20,21,22] that attempts to relate the occurrence of high rates of excessive drinking in certain occupations as evidence for high-risk occupations, this relatively large body of literature is based on many redundant citations and small samples and is suspect on methodological grounds.[20] Therefore, it is difficult to explain the reported differences in consumption between military and civilian populations on job characteristics. Examination of specific groups has yielded some general attributes that may explain some of the difference. Trice and Roman,[23] for example, found that unstructured jobs without clear goals, jobs with remote supervision and frequent travel or isolation, jobs that require drinking as a part of the work role, and jobs in competitive settings where drinking for relief is seen as justified have greater risk for drinking problems. Plant[21,24] did extensive research on the brewing industry and suggested that an individual's drinking pattern can be changed through the influence of the general level of drinking among work associates, availability of alcohol, the extent that coworkers cover up excesses, lax supervision, and job stresses, including boredom. Hingston et al[25] did not find consistent levels of association between heavy drinking and workers' job perceptions, except that stress and boredom were significantly related to amounts consumed. They suggested, however, that stress and boredom could be the way workers rationalize excessive drinking, regardless of the actual nature of their work. As stated, Whitehead and Simpkins[20] found many inconsistencies in work climate explanations for excessive drinking but were able to isolate eight structural factors that were significantly related to alcohol problems in the workplace: (1) social pressure to drink alcoholic beverages frequently, (2) peer sanction of heavy drinking, (3) recruitment of heavy drinkers in the occupational field, (4) peer sanction of drinking on the job, (5) official sanction of heavy drinking, (6) separation from normal sexual or social relationships, (7) opportunity to obtain alcoholic beverages relatively inexpensively, and (8) preponderance of young workers in the occupation. Whitehead and Simpkins found that 70% of the variance in the rate of alcohol problems could be explained by these factors. Moreover, two factors in combination—social pressure and inexpensive access—explained over two-thirds of the variance by themselves. Of these two factors, opportunity to obtain alcoholic beverages inexpensively appeared to be the most critical. Fitting these characteristics into the military context, it is not difficult to speculate that there might be relatively greater alcohol consumption among this population.

Despite the military's tendency to control drug and alcohol problems through the same disciplinary pressures, a monolithic view of drinking problems that presupposes that excessive alcohol use is voluntary and reflects immaturity cannot reconcile the phenomenon of late-onset alcoholism in adults who had been fairly indistinguishable from their military peers. The glaring flaw is the inability to explain the common phenomenon of the career soldier or sailor whose drinking became severe and disabling after 10 or 15 years of distinguished military service. It seems unlikely that any purported underlying factor of immaturity would apply to these individuals because it would have been a significant impediment to their career advancement and achievement.

How, then, are such individuals affected? In early stages, their alcoholism may be eclipsed by a myriad of medical complications of excessive drinking. Then later, because these career soldiers and sailors are too successful to fit the stereotype of the occupationally dysfunctional alcoholic, their excessive consumption is viewed as situational or voluntary, opening them to the moral imperatives of a willful misconduct model. Thus, it is critical for the clinician to appreciate that different populations may be represented in the common administrative net and to refine an individual diagnosis that correctly sorts the immature from the chemically dependent. Clearly, the DoD policy context—influenced as well by defense downsizing—impedes this objective somewhat.

Military personnel may not seek help because of real or perceived threats to their careers. That perception, observes Bray et al,[19] is not surprising in view of the emphasis of disciplinary action for drug use. Current policy is to process officers and senior enlisted personnel for discharge after the first detected drug offense but to give junior enlisted personnel a second chance to prove themselves. This policy is at odds with a concurrent DoD policy of encouraging individuals with alcohol problems to seek help, and the two are frequently confused. Thus, 58 percent of respondents to the 1988 Worldwide Survey expected disciplinary action would be taken against a person seeking treatment for an alcohol problem, and 60.9 percent expected it for a drug problem.[26] The best evidence to represent the barrier of fear is that one-third of respondents believed that those who sought help for an alcohol problem would damage their careers although military policies encourage rehabilitation. Although the healthcare provider may not be capable of changing this mass psychology, it is important to recognize its presence and its power to drive avoidance treatment-seeking and treatment-offering behavior.

The medical and psychiatric literature, however, has consistently expanded the biological understanding of addictive behavior. Many neurophysiologic research efforts have supported the notion that drug-craving behavior and repetitive drug and alcohol use may be linked to alterations in the neurochemical milieu.[27,28,29] Genetic factors are also postulated, especially in alcoholism,[30,31] particularly among Native Americans and Asians who have low levels of alcohol dehydrogenase. In addition, life-cycle studies show an increased incidence of alcohol and substance abuse in adults who have a history of attention deficit disorder as children.[32,33]

Public Law

1971 marked a turning point for military substance abuse treatment because of the enactment of specific legislation that directed the Secretary of Defense "to identify, treat and rehabilitate members of the Armed Forces who are drug or alcohol dependent."[3(p646)] This legislation, Public Law 92–129, required the military to participate in full compliance with the earlier Comprehensive Alcohol Abuse and Alcoholism Prevention, Treatment, and Rehabilitation Act of 1970,[15] better known as the Hughes Act. Signed by President Nixon, against the urging of influential Cabinet members,[34] the Hughes Act provided the country's first comprehensive national policy on alcoholism since the repeal of Prohibition. Among its provisions, it mandated alcoholism treatment and rehabilitation for federal employees, prohibited hospitals that received federal funds from discriminating against the admission and treatment of alcohol abusers and alcoholics, safeguarded the confidentiality of records of alcoholic patients, and established the National Institute on Alcohol Abuse and Alcoholism as a catalyst for fostering programs to identify and rehabilitate alcoholics with special emphasis on the workplace. Public Law 92–129 made it clear that the military also had to carry out the policies stated in the Hughes Act. It thus gave impetus to the significant expansion of alcoholism treatment programs in the military services.

In the meantime, the narcotic problems emanating from Vietnam ended with the withdrawal from Vietnam. There was also an upsurge of narcotic abuse in troops stationed in Europe during the 1970s, particularly with intravenous heroin. This drug abuse also created a hepatitis epidemic, requiring massive air evacuation of these soldiers to the continental United States.

As the substance abuse policy was implemented and expanded, military and civilian personnel were trained specifically for the ADAPCP, and treatment facilities were created, expanded, and evaluated. In addition, urine testing was implemented for the massive screening of drugs within the military. This impetus has since resulted in the successful program of prevention, control, and treatment of substance abuse as it currently exists.

DIAGNOSIS AND DEFINITIONS

Diagnosis

During the early 1900s, the U.S. Army classified drug and alcohol addiction separately from mental diseases. In other words, drug and alcohol problems without a physical or mental disease were considered as nonmedical disorders. Current policy still dictates medical and nonmedical disposition of soldiers identified with a psychoactive substance use, abuse, or dependency problem, despite the considerable evidence[28] that suggests that these disorders are genetically and physiologically based.

The U.S. Army (and all of DoD) uses the International Classification of Diseases (ICD) system. The ICD-Clinical Modification (ICD–CM) and the *Diagnostic and Statistical Manual of Mental Disorders* (3rd ed., revised, DSM III–R),[35] which is correlated with the ICD-CM, are used in the United States for diagnostic purposes.

Definitions

The following terminology is frequently encountered in substance use disorders.

- *Substance* refers to alcohol, drugs, or any chemical that, when taken, affects the physical and mental functions of an individual.
- *Substance use* refers to the consumption of alcohol or other psychoactive drugs that can have negative effects on the person's social, occupational, or physical well-being.
- *Substance abuse* is a pattern of use that results in negative consequences although these effects may not be visible or even recognized by those in the environment.[3]
- *Substance dependence* is a condition, psychological or physical, of interaction between a person and substance, characterized by a compulsion to take the substance on either a continuous or a periodic basis to experience its psychological effects or to avoid the discomfort of its absence.
- *Physical dependence* is an altered physiological state brought on by the frequent use of a substance and resulting in physiological symptoms on withdrawal. Note that one may become dependent on a substance without abusing it or being addicted to it as in cancer or chronic pain patients.
- *Psychological dependence* is substance dependence without the physiological evidence of dependence.
- *Tolerance* is the altered physiological state produced by the continuous use of a substance with the declining effect of the given dose.[3,36]

Dependence Syndrome

The *dependence syndrome* associated with psychoactive substances is the hallmark of these addictive disorders. It is multidimensional with biological, social, and behavioral components. The *loss of control* over the substance use is the cardinal feature of this syndrome. The syndrome elements are as follows:

- Substance use takes on a regular schedule of almost continuous or daily use.
- Substance use becomes a higher priority than any other activities despite negative consequences.
- Increased tolerance develops.
- Withdrawal symptoms occur.
- The substance is used to avoid withdrawal.
- A compulsion to use the substance develops.
- Readdiction liability is possible.

Most of the above syndrome elements have been incorporated in the current DSM III–R criteria for psychoactive substance dependence. Because the military services apply the DSM III–R criteria for diagnostic purposes, it is essential that familiarity with the criteria is established. See Exhibit 5–1.

Although *tolerance* and *withdrawal* are symptoms that are listed in the DSM III–R criteria for dependence, these two symptoms are not required to make the diagnosis of dependence as had been in the original DSM III[37] system. To diagnose dependence, it is necessary to fulfill only three of the nine DSM III–R criteria. In addition, social and occupational impairment has also been deemphasized as being essential in the current DSM III–R diagnosis of either dependence or abuse.[38]

DETERMINANTS OF SUBSTANCE ABUSE

Individual Determinants

The use and abuse of psychoactive substances, along with the dependence syndrome, are multidetermined. The military population being a subsample of the general population is made up of individuals of various ages, personalities, and backgrounds. They thus share the biological, psychological, and social vulnerabilities of the general population. The individual determinants are significant because the constitutional vulnerabilities are present within the soldier and, given a set of circumstances, an emergence of the substance abuse disorder can occur.

Although polydrug abuse has not been conclusively linked to genetic factors, studies in alcoholism have shown evidence of genetic linkage.[32] These studies indicate that a child of an alcoholic has a greater risk of developing alcoholism than a child of nonalcoholic parents, even when adopted by nonalcoholics at birth.[31,39] There has also been noted physiological differences between children of alcoholics and those of nonalcoholics in their biological response to alcohol and other sedatives in their central nervous system function.[28]

Personality appears to play a more important role in the genesis of polydrug abuse than in alcoholism. Drug abusers frequently display severe

EXHIBIT 5–1

DSM III–R DIAGNOSTIC CRITERIA FOR PSYCHOACTIVE SUBSTANCE DEPENDENCE AND ABUSE

I. Dependence

A. At least three of the following:

1. Substance often taken in larger amounts or over a longer period than the person intended
2. Persistent desire or one or more unsuccessful efforts to cut down or control substance use
3. A great deal of time spent in activities necessary to get the substance, take the substance, or recover from its effects
4. Frequent intoxication or withdrawal symptoms when expected to fulfill major role obligations at work, school, or home, or when substance use is physically hazardous
5. Important social, occupational, or recreational activities given up or reduced because of substance use
6. Continued substance use despite knowledge of having a persistent or recurrent social, psychological, or physical problem that is caused or exacerbated by the use of the substance
7. Marked tolerance: need for markedly increased amounts of the substance (at least 50% increase) to achieve intoxication or desired effect, or markedly diminished effect with continued use of the same amount
8. Characteristic withdrawal symptoms
9. Substance often taken to relieve or avoid withdrawal symptoms

B. Some symptoms of the disturbance have persisted for at least 1 month or have occurred repeatedly over a longer period of time.

II. Abuse

A. A maladaptive pattern of psychoactive substance use indicated by at least one of the following:

1. Continued use despite knowledge of persistent or recurrent social, occupational, psychological, or physical problems that are caused or exacerbated by use of the psychoactive substance
2. Recurrent use in situations when use is physically hazardous

B. Some symptoms of the disturbance have persisted for at least 1 month or have occurred repeatedly over a longer period of time.

C. Never met the criteria for psychoactive substance dependence for this substance.

personality disorders of the antisocial or borderline type. Psychological and personality characteristics of drug-abusing persons most often have been reported as impulsive and novelty seeking.[39]

Social maladjustment and environmental deprivation likewise are significant as determinants of substance abuse. This finding is more true with polydrug abusers.[40]

Environmental Determinants

Substance abuse like any other behavior is the product of an individual interacting with his environment. In any organizational management of substance abuse, it is therefore essential to understand the environment in which the disorder occurs. The military environment has its unique stressors, which are experienced by all but to which each soldier's reaction differs depending on individual strengths. Young soldiers tend to face insurmountable obstacles to a sense of personal identity and unit affiliation by the high level of turbulence in the units, the geographical separation from friends and family, and the psychological isolation from officers, noncommissioned officers, and the surrounding community.

Excessive drinking has been associated with military personnel, and active duty has been considered to be a high-risk occupation for alcoholism. That the military environment contributes to alcohol use and abuse has been frequently cited.[1,2,3,17,19] Studies have also indicated little change in patterns of alcohol use over the years.[3] In a survey among military personnel, there was a definite relation between stress at work and alcohol consumption.[26]

It has been noted that the pattern of substance use among soldiers is determined less by pharmacological and personality variables and more by the circumstances, such as substance availability, peer pressure, and need for affiliation in an environment in which social supports tend to be lacking and in which loneliness and isolation abound.[41,42] Drugs have been used as a way of "bolstering self-esteem through identification with a group, to reduce anxiety, and to provide themselves with an interpersonal relationship."[43(p448)]

Combat, the most significant stressful situation in the military, generally tends to increase substance use. A study of veterans of the Korean and Vietnam conflicts indicated "a significant association between combat exposure and excessive alcohol use."[44(p572)] Many veterans of the Vietnam conflict began using heroin during their tour of duty for relief of fear and tensions of war. Abuse of heroin, cannabis, and alcohol by combat soldiers was not usual while in the field in close proximity with the enemy but rather was usual while back at the fire base or on rest and recreation. Apparently, the desire for survival mobilized peer pressure to keep soldiers alert while on patrol. For other soldiers, boredom and the lack of meaningful activity contributed to substance use.[45]

Availability

There can be no widespread substance abuse without its availability. This situation was clearly demonstrated during the Vietnam conflict when the use of narcotics dramatically increased due to its availability and low cost. In addition, many who were regular drinkers, including some who had drinking problems, switched to opiates and then became opiate dependent. After the Vietnam conflict, opiate use decreased, and alcohol use again became ascendant.[46] A study of soldiers returning from the Republic of Vietnam (RVN) in 1971 disclosed "less than 1% ever addicted to narcotics before arrival in RVN; while in RVN, 1/2 of them used narcotics and 1/5 reported opiate addiction. After their return to the US, usage and addiction decreased to pre-Vietnam levels."[47] Similarly, the 1990 to 1991 Persian Gulf War saw an absence of alcohol problems because of strictures against importation of alcohol into Islamic countries.

Organizational Determinants

The level of stress present within the unit impacts on its members significantly. As a result of leadership difficulties or organizational problems, the soldiers in the unit can experience a significant amount of discontent, frustration, and poor morale. Problems in behavior among the troops rise significantly, and substance abuse rates tend to rise accordingly. Therefore, in any situation in which significant substance abuse is determined, a command consultation with the unit is indicated, and organizational functioning needs to be assessed. Primary preventive measures could significantly reduce the abuse rates in dysfunctional units.

CURRENT THEORIES

Biopsychosocial

Soldiers may take substances for many reasons. These reasons include curiosity, peer pressure, and the desire to diminish dysphoric feelings or experience euphoriant feelings. Drug use among young soldiers is generally experimental and tends to be confined to social situations that often provide a focus for group interactions and identity.[1] This type of substance use is quite different from regular use or dependence.

Today, the biopsychosocial theory is the dominant concept in alcoholism. The theory postulates that certain susceptible individuals are more likely to develop alcohol dependence because of biological (genetic), psychological, (depression), or social (peer influences) predispositional factors. Stressful life events or psychological conditions (anxiety, insomnia, depression, and so forth) precipitate increased drinking, and the drinking becomes progressive as alcohol in these susceptible individuals provides relief by producing euphoria or alleviating the dysphoria. As a consequence, primary psychological dependence is developed resulting in tolerance. Physical dependence follows with the need to drink to prevent withdrawal symptoms. The established addictive cycle is then intensified by the protracted abstinence syndrome with persistent psychological craving. Even after a period of abstinence, and this period can last many years, because the physical dependence mechanism remains, the addictive behavior becomes reactivated by alcohol ingestion.[39]

Subtypes of Alcoholism

Military experience has indicated that alcoholism is manifested in different ways among soldiers. What is frequently seen among the younger soldiers is not the same as what is seen with older soldiers. Studies[31,39] of families with alcoholism and adoption studies[28,39] have clarified these impressions by the determination of two clinical subgroups of persons with alcoholism that differ in their genetic and environmental backgrounds.[28] These subtypes imply different approaches for the management and the treatment of alcoholism in the military.

Type 1 alcoholism is the classical alcohol-dependent person with a loss of control and the compulsion to drink. Type 1 alcoholics are generally anxious or passive-dependent and drink to relieve the anxiety. They may experience prolonged and severe depressive responses to separation or loss of social attachments. For this group, mild or severe alcohol abuse occurs after the age of 25 years, and tolerance and dependence develop rapidly on drinking. They tend to display recurrent binges, guilt about drinking, and liver disorders. The disorder is more often familial than with Type 2, often with both their parents having a similar pattern. There is little or no criminality. Because of the loss of control and prominent psychological dependence, the treatment goal should be a total, lifelong abstinence. Supportive social relationships and appropriate means of relieving anxiety are also essential for recovery.[28]

Those with Type 2 alcoholism are typical alcohol abusers, characterized by the onset of moderate alcohol abuse during their teenage years (before the age of 25). They drink to seek stimulation and pleasure and present a history of frequent criminality with arrests, suicidal acts, and other acting-out behavior. Generally, there is a history of an early onset of alcohol abuse and criminality in their biological fathers. Antisocial personality characteristics are common with impulsive and aggressive behavior. They tend to be risk takers who abuse a variety of substances in addition to alcohol. The alcoholism is manifested by an inability to abstain, fighting while drinking, and drinking and driving recklessly. Women seem less at risk for the Type 2 alcoholic disorder than do men. Treatment should be heavily directed toward seeking other ways to obtain stimulation and pleasure, that is, physical activities in addition to developing self-control.[28]

IDENTIFICATION

Substance abusers are quite unlike the usual patients that a physician sees in two major respects. First, the typical medical patient is motivated by his distress and discomforts to seek relief. The drug abuser does not consider himself ill or his activity undesirable. It is only when he suffers from intoxication, withdrawal, or other effects of substance use that he is brought to medical attention, and then usually as a referral by his commander. Second, although the treatment of the physical effects of substance use is a medical responsibility, the treatment of the substance use disorder (rehabilitation) is a command responsibility.

Unlike with most other medical disorders, the pervasive existence of denial among substance abusers maintains the drug use and perpetuates the disorder. The motivation for recovery is often provided by the threat of career termination because the military services have considered continued substance abuse to be incompatible with military service.

Biochemical testing is used widely within the military services for the detection of alcohol and drug use. For alcohol, breathalyzers are a rapid means of ascertaining the level of blood alcohol present for treatment purposes; however, whenever a need arises for a legal determination of blood alcohol concentration (BAC), a laboratory analysis of the blood sample is necessary, utilizing proper procedures and a chain of custody. Usually, commanders have the authority to order such testing.

Urinalysis

Urinalysis testing is useful for detecting substance use such as cannabis, cocaine, amphetamines, phencyclidine, barbiturates, and opiates. Testing is done under strict procedures to minimize administrative errors because a soldier's career may be determined by its result. Commanders often utilize random urine testing for drugs. For both alcohol and drugs, commanders have the prerogative of ordering testing whenever there is a suspicion of use or impairment.

The physician plays a key role in the evaluation of all confirmed laboratory tests because prescribed drugs can give an erroneous impression of abuse. The physician assesses all available data, including medical records, examines the subject, and renders a diagnosis and recommendations. It is important that physicians work closely with the commander in obtaining all pertinent information before any final decision is made that the individual is or is not a substance abuser. To assist the physician, questionnaires such as the Michigan Alcoholism Screening Test (MAST)[48] and the CAGE[49] (Have you tried to **C**ut down? Are people **A**ngry when you drink? Do you feel **G**uilty about drinking? Do you take an **E**ye-opener in the morning?) are available and easily administered and scored.

A proper diagnosis of substance abuse disorder is essential in ensuring proper intervention, treatment, and follow-up. The physician should be objective in considering the needs of both the individual and the organization rather than "protecting" the person, as sometimes occurs. In addition, the primary concern of all professionals should be to encourage substance abusers voluntarily to seek assistance and to eliminate those factors that prevent this assistance.

Medical Screening

An important means of detection is available to the physician attending to "sick call." Conditions such as hepatitis, recurrent Monday "flu" syndromes, and gastritis may indicate substance abuse. Alcohol misuse can aggravate almost any of the routine complaints and findings seen in the everyday practice of medicine, particularly neurological, gastrointestinal, and cardiorespiratory symptoms. Physicians should always consider substance abuse in any recurrent or nonspecific medical conditions and recurrent injuries.

Commander's Suspicion

For commanders, the usual means of identifying alcoholism is based on performance criteria such as absenteeism, tardiness, personality changes, disinterest, argumentativeness, accidents, and sickness. This is true largely in the lower enlisted ranks. Among the higher enlisted ranks and officers, impairment is quite subtle and less conspicuous. Therefore, identification is more difficult. Here, a recognition of longer lunch breaks with a smell of alcohol on the breath may be a clue to an alcohol problem. Identification based on performance becomes an especially difficult task. The performance requirements of jobs differ, and the higher status jobs allow more variation in work performance. Furthermore, the senior service member has less immediate supervision, more privacy, and more opportunity to set his own pace and hours, and there are fewer opportunities for accidents. In addition, there is less social distance and more collegiality between the higher enlisted ranks and officers and their supervisors. These supervisors are often reluctant to acknowledge that a problem exists.

Within the DoD, any person having a blood alcohol level of 0.05 percent while on duty is considered impaired and should not continue to work. "Alcohol is a primary and continuous depressant of the central nervous system. In persons intolerant of alcohol, impairment of judgement and of recently learned, complex, and finely tuned skills begins to occur at BACs as low as 5.4 mmol per liter (0.025 percent), followed by the loss of more primitive skills and functions, such as gross motor control and orientation, at concentrations in excess of 11 mmol per liter (0.05 percent)."[50(p456)]

For troops in combat or in the field, the problem is especially critical as impairment in information processing occurs even at minimal blood levels. The ability to abstract and conceptualize is diminished along with the cognitive ability to interpret incoming information. The soldier is also less able to appreciate the potential danger or the negative consequences of a particular action because alcohol tends to cause him to act impulsively.[50]

TREATMENT

For many years, alcoholism as a treatable condition was ignored by the military as well as by the medical community. Little was known then of alcoholism as a disease. While great strides have been made in its understanding, much more needs to be understood of its mechanisms and phenomena in order to develop more effective treatment.

In the past, while the military had a variety of mechanisms for handling alcoholic dereliction of duty, it lacked treatment programs. As a result, the soldier's denial was echoed by the military because commanders seldom wished to terminate what had been a promising career. Soldiers with confirmed alcoholism were put in the same category as those with mental deficiency or psychopathic state, and they were considered to be constitutionally handicapped. "Their separation from the army under the appropriate administrative regulation was in the best interest of the soldier and the service."[51(p590)]

Alcoholism was considered a result of willful misconduct, and the punitive approach was the usual means of management. However, medical personnel felt that treatment should be offered to the afflicted soldier rather than punishment.

> Alcoholism was a difficult problem. There was often doubt whether a "drunk" belonged in the local guardhouse or in the hospital, where possible intracranial injuries for example, could be detected. A compromise solution was reached when one of the neuropsychiatric closed wards was assigned to care for such problem personnel. Acute alcoholics were admitted to this ward and then transferred to the guardhouse if no medical disorder existed. This was in accord with Army policy that regarded alcoholism as misbehavior rather than illness."[52(p814)]

For those fortunate enough to be placed on the psychiatric service, alcoholism was invariably considered to be a symptom of some underlying psychiatric disorder. Even so, long-term treatment of such a condition was unavailable in the services.

Although there was some early work done in the hospital treatment of alcoholics at various military treatment centers,[3] it was only after 1970 that a clear policy had emerged in abandoning the willful misconduct concept and that took a more humanitarian and therapeutic approach. The U.S. Army initiated its ADAPCP in 1971 on a congressional mandate.[53] The program approach was in large part a result of the policy of conservation of manpower because senior noncommissioned officers and officers represented a considerable financial and experiential investment by the military. The military services could not afford the constant replacement of highly skilled service members and the ongoing toll of impaired performance and hazards associated with substance use.[17] It had been clearly shown previously[26] that substance use correlated highly with the occurrence of physical symptoms, social disruption, and the deterioration of work performance. Providing treatment favorably affected health and performance.[54]

An effect that may not be as important in other settings but is highly significant within the military setting is that the use of a substance has the potential of modifying the relationships existing in small groups.[55] Drug use can be disruptive to unit cohesion because it can fragment the unit into disparate groups. The unit cohesion that is so vital in sustaining the soldier in battle can be compromised.[56]

Since the inception of treatment as an alternative in the management of substance abusers, programs have been made available in each military installation. The thrust has been along voluntary treatment and early intervention. Both outpatient and inpatient modalities are available and current programs match the intensity of treatment to the needs of the patient at hand. The current treatment policy is more favorable in the military for those with alcoholism. There is less tolerance for other substance abusers.[3]

Triage

The ADAPCP in the U.S. Army is a command program.[57–59] By this policy, the commander makes the decision of whether the soldier should receive rehabilitation for his substance abuse disorder. Unlike other treatment, the medical officer can recommend, but the commander makes the final decision. Generally, the commander bases his decision on the soldier's performance and his potential for further active duty, that is, the soldier's past and future contributions to the military.

The treatment of the effects of drugs and alcohol as they are manifested physically is a medical responsibility. However, once the condition stabilizes and the soldier is no longer in danger, the commander decides on whether the soldier receives rehabilitation or administrative action, including separation.

As indicated previously, substance abusers can generally be divided into the two types. Within the military, this division can be done quite easily. Considering the differences in characteristics and symptomatology, the treatment implications are enormous. Soldiers of the Type 1 group will be considered more likely to have the disease of alcoholism and thus benefit from the medical approach, that is treatment in the residential treatment facility (RTF). Soldiers of the Type 2 group would receive only limited benefits from the purely medical approach. Their management should include a significant command approach, utilizing discipline, structure, training, and administrative action.

Although there are exceptions, with a large proportion of the military population being less than 25 years old, it appears that a great majority would fall into the Type 2 group with the diagnosis of alcohol abuse. Occasionally, soldiers referred for alcohol intoxication or an alcohol-related incident may not fit into the DSM III–R criteria for alcohol abuse. This also occurs with some soldiers who test positive on urinalysis for substances. In these cases, because no definitive diagnosis can be made, the soldier is considered to have used the substance improperly. He is therefore enrolled into the education program, usually for a 30-day period. The staff may use this time to further observe and evaluate the soldier.

Treatment Strategies

Although soldiers entering into a treatment program, whether outpatient or RTF, have different degrees of the disorder with differences in need, they all require restoration and changes in their basic behavior to pursue recovery. Within the substance abuse field, there is yet no cure. For many, abstinence is the goal, and recovery is a lifelong task. The strength of one's recovery program minimizes the slips and relapses. Treatment strategies emphasize various means to avoid drinking, including taking disulfiram and attending Alcoholics Anonymous (AA) meetings. Strategies are also directed to repairing social and medical problems, restoring hope and self-esteem, and developing new interests and associations.[36] The establishment of a new social network along with substitute behavior is also critical.

For treatment to be effective, a comprehensive approach is necessary. Every area of the patient's functioning should be assessed and addressed because these individuals display multiple impairments by the time they come to treatment. These are behavioral difficulties, psychological disturbances (mood and affect), social-interpersonal impairments, and physical and cognitive dysfunctions. In addition, the adverse effect on work performance and legal difficulties, if any, need resolution.

When an abuser enters treatment, the outcome is largely dependent on the service member's motivation to remain in the service by giving up the use of substances of abuse. A service member must not only comply with the treatment plan in terms of attendance and participation, but he must demonstrate an actual change in attitude, abstention from substance abuse, and a satisfactory duty performance. With readiness for duty as the policy in the military, service members not motivated for rehabilitation are expeditiously separated. These individuals are, however, given the opportunity for treatment at a Veterans Administration medical facility within 30 days of separation.

Outpatient

The outpatient treatment modality is the first treatment intervention. The usual entrance reason is an alcohol-related incident. A psychoactive substance use disorder[60] diagnosed by medical personnel following a comprehensive clinical assessment is necessary for enrollment. The outpatient program usually consists of weekly group counseling sessions and individual sessions as necessary. Treatment plans also include AA participation and disulfiram as indicated. Narcotics Anonymous (NA) and Cocaine Anonymous (CA) may be utilized when substances other than alcohol are abused. Periodic urinalysis is also utilized to discourage the substitution of other psychoactive substances. The commander enrolls the soldier into the program on the recommendation of the professional staff. For the duration of the soldier's treatment, there is active collaboration with command. The commander provides the direction, structure, and limits that are necessary in rehabilitation. The program is especially suited for the young soldier who abuses alcohol.

Residential Treatment Facility

Inpatient treatment of alcoholism and other drug dependence is conducted in one of the many military RTFs. For those soldiers that are alcohol- or drug-dependent by DSM III–R criteria, it supplements and augments outpatient care. It is a hospital-based program of intensive therapy, lasting 4 to 6 weeks and followed by outpatient treatment for the next year. Community living milieu and intensive group therapy to overcome denial and to effect lifestyle changes are heavily utilized. Counseling and education with intensive AA/NA participation are included. If not medically contraindicated, disulfiram (Antabuse) is encouraged as an adjunct to treatment. Because of the effect of family dynamics in the treatment process, family issues are addressed and many programs include spouses and other codependents to support the rehabilitation of the individual and to prevent further enabling.[3] It is an intensive but time-limited recovery program with abstinence as its goal.

To continue the recovery process initiated in the RTF, at the time of release, a sound aftercare plan is prepared. The service member is referred back to his own military community's outpatient facility for continued care according to its outpatient format (ie, weekly counseling sessions, disulfiram therapy, and AA attendance) for the next year. Commanders are involved in the aftercare, and their support is considered essential for the service member's return to duty, compliance with treatment, and ultimately assurance of adequate rehabilitation. The year of aftercare is a probationary period during which a service member is stabilized geographically in his unit and reenlistment contracts cannot be negotiated. This is to maintain the continuity of treatment at one location as well as to allow the commander the continued assessment of the soldier. Adequate medical follow-up is also necessary during this period because of the recurrent medical problems that many alcoholics have developed over the years. In addition, because of the tendency to substitute other drugs for a previous alcohol dependency, the physician should be acutely sensitive to the use of medications by the soldier for any reason. It may be necessary periodically to subject the soldier to random urinalysis.

MANAGEMENT OF CLINICAL CONDITIONS

Of importance in the treatment and management of substance-induced disorders is an understanding of the disorder and its psychosocial aspects. Proper treatment utilizes the various psychiatric treatment modalities, including both pharmacologic and psychosocial approaches. The goal is to restore the soldier's functioning in the military milieu and correct any performance deficits. Appropriate management utilizes the support of the community, family, unit, and organization to optimize recovery. Essential in the management is the understanding of the soldier's personality and circumstances that led to the disability or illness.[61]

Two frequently encountered complications seen among soldiers are alcohol- or drug-induced intoxication and psychoses. Intoxications are acute disorders that require immediate treatment. The psychoses may be acute or chronic. The withdrawal delirium is one type that requires immediate intervention.

The standard treatment for psychosis differs in the treatment of the substance-induced psychotic disorders; however, both may include the use of neuroleptics and appropriate supportive measures. Elimination of the toxic substance and correction of metabolic diatheses is of paramount emphasis in substance-induced psychoses. The treatment of alcohol intoxication and alcohol delirium will follow. The measures utilized in these disorders can be utilized in similar conditions that are drug-induced.

Alcohol Intoxication

Among the troop population, intoxication plays a major role in the morbidity and mortality associated with accidents, homicide, suicide, and medical and surgical conditions. Intoxication or drunkenness should not be confused with alcoholism. It is seen in both alcohol abuse and alcohol dependence. Intoxication is often defined, especially in relation to driving offenses as a BAC of 100 mg per 100 ml of blood.

> A standard drink—defined as 44 ml (1.5 oz) of distilled liquor (80 proof, or 40 percent alcohol by volume), 360 ml (12 oz) of beer (5 percent alcohol) or 150 ml (5 oz) of wine (12 percent alcohol)—contains about 15 g of alcohol, and in a 70-kg person the ingestion of one such drink will result in a peak blood alcohol concentration of approximately 4.3 to 8.7 mmol per liter (0.02 to 0.04 percent), depending on the rates of ingestion and absorption. Alcohol is metabolized and eliminated from the body at an average rate of about 8 g per hour; thus, for each standard drink consumed, approximately two hours are required for the blood alcohol concentration to fall to near zero, though slow rates of absorption may prolong the tail of the elimination curve beyond two hours."[50(p456)]

Sporadic, deliberate intoxication and voluntary heavy drinking (drunkenness) must be distinguished from the disease of alcoholism or alcohol dependence. Drunkenness is usually a hallmark of an alcohol abuser, but a history of repeated episodes points to dependence.

Alcohol intoxication varies in degrees and may be associated with abuse of other substances. Usually, the pure alcohol intoxication tends to be uncomplicated, and recovery is fairly rapid. Because of the social and other supports that are not available in barracks living, soldiers are often hospitalized briefly to avoid any unforeseen complications and to ensure safe recovery.

The usual signs of intoxication are slurred speech, nystagmus, hyporeflexia, unsteady gait, incoordination, flushing, somnolence, and drowsiness. A strong alcoholic breath is usually apparent but may be absent if unperfumed vodka has been ingested. Effectively treated with bed rest, recovery is fairly rapid. To control excitement or violence, careful restraint may be needed. The use of medications is controversial because deaths have occurred with additional sedation and important neurological signs may be masked.

Severe intoxications (alcohol overdose) present potential respiratory, cardiovascular, and central nervous system complications, including coma. There is also the possibility of unpredictable behavioral manifestations. Because the primary approach to the management of these individuals is life support, these cases should be managed in the hospital intensive care unit.

Severe intoxication is seen most often among young soldiers in a foreign country who, unfamiliar with the alcohol content of the local beverages, consume a significant quantity in a short period of time. It can also occur in binge drinkers who drink enormous quantities of alcohol rapidly. Because drugs may also be involved, it is necessary to obtain not only a BAC but also a drug screen. Because identification of the specific substances may not be immediately available, familiarity with substances available in the local community is helpful. An example in South Korea is Soju, a beer with a high-alcohol content.

Optimal management and treatment presuppose that the clinician has a clear appreciation of the clinical situation, including an adequate history and physical examination. Appropriate laboratory support is also essential. However, when a soldier is brought in by the military police or by ambulance, reliable and accurate information may be lacking. It is often necessary to start treatment immediately on a high index of suspicion as to the psychoactive substances involved.

Case Study 1

A 20-year-old serviceman with 8 months of active duty was brought to his medical treatment facility by the military police for treatment of a head laceration following his apprehension for fighting at the club. When seen, he was intoxicated with a BAC of 0.15 mg% of alcohol and was hostile and belligerent. For the treatment of his wound and for observation, he was admitted into the base hospital. He recovered from the incident uneventfully over the next day. Past history indicated that he had been drinking for the past 5 years and was apprehended a year ago for driving while intoxicated. He entered the army at the insistence of his parents and because he had no job. Since arrival at his unit, he has had two incidents of fighting while intoxicated and was charged twice for disobeying orders. He had also tested positive for cannabis a month ago. On release from the hospital, he was enrolled in the outpatient program by his commander. Attendance at the group sessions was erratic, and when he attended, he minimally participated. When confronted, he became hostile and defensive. He refused disulfiram, allegedly because he had no intention of quitting alcohol. A repeat of his urine drug screen a few weeks later again was positive for cannabis. Because of his failure to benefit from treatment and the continued use of an illegal substance, he was disenrolled from the program by his commander and separated administratively from the service.

Comment: Soldiers who have had alcohol and drug problems before entering on active duty often experience a relapse during their term of service. Motivation for treatment is perhaps the best predictor of success. The individual in the above case study had no motivation to stop drinking.

Case Study 2

A 21-year-old serviceman with 2 years of active duty was brought to the base dispensary after he passed out at the local bar. He had been in Korea a week when he decided to try the clubs with his fellow soldiers. At their insistence, he had two bottles of Soju, a Korean drink, and four bottles of beer over a period of 2 hours. When seen at the hospital, he was drowsy but responsive. BAC was 0.25 mg% for alcohol. He was admitted into the hospital for observation. The recovery was uneventful, and he required no medications. Continued observation indicated no emergence of tremors or withdrawal symptoms. Additional history indicated that the patient had been drinking for the past 4 years and that at his last duty post he had been cited for driving while intoxicated. He usually drank on weekends with fellow soldiers and had been drunk on several occasions at parties. Following his release from the hospital, he was enrolled in the outpatient program by his commander because he was generally considered a good soldier. He received weekly group counseling, attended the local AA meetings, and complied with the program requirements for the 6 months of his enrollment. During treatment, there was active command collaboration and consultation. The soldier was well aware of potential administrative action, including separation, should he fail to progress in the program. He successfully completed the program and remained free of any alcohol-related incidents for the next year when he was honorably discharged on his expected termination of service.

Comment: The above case study illustrates a successful outcome of a soldier placed in the outpatient treatment program. It is estimated that 60% of those enrolled in the outpatient program are successfully rehabilitated.[62]

Case Study 3

A 42-year-old Sergeant First Class returned from deployment to Panama to find his wife had begun having an affair with a neighbor and wanted a divorce. The soldier, originally from New York City, returned home on leave to be with his family of origin for support and solace. On a dare, he used crack cocaine and noted that this drug helped with his feelings of dysphoria surrounding the breakup of his marriage. When he returned to his duty station, the soldier moved to an apartment in town and began using crack cocaine on a regular basis. His work performance declined and he tested positive on a random urine drug screening.

During his referral to the ADAPCP, a psychiatric evaluation confirmed the presence of an adjustment disorder with depression. He readily engaged in outpatient counseling and his command began processing his separation.

The soldier received 8 months of drug abuse counseling before being separated from the service. One year after separation, he was still doing well and had found another job in the defense industry.

Comment: Despite the regulation that mandates separation because of drug use, soldiers can still receive benefits from evaluation and treatment while awaiting separation.

Alcohol Withdrawal

The objectives in treating alcohol withdrawal are the relief of discomfort, prevention or treatment of complications, and preparation for rehabilitation. Withdrawal symptoms usually occur in persons that have developed tolerance and are alcohol-dependent in contrast to abusers of alcohol. Withdrawal syndromes are usually seen in situations of voluntary abstinence, in treatment centers where the soldier is being treated for an intercurrent disease or trauma, in custody of military police, or during troop movements. Although cessation of drinking is the usual cause of the emergence of the withdrawal syndrome, it can be precipitated by reduced consumption or by any intercurrent illness, particularly infectious diseases. Because of inability to control their drinking, these individuals may display impairments in performance, and social relations, legal difficulties, and medical complications.

In the case of depressant drugs (alcohol, barbiturates, sedatives, or hypnotics) untreated withdrawal can be lethal. With narcotics, the withdrawal, although uncomfortable, is seldom lethal in a healthy individual.

Good management requires an adequate knowledge of the overall medical condition of the patient. Before withdrawal, medical conditions should be stabilized, including dehydration, infections, or trauma that requires treatment.

Detoxification is the first step in the treatment of addiction; the ultimate goal is recovery through a continuing treatment program. It should be performed in an adequate treatment setting, preferably a hospital setting, because convulsions and delirium can occur. Symptoms of withdrawal can begin as early as 8 hours or as late as 72 hours after the last drink. Information useful in the treatment of the alcohol withdrawal syndrome is the drinking history (duration, amount and pattern to ascertain the degree of tolerance, and blackouts), the history of signs and symptoms of physical dependence, (early morning shakiness, nausea, and nightmares relieved by drinking), and the manifestations of previous withdrawal, particularly DTs and seizures.[61]

The withdrawal syndrome ranges from mild to severe. The mild withdrawal syndrome is usually self-limited, resembling a hyperadrenergic state. It is manifested by anxiety, tremors of hands, diaphoresis, tachycardia, systolic hypertension, mild nausea, and sleep disturbance. It typically appears within 12 to 24 hours after the cessation of drinking, and the duration is usually 3 to 4 days.[61] Many of these patients require only observation, reassurance, and comfort with little or no medication. When in the field, these cases can best be managed in a setting that can render supportive care, such as hydration, nutrition, rest and sleep, reassurance, and orientation. However, for those that have a long history of drinking and evidence of dependence, this may be risky because they can easily progress in symptomatology and there is more risk of complications.

The severe form of withdrawal, with DTs is characterized by a symptom complex of profound confusion, disorientation, hallucinations, agitation, and autonomic hyperactivity. It appears 3 to 4 days after the cessation of drinking and resolves in the next 5 days with adequate treatment. The dangers are hyperpyrexia, dehydration, and electrolyte imbalance.[36]

The withdrawal syndrome requires prompt treatment and continual close attention to avert complications. The possibility of simultaneous withdrawal from other drugs should always be considered. For this reason, serum or urine drug screen as well as corroborative information is essential for proper management. Besides DTs, the other complications are seizures, dementia, and hallucinosis. The amount of medications needed to control withdrawal varies greatly among patients. Although many sedative-hypnotic drugs have been used to treat the withdrawal syndrome, the long-acting benzodiazepines, chlordiazepoxide and diazepam are currently the most widely used.[62] These benzodiazepines have the advantage of being cross-tolerant with alcohol, and their long half life is usually an advantage. Model detoxification procedures are described in Exhibit 5–2.[63,64]

The usual detoxification procedure calls for the administration of adequate doses of benzodiazepines. For mild to moderate withdrawal, the patient is initially given 50 to 100 mg of chlordiazepoxide or 5 to 10 mg of diazepam by mouth or intravenously. Close observation with attention to the signs of withdrawal and subjective complaints guide the use of additional medications.[36] Objective findings to monitor are sweating, hyperreflexia, tachycardia, confusion, agitation, body temperature, and blood pressure. A flow sheet monitoring the patient's condition and medications given greatly aids in management. The Clinical Institute Withdrawal Assessment for Alcohol (CIWA–A) is a reliable instrument that is available to assess the severity of alcohol withdrawal.[65,66] Withdrawal symptoms are rated, and the scores are helpful in titrating medications. Healthcare workers can be easily taught this scale to assess symptomatology and to monitor progress. However, the clinical evaluation still takes precedence over any test or scale in the final analysis of the treatment.

Following the adequate administration of the benzodiazepine during the first day or two, subsequent doses can be reduced rapidly because of the long half life of the drug. Uncomplicated detoxification is usually accomplished in 3 to 6 days.

The most severe type of withdrawal, DTs, requires the closest medical attention. In these cases, diazepam intravenously is often used; 10 mg may be given initially, followed by 5 mg every 5 minutes until a calming effect is achieved. Because diazepam and its major active metabolite have very long half lives (about 36 hours), additional medication may not be required. Persistent hallucinations, delusions, and agitation may require neuroleptics.

The absorption of diazepam in intramuscular form is quite unreliable, and therefore, patients should be given oral diazepam or chlordiazepoxide as soon as they are able to tolerate oral medications.

Combined treatment involving a benzodiazepine and a sympathetic blocking agent, such as clonidine, is emerging as a means of enhancing the effects of the standard benzodiazepine therapy of alcohol withdrawal.[29] Clonidine alleviates the hyperadrenergic state but does not protect against seizures.

Antipsychotics are not indicated for the treatment of withdrawal unless hallucinations, delusions, or severe agitation persist, in which case they should be added to the benzodiazepine. Haloperidol is often used for this purpose, but care should be taken to prevent extrapyramidal syndromes including neuroleptic malignant syndrome.

Abstinence Syndromes

Abstinence syndromes include acute alcohol withdrawal described above and other symptoms that can be protracted. These chronic symptoms point to a persistent hyperadrenergic state that may last 6 to 12 months. Persistent insomnia, anxiety, and depression can contribute to the risk of relapse by tempting the patient to seek relief with alcohol. Electrophysiological evidence for the existence of protracted abstinence in detoxified alcoholics has been demonstrated.[39] Alcohol consumption by an abstinent alcoholic may elicit withdrawal-like symptoms because of persistent latent central nervous system hyperexcitability. In some alcoholics with persistent hyperadrenergic states, antidepressants have proved useful.[67]

Drug Abuse

Abusers of illegal substances are not tolerated in the military and therefore are less often the subjects of treatment. However, the military drug and alcohol clinics do provide outpatient treatment to the lower enlisted personnel for those who abuse substances other than alcohol. Senior enlisted personnel and officers are often processed for separation because they have undermined a public trust.

Withdrawal from amphetamine and cocaine usually causes some physical distress but is self-limited. Life-threatening events are usually associated with use including fatal arrhythmias, seizures, and cerebrovascular accidents. A drug-free environment, symptomatic treatment, and psychological support are usually sufficient. However, suicidal depressions and paranoid psychosis may be manifested or emerge on withdrawal, requiring vigorous psychiatric care. Because of the usual severe underlying social and personality disorders encountered in drug abusers, treatment is necessarily complex and prolonged. A narcotic withdrawal procedure is described in Exhibit 5–3. The withdrawal from sedatives and hypnotics is very similar to that from alcohol, and the same procedure is applied with some modification. Exhibit 5–4 describes the procedure.

Withdrawal from cannabis (marijuana, hashish) is usually uncomplicated, requiring no medical intervention. Similarly "coming down" from a hallu-

EXHIBIT 5–2

MODEL ALCOHOL WITHDRAWAL PROCEDURE

I. Purpose: To prevent medical and withdrawal complications such as organic brain syndrome, vitamin deficiency, neuropathic and encephalopathic disease, and aggravation of existing medical problems. Withdrawal symptoms can begin within hours of the last drink but may not emerge until up to 7 days.

II. Medications: All medications, if possible, should be given orally to avoid activating psychological needs and symbolism of injections. Doses are based on the average (70 kg) person. Higher or lower amounts should be based on actual physical status.

A. Vitamins: Initially it is important to start the debilitated patient on parental vitamins (ie, thiamine HCL,[1] Berocca parental nutrition) immediately on admission to avoid the possibility of one of the permanent organic brain syndromes or peripheral neuropathies. However, if oral intake is adequate, high doses of oral vitamins should be used for the first week. After than, an adequate diet should suffice.

1. Berocca parental: 4 ml intramuscular (IM) (for 1 or 2 doses).
2. Vitamin K: 5 to 10 mg IM (for 1 or 2 times if prothrombin time is prolonged more than 3 seconds beyond the control).
3. Thiamine HCL: 100 mg IM. Start P.O. vitamins as soon as possible.
4. Ascorbic acid: 500 mg per day.
5. Pyridoxine HCL: 100 mg per day.
6. Folic acid: 1 to 5 mg per day x 5 days.
7. Multiple vitamins: 1 twice per day.
8. Thiamine: 100 mg 3 times per day.

B. Tranquilizers: Type should be based on several factors of which physician's experience, drug, and patient characteristics are of paramount importance. These can be used during the first few days of detoxification if needed. Care should be taken not to overuse tranquilizers or other sedatives in the acute intoxication phase or with markedly elevated alcohol blood levels (eg, 100 to 150 mg/dl or above). Benzodiazepines are the drugs of choice, but major tranquilizers can be used if necessary. If IM benzodiazepines are needed, use lorazepam (Ativan).

1. Diazepam (Valium): Initial loading dose of 5 to 20 mg P.O. every 1 hour until symptom-free and mildly sedated. Usually 1 to 3 doses over 6 hours are needed but may require up to 12 doses over 48 hours. Determination of the need for continue dosing should be made 45 minutes after the previous dose. After symptoms are controlled, no more is needed because of its long half life.
2. Chlordiazepoxide (Librium): Similar to diazepam but scheduled especially if less sedation is desirable. Doses of 50 to 100 mg every 1 to 1.5 hours.
3. Lorazepam (Ativan): 2 to 4 mg IM as above if oral medication cannot be tolerated or IM medication is required. 1 mg of lorazepam is equivalent to about 5 mg of diazepam.
4. Haloperidol (Haldol): 2 to 5 mg oral or IM every 4 hours or more often for persistent psychosis.
5. Diphenhydramine (Benadryl): 25 to 50 mg IM STAT[2] for EPS,[3] followed by any oral anti-Parkinsonian agent if major tranquilizer is utilized and EPS develops.
6. Other major and minor tranquilizers can be used depending on clinical experience.

C. Sleeping medications: Should be avoided. Additional diazepam may be given in some cases.

D. Anticonvulsive medications: Should not be used routinely but used only if seizures have been a factor in the past. If a severe withdrawal has resulted in seizure-like activity despite diazepam use, the following can be used for 7 to 10 days:

1. Phenytoin (Dilantin): 200 mg IM, then:
2. Phenytoin: 100 mg, 4 times per day P.O. Do not exceed blood levels of 1 to 2 mg/dl therapeutic range.
3. Note that even with IM dosing, therapeutic levels usually take several days.

EXHIBIT 5–2 (*continued*)

MODEL ALCOHOL WITHDRAWAL PROCEDURE

E. Antihypertensives: Elevated blood pressure is common in alcohol withdrawal and may revert to normal after detoxification. Aldomet, beta-blockers, and calcium channel blockers may be used for dangerous elevations.

F. Intravenous fluids: Only if severe dehydration, orthostatic hypotension, hemoconcentration, vomiting, or debilitation. The rapid administration of 1 to 2 liters of balanced intravenous fluids with vitamins added, infused over several hours should reduce morbidity.

III. Laboratory Tests:

A. Within 24 hours or sooner: Initial blood alcohol, blood sugar, CBC[4] (to include mean blood cell volume, MCV[5]), urine analysis, (including drug screen), liver screen (at least SGOT,[6] SGPT,[7] LDH,[8] alkaline phosphatase, bilirubin, albumin), serology, chest X-ray (posterior, anterior, and lateral). A MCV increase may indicate folate deficiency, liver disease, or reticulocytosis.

B. Blood antibodies for human immunodeficiency virus (HIV).

C. Electoencephalogram and electrocardiogram should be done initially only if clinically indicated and are best repeated after 7 to 10 days of return to a fairly normal physiological status.

D. Other tests to consider: electrolytes (sodium, potassium, chloride), blood urea nitrogen, creatinine, amylase, bromsulphthalein (for hepatocellular damage), fasting and 2-hour postprandial blood sugar, sputum for culture, and sensitivity.

IV. Nursing Care:

A. Vital signs:

1. TPR[9] and blood pressure four times per day for 3 days, then routine. Pulse and blood pressure, supine then after 3 minutes standing, for 48 hours, then routine.

2. Weight: Admission and then 2 or 3 times per week.

B. Diet: Initially patients may need assistance, encouragement, and direction in obtaining an adequate diet.

1. Fluids: Large oral intake is necessary because of various degrees of dehydration. Orange juice is a good source of potassium. Supplemental magnesium may be needed.

2. Supplementary feedings, if indicated.

C. Orientation: Patients should be oriented and familiarized to the unit. Orientation and mental status should be checked and noted daily.

1. HCL—hydrochloride
2. STAT—immediate
3. EPS—extrapyramidal symptoms
4. CBC—complete blood count
5. MCV—mean corpsular volume
6. SGOT—serum glutamic oxaloacetic transaminase
7. SGPT—serum glutamic pyruvic transaminase
8. LDH—lactic dehydrogenase
9. TPR—temperature, pulse rate, respiratory rate

cinogen "trip" usually requires a knowledgeable person to "talk down" the patient and prevent him from coming to harm. Phencyclidine and atropine-like poisoning may require more intensive medical intervention.

Case Study 4

A 34-year-old serviceman with 14 years of active duty was brought to the station hospital because he seemed "keyed-up" and restless on duty. He claimed to have had his last drink 3 days ago. This service member presented a history of drinking the past 18 years. He had previously experienced blackouts or periods of amnesia after drinking. He was hospitalized twice in the last 10 years for alcohol withdrawal symptoms when he was unable to obtain alcohol during field exercises. Following the last withdrawal episode 6 months ago, he was placed in the RTF and was recently returned to duty with follow-up treatment at his local ADAPCP. He discontinued disulfiram a month ago and started to drink because of work stress.

On admission, he was placed on the alcohol detoxification protocol because he was grossly tremulous and

EXHIBIT 5–3

MODEL SPECIFIC SEDATIVE/HYPNOTIC WITHDRAWAL PROCEDURE

Generally, most of the alcohol standing operating procedure applies.

1. Tranquilizer withdrawal: For oral drugs use diazepam. If IM needed, use lorazepam; 1 mg lorazepam equals 5 mg diazepam.
   a. Loading dose: 10 to 20 mg diazepam or 2 to 5 mg lorazepam IM.
   b. Maintenance dose: Repeat dose every hour over next 6 to 48 hours until symptom-free and mildly sedated. Determine next dose after 45 minutes of previous dose. Once stability is achieved, no further diazepam is needed because of its long half life.
2. Barbiturate withdrawal: Check for level of tolerance with use of short-acting drug. Thereafter, a long-acting drug can be used for withdrawal.
   a. Test dose: Pentobarbital. 50 to 200 mg P.O. every 1/2 to 1 hour over 6-hour period to point of intoxication: ataxia, nystagmus, slurred speech. If less than 100 to 200 mg produces intoxication, then a detoxification schedule is not needed.
   b. Stabilization dose: the 6-hour test dose is given 4 times per day for the next 1 to 3 days. Phenobarbital 30 mg can be substituted for 100 mg pentobarbital and given once or twice per day because of its long half life.
   c. Withdrawal dose: Decrease 100 mg pentobarb or 30 mg phenobarb, or less, per day over the next 10 to 20 days. If withdrawal symptoms occur, reduce dose more slowly. Consider blood and urine for barb levels and other drugs.

diaphoretic. Over the next few hours, he became increasingly confused, agitated, and aggressive. He displayed disorientation for time and place, felt that he was in prison, and saw "bugs" around the bed. He also felt that he was being poisoned. He loudly insisted that he was innocent and wished to leave. Following a week of hospitalization during which time large doses of benzodiazepine were administered along with haloperidol to treat his delirium, he recovered from the episode with spotty recollection of the events. Because of his poor compliance to treatment and recurrent drinking, he was administratively separated from the service.

EXHIBIT 5–4

MODEL NARCOTIC WITHDRAWAL PROCEDURES

Procedure is the same as for alcohol, except administer additional medications to control physical symptoms.

1. Narcotic withdrawal: A narcotic antagonist will start the withdrawal abruptly or reverse an acute overdose. Methadone and clonidine can be used to prevent withdrawal symptoms although withdrawal by itself is not life-threatening.
   a. Acute overdose: Naloxone 0.4 mg IM, intravenously or subcutaneously every 5 minutes until awake. Usually 2 to 3 vials are adequate. Note that the short half life of naloxone requires repeated dosing.
   b. Initiate withdrawal dose: As above but less frequent to produce physical withdrawal symptoms.
   c. Methadone dose: This long-acting narcotic can be used for withdrawal.
      (1) Initial dose: 15 to 20 mg P.O.
      (2) Withdrawal dose: Repeat dose when symptoms return over 24 hours. Reduce daily dose by 5 to 10 mg per day.

Comment: This is not the typical outcome of those soldiers enrolled in the RTF. The great majority of them are motivated for treatment and respond positively with a successful completion of the program (eg, Case Study 3). However, there are individuals that are unable or unwilling to break through the denial and to confront their disorder. Thus, they end up as treatment failures with their consequences. Because there are no means to clearly predict the patient's response to treatment before admission to an RTF, the first 2 weeks as an inpatient are critical in terms of assessing the potentials for treatment and outcome. Here, commanders are involved in the decision of continuing treatment or not. In most cases, a failure in treatment in the RTF, like a failure of outpatient treatment, leads to an administrative separation from the service.

Case Study 5

A 28–year-old serviceman with 10 years of active duty was referred to the base medical treatment facility when his commander noted irritability and an alcoholic breath.

Examination indicated the soldier to be intoxicated with a BAC of 0.10 mg% of alcohol and mild incoordination. He presented a history of drinking since he entered the Army at age 18. He had arrived overseas 2 months previously. Six years ago, he completed the outpatient program following a drinking while intoxicated incident. Knowing from past experiences that he had a tendency to lose control of his drinking, he generally refrained from alcohol use until he arrived overseas. On arrival here, his unstable marital relationship collapsed, and he also experienced significant job stresses. He succumbed to peer influences as in the past, and soon he was consuming alcohol several times a week. He unsuccessfully attempted to decrease his drinking. Recently, he had experienced blackouts.

The service member was placed under observation. Over the following 24 hours he became increasingly tremulous and agitated. He also displayed tachycardia, sweating, mild blood pressure elevation, and nausea. Medications were given, and his condition was monitored for the next few days. He recovered uneventfully. On the recommendation of the medical officer, he was enrolled in the RTF (Track III) by his commander because he had been a "good performer" until recently. He complied with the program requirements, elected to take disulfiram, and appropriately confronted his long-standing substance disorder. He regularly attended the AA meetings and displayed a definite motivation toward rehabilitation. On the successful completion of the inpatient phase, he returned to duty and continued treatment as an outpatient. Follow-up 8 months later indicated that the soldier was doing well on duty and had remained abstinent.

Comment: Some soldiers with 8 to 15 years of active service turn to alcohol or drugs in the midst of personal or career crises. The above case exemplifies the commander's concern for his soldier and the therapist's attentiveness to the patient's life circumstances.

TREATMENT MODALITIES

Counseling

Therapeutic groups and group therapy are the principal treatment modalities for alcoholism. Individual counseling is of limited use in a disease that is best treated by peer group support and group counseling.[68] When individual sessions are used, it is to provide the initial support, confrontation, ventilation, and resolution of the immediate crisis. These sessions are basically used to prepare the individual for group counseling and AA. In both types of counseling, the here-and-now approach is utilized with the focus on abstinence. Exploration as to reasons for drinking are avoided. The counseling is done in a supportive confrontational manner, especially in dealing with the strong denial of the patients.

The peer group provides the extremely necessary support and a system of dealing with anxiety, isolation, loneliness, anger, and rejections. These therapeutic groups serve as a place for patients to learn about alcoholism, benefit from fellow patients in different stages of recovery, and obtain help from members for specific problems.

Alcoholics Anonymous and Other Self-Help Groups

Founded more than 50 years ago by two men seeking a means to remain abstinent, AA has continued to be the most potent of all resources to help those with alcoholism. It is considered a bona fide treatment modality by the military and is used extensively by both outpatient and inpatient programs. AA is the organization that a soldier must largely depend on for his continued recovery. Its basic beliefs are embodied in the well-known 12 steps.[69]

The AA program is a spiritual way of life without any creed or dogma. It is compatible with any program of recovery and is a vital adjunct to the management of alcoholism. AA has always viewed alcoholism as a disease and has considered abstinence as the only realistic goal. It teaches its members to resist the strong internal and external pressures to drink by living one day at a time. For many years before the establishment of any military treatment program, AA was the only source of "treatment" available. Soldiers who were motivated and who participated seemed to obtain the help that they sought.

Alcoholism is a lifelong disorder; therefore, for continued support and recovery, the individual should become dependent on the AA program rather than any particular individual or agent. AA groups provide hope, a social network to remain abstinent, a crisis response system, and a worldwide organization with many members and local branches. For many, the missing of AA meetings usually leads to a relapse.

Conceptualized in a similar manner, NA is currently available for those that abuse or are dependent on other substances. Al-Anon and Alateen work in conjunction with AA to assist family members of those with alcoholism to help themselves and their addicted member by providing education, support, and needed interventions. A relatively new organization, Adult Children of Alcoholics (ACOA), is helpful for those whose parents had alcoholism. For those who are atheists or who eschew a dependent role, a new organization based on Ellis' Rational Emotive Therapy and cognitive therapy is emerging. These groups supply peer support similar to AA.

Disulfiram

No medication by itself should be considered the treatment for alcoholism. There are medications, however, that can serve as adjuncts to treatment. Disulfiram (Antabuse) is one that is used extensively in the recovery programs of both outpatients and inpatients with good success.[70] In military treatment centers, although encouraged, it is not made a requirement. It is only prescribed with the patients's full knowledge and consent. Offered to help one resist the impulse to drink, it is compatible with other forms of alcoholism treatment. Although short-term use of disulfiram should be the intent while the person solidifies his recovery program, this medication has been used for 1 year or more in those that have required this support.

Disulfiram should not be used in those with significant liver disease or those that are unable to stop the use of alcohol. Other methods should be utilized to encourage abstinence. Before prescribing disulfiram, the physician should review its precautions, contraindications, and drug interactions.

Disulfiram works by blocking the enzyme aldehyde dehydrogenase, which is necessary for the breakdown of acetaldehyde. On ingestion, alcohol is metabolized in the liver to acetaldehyde. Disulfiram causes the accumulation of acetaldehyde, which produces the "alcohol-Antabuse reaction." This *reaction* is manifested by nausea, flushing, dysphoria, dyspnea, hypertension, headache, and sometimes emesis and syncope. In rare instances in which the individual has cardiovascular or cerebrovascular disease, heart failure, stroke, and death are possible. Very rarely disulfiram may produce an acute brain syndrome mimicking intoxication. This occurs in about one in 1,000 patients and usually on higher doses (500 mg).[70] It is fully reversible with discontinuance of disulfiram. Careful monitoring of patients on disulfiram is essential because it is not an innocuous drug.

Patients starting disulfiram need to be free of alcohol for at least 1 full day. The usual procedure is to prescribe a loading dose of 500 mg for a few days and then a daily maintenance dose of 250 mg. Because taking alcohol in any form may cause a reaction, before starting this medication, patients need to be instructed on the foods and products containing alcohol. Medication in elixir form should be avoided unless it specifically is labelled nonalcoholic. Sensitive persons may react to aftershave lotion, mouthwashes, or external agents containing alcohol usually through inhalation. Because disulfiram accumulates in the body, patients may have some reaction to alcohol up to 2 to 3 weeks after the last dosage if they resume drinking. Because some complain of drowsiness after taking disulfiram, the dosage can be taken before sleep rather than during the day. Other minor complaints are of a metallic or garlic taste in the mouth and mild indigestion. The former disappears in a week or so, and the latter can be controlled by taking disulfiram with food. For those allergic to disulfiram, metronidazole (Flagyl) is an alternative medication that also blocks aldehyde dehydrogenase. Metronidazole and disulfiram should not be taken together.

Psychiatric Comorbidity

A variety of clinically significant psychiatric disorders can coexist with alcohol dependence. These disorders confer a poorer prognosis in treatment and modification of treatment with additional psychotherapeutic approaches, and pharmacologic agents may be necessary. To diagnose and treat these disorders, it is essential that these soldiers are also seen at the local mental health facility or by the division psychiatrist. Depression is the most common associated mental disorder among those with alcoholism. Depressive symptoms commonly seen in alcohol withdrawal frequently remit spontaneously with time. For depression that persists beyond the period of acute withdrawal, a tricyclic antidepressant or heterocyclic antidepressant is the usual drug of choice. These medications are usually appropriate for chronic anxiety and panic attacks of the hyperadrenergic state also.

Because comorbid disorders contribute to the deficient behavior and functioning of one with alcoholism, the treatment of concomitant pathology is essential. Psychotropic medications may be indicated to treat the negative states that contribute to relapse.[38] These medications include antidepressants, lithium, antipsychotics, and antianxiety agents. It is necessary to assess the response and continued indications in follow-up. The antianxiety agent of choice is buspirone because it is not addictive and does not increase alcohol brain depression.

PREVENTION AND CONTROL

Current Data

The efforts since 1971 in decreasing substance abuse among military personnel have resulted in significant gains in the 1980s. Worldwide studies[18] during the past 10 years have indicated a general decline in both drug and alcohol use. However, the reduction in drug use has been much more substantial than has alcohol reduction.[17] "Drug use among military personnel declined dramatically between 1980 and 1988 and is now the lowest since the survey series began. The declines are probably partially related to similar declines among civilians, but they also demonstrate the continuing effectiveness of military efforts to eliminate drug use among military personnel."[26(pxix)]

Although the abuse of psychoactive drugs may have been significantly curtailed by the current military preventive and control measures,[26] alcohol, by its availability and widespread use, continues to create a problem among its users. "In 1988, about 83 percent of military personnel were current drinkers, with about two thirds being moderate to heavy drinkers and 8.2 percent being heavy drinkers."[26(p13)] "Drinking levels are positively related to serious consequences. Heavy drinkers experience the most consequences."[26(p35)]

Recent epidemiological studies indicate an increasing consumption of alcohol in the general population, and the prevalence of alcoholism seems to be increasing as well. In those that are susceptible, the risk of alcoholism is greater, with the age of onset being earlier than in the past.[28] This phenomenon would impact on the military services in a significant manner because the bulk of the service members are young people.

In the military services, current alcohol and drug use seems to be concentrated among the younger, less-educated, unmarried, junior and midcareer enlisted personnel.[71] It has also been noted that "alcohol-related serious consequences, productivity loss, and alcohol dependence are substantially higher among E1 to E3 pay grades; for any negative effects and alcohol dependence, rates for E1 to E3s are almost twice as high as E4s to E6s and for productivity loss, about 10 percentage points higher."[26(p33)] It seems essential that the current programs be continued to maintain the gains of recent years.

Biochemical Testing

Random urinalysis for substances has been important not only to identify abusers as early as possible, but also to serve as a deterrent to the use of substances by troops. The techniques of biochemical analysis as well as the administrative procedures in running a secure testing program have been significantly refined to minimize false-positives. A urine positive rate up to 2% has been considered acceptable within the troop population as evidence of adequate surveillance and control. A rate higher than this would be of some concern as to the adequacy of control measures. Identification of drug abusers as early as possible is considered important to not only restrain their own drug use, but to curtail the spread of drug use to others in the unit.[72]

Only results reported from the large certified laboratories can be counted on as legal evidence; any testing done in the field is still considered inaccurate. For purposes of assessment and treatment, these field test results may be useful but not beyond that. Likewise, breathalyzers are very useful in the field for the determination of alcohol in the blood, but their use is limited to medical management. Recently, drug testing has included cannabis, cocaine, phencyclidine (PCP), opiates, and amphetamines where use of these substances is suspected. The presence of medicinals, such as opiates and amphetamines, on urine drug screens create special problems; therefore, written procedures are available to the physician (medical review officer) in evaluating these cases.

Education

In any preventive program, education remains the key, and this cannot be overemphasized in the area of substance abuse. Disciplinary action and treatment are means of dealing with abusers of substances, but primary prevention depends on the educational efforts promoted by command. A variety of means are available to command to do this. Alcohol and drug preventive educational sessions are usually included during annual training with support from the installation Alcohol and Drug Counseling Center.

Deglamorization of Alcohol

Deglamorization appears to have done its part in the reduction of alcohol use and abuse in recent years. Military social activities no longer emphasize drinking, and even penalties are awarded in situations in which drinking is promoted. The health promotion efforts of the DoD definitely seem to have a positive impact on the current attitude toward alcohol and drug use not only in the workplace, but also at all other times.

In addition, the driving while intoxicated program, with commanders being notified and being involved in some administrative action, appears to serve as a positive deterrent. Because prevention and control are a command responsibility, commanders should be familiar with the administrative and medical resources at hand to accomplish the mission of maintaining the unit's health and readiness.

OPERATIONAL CONSIDERATIONS

The Combat Medical Provider's Tasks

Substance abuse disorders have a special interest to military medicine and, in particular, to those in the combat environment. The unique problem for the combat care provider is that while he can expect to deal with the consequences of abuse, he must improvise a solution without the familiar structure of the employee assistance model that is commonly available throughout the DoD in peacetime. Given the elevated base rates for substance misuse under conditions of excessive combat stress, before reaching a diagnosis of substance dependence, he must guard his index of suspicion by avoiding criteria based on amounts consumed. The problem is that the threshold of abuse (as defined chiefly by consumption level) may rise above the norms to which the clinician is accustomed. Moreover, his clinical objectives are defined by the short-term focus of manpower conservation to return the patient to duty, rather than the long-term goal of occupational rehabilitation. His immediate concerns are detoxification and observation for acute withdrawal syndromes, with less attention given to the soldier's rehabilitation.

Three predictions appear likely: first, the combat clinician will treat an increased number of overuse cases than he would typically encounter in peacetime practice; second, there will be no greater incidence of substance dependence disorders than normally occurs (3 to 5% in the military population);[26] and third, dependence disorders will be more difficult to confirm because of increased consumption and the pressures to return expeditiously as many patients as possible to duty. That is, the sensitivity and specificity of his clinical decisions will be markedly affected by the aberrant consumption patterns of wartime.

Limiting Interference

This presents the greatest clinical dilemma: it is no less important to obtain correct and timely treatment of the alcoholic or drug-dependent soldier during wartime, regardless of the difficulty in detection. In the midst of interference created by increased consumption of alcohol and adventitious use of illicit substances, how can the clinician improve his ability to identify the patient who should receive a definitive rehabilitation for a substance dependence disorder? The answer—he must emphasize command consultation with the goal of encouraging the primary prevention of substance use through command policies that deglamorize excessive alcohol consumption and assist abstinence from illicit drugs through detection and administrative sanctions (to include judicial avenues).

Recognizing that the exaggerated consumption he observes is symptomatic of the stressful environment, he may assist the commander to lower the stress by facilitating increased cohesion, communication, and group support to dissipate some of the excess tension. Finally, he can make the commander aware that he may have the strongest influence over excessive consumption because key factors to excessive use are social pressure to drink and inexpensive alcoholic beverages. In fact, social pressure and inexpensive access may explain two-thirds of the difference between various occupational groups considered at high risk for drinking problems.[20]

Setting The Stage For Rehabilitation

In a combat environment, the clinician should not anticipate that he will have the luxury of sending many (if any) with chronic alcoholism away for rehabilitation. Most of his efficacy must be directed toward the acute condition and his clinical role in setting the stage for later definitive treatment. He can do this in several ways. First, he can provide the patient with an unequivocal diagnosis of substance abuse when the facts support it. Not uncommonly, a patient has been released after detoxification without a frank discussion between doctor and patient about his alcoholism. The cofounder of the Navy's rehabilitation system received no less than seven postretirement hospitalizations before anyone mentioned the connection between the detoxification and substance abuse.[73,74] In addition, one must document all the facts as they are revealed in the history so that future providers can follow a trend. This sets the stage for later intervention.

SUMMARY AND CONCLUSION

Among newly inducted young service members, there usually is an increased use of a substance, namely alcohol, in the new military setting. This may be to alleviate the anxiety of being in a stressful situation as well as exercising the new found freedom away from home. In addition, illicit drug use that may be associated with alcohol use can emerge.

Because the experiment with Prohibition was a failure, alcohol will always be with us. Thus, there will always be service members who will develop abuse and dependence disorders. Likewise, drugs of whatever nature, such as cannabis, phencyclidine, cocaine, amphetamines, opiates, or designer drugs, will periodically emerge to threaten and undermine the health and readiness of troops.

Since 1971, the military services, with their resolve to deal with substance abuse among their ranks with intensive programs of prevention, control, and treatment, have been rewarded with almost a total eradication of illegal drug use and a decreasing alcohol consumption. The command-centered substance abuse program with support from the medical services has been highly successful. The continued success of the substance abuse program will depend on the viability of the existing structure and relationship with command.

Whether in peace or in war, substance abuse is a problem that requires monitoring and surveillance. In addition, substance abuse cannot be separated into a command or a medical problem. Because the emergence and the maintenance of substance abuse are multidetermined, like any behavior, the management and disposition are highly complex and require both administrative and medical elements.

REFERENCES

1. Ingraham LH. *The Boys in the Barracks*. Philadelphia: Institute for the Study of Human Issues; 1984.
2. Rock NL. Military Alcohol and Drug Abuse Program: Old problems—new program. *Med Bull US Army Europe*. 1973;30(4):87–93.
3. Harig PT. Substance abuse programs in military settings. In: Gal R, Mangelsdorff AD, eds. *Handbook of Military Psychology*. London: John Wiley and Sons; 1990: 635–655.
4. Morton AS, Cook RF. *An Assessment of Alcohol and Drug Education/Prevention Programs in the United States Army*. Alexandria, Va: US Army Research Institute; 1973. ARI Research Problem Review 73-3.
5. *US Senate Hearings Before the Special Subcommittee on Alcoholism and Narcotics*. Ninety-first Cong; Drug and alcohol abuse in the military, pp. 10–87. Washington, DC: GPO; 1970.
6. Walters LS. *A Contest Without a Loser: The Development of the Navy's Alcohol Rehabilitation Program*. Monterey, Calif: Naval Postgraduate School; 1981. Thesis.
7. Krebs JM. *New Directions for Army Drug and Alcohol Abuse Control*. Carlisle, Pa: US Army War College; 1975. NTIS Document AD-403 565.
8. Koshes RJ, Shanahan J. Progress in the treatment of cocaine and crack addicts. *Milit Med*. 1990;155:A12.
9. Farley WJ. Addiction and the anesthesiologist. *Straight Forward: The Official Publication of the Physician Rehabilitation Program of the Medical and Chirurgical Faculty of Maryland*. 1994;5(2):1–2.
10. Shiplet ME. Alert: The abuse of fentanyl. *Straight Forward: The Official Publication of the Physician Rehabilitation Program of the Medical and Chirurgical Faculty of Maryland*. 1994;5(2):6–7.

11. US Department of the Army. *Quality Assurance Administration*. Washington, DC: DA; 1989; Chapter 7, Impaired Health Care Provider Program. Army Regulation 40–68.

12. Richards RL. Mental and nervous disorders in the Russo-Japanese War. *Milit Surgeon*. 1910;26(2):177–193.

13. Glass AJ. Army psychiatry before World War II. In: *Zone of Interior*. Vol. 1. In: Glass AJ, Bernucci RJ, eds. *Neuropsychiatry in World War II*. Washington, DC: GPO; 1966: Chap 1.

14. Brill NQ. Hospitalization and disposition. In: *Zone of Interior*. Vol. 1. In: Glass AJ, Bernucci RJ, eds. *Neuropsychiatry in World War II*. Washington, DC: GPO; 1966: Chap 9.

15. The Comprehensive Alcohol Abuse and Alcoholism Prevention, Treatment, and Rehabilitation Act. Pub L No. 91–616. 1970.

16. US Department of Defense. *Health Promotion*. Washington, DC: DoD; 1986. DoD Directive 1010.10.

17. Allen J, Mazzuchi J. Alcohol and drug abuse among American military personnel: Prevalence and policy implications. *Milit Med*. 1985;150:250–255.

18. Burt MR, Bliegel MM, Carnes Y, Farley EC. *Worldwide Survey of Nonmedical Drug Use and Alcohol Use Among Military Personnel*. Bethesda, Md: Burt Associates; 1982.

19. Bray RM, Marsden ME, Herbold JR, Peterson MR. Progress toward eliminating drug and alcohol abuse among US military personnel. *Armed Forces and Society*. 1992;18(4):476–496.

20. Whitehead PC, Simpkins SJ. Occupational factors in alcoholism. In: Kissin B, Begleiter H, eds. *The Pathogenesis of Alcoholism: Psychosocial Factors*. New York: Plenum Press; 1983: 405–496.

21. Plant MA. Occupations, drinking patterns and alcohol-related problems. *Br J Addict*. 1979;74:267–273.

22. Vaillant GE. The etiology of alcoholism. In: *The Natural History of Alcoholism*. Cambridge, Mass: Harvard University Press; 1983: Chap 2.

23. Trice HM, Roman PM. *Spirits and Demons at Work: Alcohol and Other Drugs on the Job*. Ithaca, NY: Cornell University Press; 1972.

24. Plant MA. Occupations and alcohol-related problems. *Br J Alcohol Alcoholism*. 1979;14:119–120.

25. Hingston R, Mangioney T, Barret J. Job characteristics and drinking practices in the Boston metropolitan area. *Q J Stud Alcohol*. 1981;42:725–738.

26. Bray RM, Marsden ME, Guess LL, Wheeless SC, Iannacchione VG, Keesling SR. *1988 Worldwide Survey of Substance Abuse and Health Behaviors Among Military Personnel*. Research Triangle, North Carolina: Research Triangle Institute; January 25, 1989: Report RTI/4000/06–02FR.

27. Docherty JP. Personal Communication, 1992.

28. Cloninger CR, Dinwiddie SH, Reich T. Epidemiology and genetics of alcoholism. In: Tasman A, Hales RE, Frances AJ, eds. *Review of Psychiatry*. Washington, DC: APA Press; 1989: 293–308.

29. Kranzler HR, Orrok B. The pharmacotherapy of alcoholism. In: Tasman A, Hales RE, Frances AJ, eds. *Review of Psychiatry*. Washington, DC: APA Press; 1989: 359–379.

30. Donovan JM. An etiologic model of alcoholism. *Am J Psychiatry*. 1986;143(1):1–11.

31. Crowe L. Alcohol and heredity: Theories about the effects of alcohol use on offspring. *Soc Biol*. 1985;32(3–4):146–161.

32. Mannuzza S, Klein RG, Bonagura N, Konig PH, Shenker R. Hyperactive boys almost grown up. II. Status of subjects without a mental disorder. *Arch Gen Psychiatry*. 1988;45(1):13–18.

33. Manshadi M, Lippmann S, O'Daniel RG, Blackman A. Alcohol abuse and attention deficit disorder. *J Clin Psychiatry*. 1983;44(10):379–380.

34. Burney GL. *NIAAA Remembers: Milestones in the History of the Alcohol Field*. Rockville, Md: National Institute of Alcohol Abuse and Alcoholism; 1988.

35. American Psychiatric Association. *Diagnostic and Statistical Manual of Mental Disorders*. 3rd ed. Revised. (DSM III–R). Washington, DC: APA; 1987.

36. Vaillant GE. The alcohol-dependent and drug-dependent person. In: Nicholi AM, Jr., ed. *The New Harvard Guide to Psychiatry*. Cambridge, Mass: Harvard University Press; 1988: 700–713.

37. American Psychiatric Association. *Diagnostic and Statistical Manual of Mental Disorders*. 3rd ed. Revised. (DSM III). Washington, DC: APA; 1980.

38. Rounsaville BJ, Kranzler HR. The DSM III–R Diagnosis of Alcoholism. In: Tasman A, Hales RE, Frances AJ, eds. *Review of Psychiatry*. Washington, DC: APA Press; 1989: 323–340.

39. Meyer RE, Barbor TF. Explanatory models of alcoholism. In: Tasman A, Hales RE, Frances AJ, eds. *Review of Psychiatry*. Washington, DC: APA Press; 1989: 273–292.

40. Helzer JE, Robins LN, Davis DH. Antecedents of narcotic use and addiction: A study of 898 Vietnam Veterans. *Drug Alcohol Depend*. 1976;1(3):183.

41. Nace EP, Meyers AL, Rothberg JM, Maleson F. Addicted and nonaddicted drug users; A comparison of drug usage patterns. *Arch Gen Psychiatry*. 1975;32(1):77–80.

42. Newby JH. Small group dynamics and drug abuse in an army setting: A case study. *Int J Addict*. 1977;12(2–3):287–300.

43. Bey DR, Zecchinelli VA. Marijuana as a coping device in Vietnam. *Milit Med*. 1971;136(5):448–450.

44. Branchy L, Davis W, Lieber CS. Alcoholism in Vietnam and Korean veterans: A long term follow-up. *Alcoholism*. 1984;8(6):572–575.

45. Hawthorne BJ. Job dissatisfaction: A job related issue. *Drug Forum*. 1978;6(2):187–195.

46. Goodwin DW, Davis DH, Robins LN. Drinking amid abundant illicit drugs: The Vietnam Case. *Arch Gen Psychiatry*. 1975;32(2):230–233.

47. Robins LN, Helzer JE, Davis DH. Narcotic use in Southeast Asia and afterward: An interview study of 898 Vietnam returnees. *Arch Gen Psychiatry*. 1975;32(8):955–961.

48. Selzer ML. The Michigan Alcoholism Screening Test: The quest for a new diagnostic instrument. *Am J Psychiatry*. 1971;127:89–94.

49. Ewing JA. Detecting alcoholism. *JAMA*. 1984;252:1905–1907.

50. Modell JG, Mountz JM. Drinking and flying—The problems of alcohol use by pilots. *N Engl J Med*. 1990;323(7):455–461.

51. Kaufman MR. Central Pacific area. In: *Overseas Theaters*. Vol 2. In: Glass AJ, ed. *Neuropsychiatry in World War II*. Washington, DC: GPO; 1973: Chap 15.

52. Flumerfelt JM. The Middle East theater. In: *Overseas Theaters*. Vol 2. In: Glass AJ, ed. *Neuropsychiatry in World War II*. Washington, DC: GPO; 1973: Chap 21.

53. Pub L No. 92–129, 10 USC § 1071 28 September 1971.

54. Kolb D, Baker DG, Gunderson EK. Effects of alcohol rehabilitation treatment on health and performance of Navy enlisted men. *Drug Alcohol Depend*. 1983;11(3–4):309–319.

55. Ingraham LH. "The Nam" and "the world": Heroin use by U.S. Army enlisted men serving in Vietnam. *Psychiatry*. 1974;37(2):114–128.

56. Sodetz FJ. *A Research Perspective on Drug and Alcohol Use in the Army*. Washington, DC: Walter Reed Institute of Research; 1983. Report WRAIR–NP–83–3.

57. US Department of the Army. *Alcohol and Drug Abuse Prevention and Control Program*. Washington, DC: DA; 1988. Army Regulation 600–85.

58. US Departments of the Army, the Navy, the Air Force. *Drug Abuse (Clinical Recognition and Treatment, Including the Disease Often Associated)*. Washington, DC: GPO; 1973. TB MED 290, NAVMED P–5116, AFP 160–33.

59. Watanabe HK. The Alcohol and Drug Abuse Prevention and Control Program: The Walter Reed experience. Presented at the Military Section of the World Psychiatric Association Regional Meeting; September 25–27, 1987; Buenos Aires, Argentina.

60. Reid WH. *Treatment of the DSM III Psychiatric Disorders*. New York: Brunner/Mazel; 1983.

61. Lewis DC, Senay EC. A specific approach to the treatment of drug and alcohol abusing patients. In: Buchwald C, Katz D, Callahan JF, eds. *Treatment of Drug and Alcohol Abuse*. New York: State University of New York; 1981: 29–39.

62. Holloway HC, Hales RE, Watanabe HK. Recognition and treatment of acute alcohol withdrawal syndromes. *Psychiatr Clin North Am*. 1984;4:729–743.

63. Rock NL, Donley PJ. Treatment program for military personnel with alcohol problems. Part II. The Program. *Int J Addict*. 1975;3:467–476.

64. Rock NL. Treatment of children and adolescents with substance abuse disorders. In: Simeon JG, Furguson HB, eds. *Treatment Strategies in Child and Adolescent Psychiatry*. New York: Plenum; 1990: 107–112.

65. Sellers EM, Naranjo CA, Harrison M, Devenyi P, Roach C, Sykora K. Diazepam loading: Simplified treatment of alcohol withdrawal. *Clin Pharmacol Ther*. 1983;34:822–826.

66. Shaw JM, Kolesar GS, Sellers EM, Kaplan SA, Sandor P. Development of optimal treatment tactics for alcohol withdrawal: I. Assessment and effectiveness of supportive care. *J Clin Psychopharmacol*. 1981;1:382–389.

67. Jones FD. Personal Communication, 1991.

68. Zuska JJ, Pursch JA. Long term management. In: Gitlow SE, Peyser HS, eds. *Alcoholism: A Practical Treatment Guide*. New York: Grune and Stratton; 1980: 131–163.

69. *Alcoholics Anonymous*. 3rd ed. New York: Alcoholics Anonymous World Series, Inc.; 1976.

70. Gitlow SE. Appendix D: Antabuse. In: Gitlow SE, Peyser HS, eds. *Alcoholism, A Practical Treatment Guide*. New York: Grune and Stratton; 1980: 273–278.

71. Bray R, Marsden ME, Guess LL, Herbold JR. Prevalence, trends, and correlates of alcohol use, non-medical drug, and tobacco use among U.S. military personnel. *Milt Med*. 1989;154:1–11.

72. Nace EP, Meyers AL, Rothberg JM. Addicted Viet Nam veterans: A comparison of self-referred and system-referred samples. *Am J Psychiatry*. 1973;130(11):1242–1245.

73. Zuska JJ. Beginnings of the Navy program: Alcoholism. *Clin Experimental Research*. 1978;2:352–357.

74. Pursch JA. From quonset hut to naval hospital: The story of an alcoholism rehabilitation service. *J Stud Alcohol*. 1976;37:1655–1665.

Chapter 6

HOMICIDE AND SUICIDE IN THE MILITARY

CHARLES P. MCDOWELL, PH.D.,* JOSEPH M. ROTHBERG, PH.D.,† AND R. GREGORY LANDE, D.O.,‡

*Senior Investigative Consultant, Headquarters, Air Force Office of Special Investigations, Bolling Air Force Base, Washington, D.C. 20332–6001.

†Research Mathematician, Department of Military Psychiatry, Walter Reed Army Institute of Research, Washington, D.C. 20307–5100

‡Lieuntenant Colonel, Medical Corps, U.S. Army; Chief, Outpatient Psychiatry Service, Walter Reed Army Medical Center, Washington, D.C. 20307–5001

INTRODUCTION: VIOLENT DEATH

Violent death is a historic by-product of the profession of arms. Killing the opponent's soldiers is not the goal of warfare in and of itself, although inflicting casualties on the enemy is one means of achieving the purpose of war. The objective of combat is to reduce the enemy's ability to wage war and thereby hasten the defeat of his political leadership. Within the military, the job of inflicting casualties is limited to certain specialties; the remainder of the military organization provides support. Even though the proportion of combat to support personnel (the tooth-to-tail ratio) is quite large in favor of the latter, all members of the military learn to kill when they go through basic training, which teaches them basic combat skills and military discipline.

Killing in the military context is bounded by law, treaty, and custom as to time, place, method, and who may be properly targeted as victims. Killing is neither arbitrary nor capricious, and those who would make it so within the military are commonly regarded with disdain by professional soldiers. Murder and suicide are both clearly outside the realm of acceptable military conduct; and although they occur with relative infrequency in the military, each is a significant social problem in its own right. The death of a military member because of homicide or suicide is a tragic personal loss. The victims are denied the richness of a full life; their immediate survivors inherit a bitter residual of shame, anger, guilt, and confusion; and the military loses the productivity of their labor. These deaths are also disruptive to the military in other ways because of the impact they have on morale. Finally, these deaths leave friends and coworkers confused and upset. Violent nonaccidental deaths are also expensive. The direct cost of death benefits and the loss of investment and the cost of replacement make these deaths much more than personal tragedies. This chapter addresses some features of murder and suicide as they occur within the military and explores their respective dynamics.

HOMICIDE

Taking another person's life is arguably the most ancient of crimes. The earliest Judeo-Christian reference to homicide is probably the biblical reference to the death of Abel by Cain in the first book of the Old Testament (Genesis IV:8). The killing of another has historically been a major crime and an inherent wrong in and of itself. There are, however, different kinds of killing, and homicide is a generic term that encompasses a wide range of behaviors, not all of which are unlawful.

The evolution of law is a slow process that reflects emerging sociocultural change. Religion has played a prominent role in shaping behavioral restraints. The Old Testament "eye for an eye" response was softened considerably by the "turn the other cheek" New Testament advice. Legal thinking sanctioned this humane approach by defining criminal behavior as requiring two elements. The *actus rea* and the *mens rea* are the historical vestiges of religion modifying the prosecution of criminal acts. The *actus rea* refers to the physical components of a crime, while the *mens rea* involves the emotional state of the perpetrator. Varying degrees of moral culpability are assigned based on the nature of the perpetrator's mental state. A cold, calculated homicide will ensure a greater social penalty than an accidental, negligent death. Consideration of the *mens rea* in criminal prosecutions is responsible for the introduction of mental health professionals into the courtroom.

According to the Centers for Disease Control (CDC),[1] in 1983, homicide was the 11th leading cause of death in the United States; however, that ranking varied by race and age. It was the fifth leading cause of death among blacks (but the leading cause of death among black males ages 15 to 34 years). Homicide was the 14th leading cause of death among whites.[1] The CDC has identified a number of common patterns in civilian homicides as follows:

- Males are more likely to be homicide victims than females.
- Homicide rates are highest among young adults (with the highest rates among those between 20 and 34 years of age).
- Most homicide victims are killed by firearms (most of which are handguns).

- More than one-half of all homicide victims are killed in the course of an argument or some other nonfelony circumstance, and only a small proportion are killed by assailants perpetrating another crime.
- One-half of all homicide victims know their killers.
- A greater proportion of female homicide victims are killed by family members than male homicide victims; conversely, a greater proportion of male than female homicide victims were killed by acquaintances or strangers.
- Homicide rates are highest in the West.

The most recent law enforcement data on homicide are contained in the Federal Bureau of Investigation's (FBI's) *Uniform Crime Reports* (UCR),[2] which reports that in 1991, the total number of murders in the United States was estimated at 24,703, or 1% of all reported violent crimes. Not only was the number of murders in 1991 high, it rose 4.3% over 1990 and was 8% higher than the 1982 rate. According to the FBI, the overall murder rate in 1990 was 9.8 per 100,000 population (in metropolitan areas it was 11 per 100,000). In 1992, there were 15,377 reported murders involving a firearm. From 1987 through 1992, the number of firearm-related criminal acts increased by 55%. Each year, about 40,000 new firearm reports are added to the previous year's total.[3] UCR data consistently support the CDC findings. For example, in 1990, about 78% of the murder victims were males, and 90% were 18 years of age or older. Almost one-half of the murder victims were black.

Under the Uniform Code of Military Justice, criminal homicides fall into two broad categories: murders and manslaughters, which differ in several ways. Murder, under military law, takes place when a member "unlawfully kills a human being when he (1) has a premeditated design to kill; (2) intends to kill or inflict great bodily harm; or, (3) is engaged in the perpetration or attempted perpetration of burglary, sodomy, rape, robbery, or aggravated assault."[4(p71)] A voluntary manslaughter, on the other hand, is committed when a military member "with an intent to kill or inflict great bodily harm, unlawfully kills a human being in the heat of passion caused by adequate provocation."[4(p74)] An involuntary manslaughter occurs when a military member, without intent to kill or inflict great bodily harm, "unlawfully kills a human being (1) by culpable negligence or (2) while perpetrating or attempting to perpetrate an offense other than a burglary, sodomy, rape, robbery, or aggravated arson."[4(p74)]

The difference between murder and manslaughter lies in intent and circumstances. In assessing the moral culpability of an accused service member, the mental state of the perpetrator is considered. The jury (or panel of members in the military) is given specific instructions by the judge. This legal guidance helps the jury evaluate and weigh the testimony. When one looks at legal distinctions (which are many and complicated), it is easy to overlook the fact that most murders and manslaughters are also human dramas that have antecedent conditions and personal outcomes. Because military members have the same vices, passions, weaknesses, and foibles as their civilian counterparts, it should come as no surprise that some of them also commit murder and manslaughter. The question then becomes whether or not the military context either abets this process or diminishes its likelihood. Unfortunately, there are little systematic data on homicides within the military.

The military community encompasses several features associated with high-risk homicide victimology: it is composed primarily of young adult males, nearly all of whom have been trained in the use of firearms. The military (particularly the army) also has a significant minority population. However, the military is not a random sample of the civilian population. Those who enter the military are screened for physical and mental fitness. They must also meet minimum education requirements, have no significant criminal record, and successfully complete basic training. In other words, the military is a selective environment, and to an undetermined extent, it probably screens out many who would be at high risk as either homicide victims or offenders.

The information that follows, including the case studies, is based on the Headquarters, U.S. Department of the Air Force Office of Special Investigations ongoing analysis of all known homicides involving active duty members of the U.S. Air Force between January 1, 1981, and December 31, 1991. This chapter provides the preliminary disclosure and publication of these statistics. The U.S. Air Force may or may not be representative of the other armed forces, but these finding at least suggest the broad nature of homicides within the military. A word of caution is in order. Although the identification of active duty military homicide victims is simple, information on military offenders is much more problematic. It is easier to count homicide victims than those who killed them simply because not all homicides are detected and not all logical suspects are identified. Although the data on military offenders are valid, they are probably not exhaustive and must therefore be regarded as representative rather than definitive.

Active Duty Victims

Although the air force homicide victims fell into discrete categories based on legal definitions, a precautionary note is in order. Crimes are both factual and legal events, and the two are not always the same. For example, in reality, a given homicide might actually be a murder but as a matter of prosecutorial convenience be defined by legal authorities as a manslaughter. The air force homicides in this chapter were classed according to their factual nature although they may have subsequently been adjudicated "downward" as something else.

The largest proportion of the homicides were murders, of which 82 (or 70%) were intentional (Table 6–1). The motives for these murders varied; some cases are hard to fathom, while others seem painfully ordinary. For example:

Case Study 1

A 26-year-old civilian went to the residence of a 22-year-old single male E–4 to smoke some marijuana. When the E–4 refused to let him in, the civilian set the house on fire, killing the E–4.

Case Study 2

A 21-year-old single male E–3 was employed off-duty as a part-time clerk in a convenience store. Two males entered one evening and robbed the store. As the E–3 ran after them with a baseball bat, one of the robbers turned and fatally shot him in the chest with a .357 revolver.

Case Study 3

A 21-year-old single male E–3 was living in a trailer with his girlfriend, the daughter of a retired military member. Another resident of the trailer park entered their home one evening and after tying up the E–3, raped his girlfriend. He then forced the girlfriend to watch him while he shot the E–3 in the forehead, and then he killed her as well. The offender was the son of a retired military member and was also suspected of killing five other people. He was sentenced to death.

Nationally, 43% of stranger killings are associated with another crime (usually a robbery).[2] The proportion of military murder victims associated with other crimes was considerably lower: 18%. The low number of robberies involving military victims probably stems from the fact that military facilities are seldom robbed and relatively few military members work off-duty, especially in the kinds of places likely to be robbed. The other category of crime in which a military member is most likely to be a homicide victim is rape, but only 9% of the military murder victims were killed during the course of a rape (4 of the 11 victims were killed during the course of a homosexual rape).

In general, aggravated assault and homicide are similar in many respects, and many homicides are actually "overly successful" assaults. This was clearly the case in many of the military manslaughters. Although they represent a diverse category of violent events, there is a painful consistency among them, as the following cases illustrate:

Case Study 4

A 30-year-old married male E–5 got into an argument in a bar with another patron over a woman. As the argument escalated, the E–5 hit the patron over the head with a beer bottle and then pushed him head-first into the

TABLE 6–1

ACTIVE DUTY AIR FORCE HOMICIDE VICTIMS (1981–1991) BY CATEGORY OF INCIDENT

Category			Number	(%)
Justifiable Homicide			3	(2)
Manslaughter			74	(38)
Vehicular		12		
Involuntary		9		
Voluntary		53		
Murder			117	(60)
Murder		68		
Murder/Suicide		10		
Murder (Terrorist)		4		
Felony Murder		35		
Arson	3			
Rape—Heterosexual	7			
Rape—Homosexual	4			
Robbery	21			
Unknown			1	
Total			195	(100)

bar. The patron became enraged, pulled out a pistol, and shot the E–5.

Case Study 5

After a 39-year-old married male E–5 assaulted his wife, she retreated into her bedroom with their children and locked the door. When the E–5 broke the door down, she shot him in the chest with a .22 rifle.

The average age of military homicide victims was 27 years (which is 6 years lower than the national average for homicide victims); however, averages can be misleading. The lower average age for military victims is probably attributable to the age distribution of the active duty population. As military members reach their early- to midthirties, their numbers diminish rapidly. Among the military homicide victims, a slightly higher proportion was married than single. The marital status of the victims is shown in Table 6–2.

The relationship between the victim and the offender is a critical component in the homicide equation, and Table 6–3 outlines the victim-offender relationships in homicides involving active duty victims. In their study of 508 Detroit homicides, Daly and Wilson[5] found that 25% were committed by relatives, a finding virtually duplicated in the military sample. However, Daly and Wilson further distinguished between genealogical (blood) relatives and affinal (marital) relationships and found that 6.3% of the Detroit homicides involved blood relatives. Among the military victims, 4% were blood relatives. Both findings are consistent with those of Wolfgang,[6] whose analysis of homicides in Philadelphia between 1948 and 1952 revealed that 136 of the 550 (25%) people killed by known assailants were the victims of relatives.

Daly and Wilson's[5] study of homicides in Detroit found that cohabitants who were not blood relatives of the killer were 11 times more likely to be killed than cohabitants who were related by blood and that the principal victims were spouses. This finding is confirmed in the U.S. Air Force homicide study, in which 82.6% of the relatives killed were spouses. It is worth noting that among the military victims, 24 wives killed their military husbands, accounting for over one-half of the homicides by relatives. Women who kill their husbands in society as a whole generally argue that the act was in self-defense against abusive husbands who are threatening either them or their children. The following cases illustrate this point:

TABLE 6–2

ACTIVE DUTY AIR FORCE HOMICIDE VICTIMS (1981–1991) BY MARITAL STATUS OF VICTIM

Status		Males		Females	Total	(%)
Single		74		10	84	(43)
Married		78		21	99	(51)
Separated	6		5			
Not Separated	72		16			
Divorced		9		3	12	(6)
Total		161		34	195	(100)

TABLE 6–3

ACTIVE DUTY AIR FORCE HOMICIDE VICTIMS (1981–1991) VICTIM-OFFENDER RELATIONSHIP

Victim-Offender		Number	(%)
Relatives		46	(24)
Child vs Parent	4		
Husband vs Wife	14		
Wife vs Husband	24		
Other Relative	4		
Intimates		19	(10)
Ex-Husband	1		
Ex-Wife	1		
Lovers	17		
Acquaintances		77	(39)
Acquaintance	12		
Coworker	21		
Date	1		
Friend	19		
Roommate	2		
Sex-Related	16		
Drug-Related	6		
Strangers		52	(27)
Unknown		1	—
Total		195	(100)

Case Study 6

A 33-year-old married (but separated) male E–6 was in his car with his estranged wife (whom he had physically assaulted in the past). As they were discussing their future plans, he became angry and assaulted her. After threatening to kill her, he reached for a gun under the seat, but she pulled hers out of her purse first and shot him four times.

Case Study 7

A 38-year-old married male E–6 had a history of spouse abuse and sexual abuse of his children (in one instance he attempted to drown the female companion of his daughter after she rejected his sexual overtures). He got into a heated argument with his wife during which he told her that he was going to kill her. As he went to get his pistol, she grabbed a .22 rifle and shot him instead.

An important part of the relationship between these victims and their offenders is their connection with the military. Slightly more than one-half of the victims (108 or 55%) were killed by civilians who had no affiliation with the military. Of the remainder, 32 (or 16%) were killed by their own family members, and 49 (or 25%) were killed by other active duty military members. One victim was killed by a retired military member, and in five cases, the affiliation of the killer was not determined. Overall, 42% of the victims were killed by individuals having some affiliation with the military community. In addition, 164 (or 84%) of the military homicide victims were killed off their military reservations and outside the military context. It stands to reason that the killings committed by civilians would take place offbase, and because many of the remainder arose from interpersonal transactions, it was likely that they would also take place offbase (but usually in or near the victim's residence). Not surprisingly, 56 (or 29%) of the killings were sex-related in some way. The majority of the sex-related cases (41 or 73%) involved heterosexual events, and 13 (or 23%) involved homosexual episodes. The age-gender relationship between the victims and their killers is shown in Table 6–4.

Table 6–5 shows the distribution of military victims by their grade. The vast majority (182 or 93%) were enlisted personnel, with the highest proportion (71%) falling between the grades of E–3 and E–5 (corresponding to the 66% of the air force enlisted personnel in grades E–3 to E–5). It is noteworthy that among the officer victims, all 13 were in the bottom-three commissioned grades: second lieutenant (O–1) through captain (O–3). These three grades have 63% of the air force officers.

The majority (161 or 83%) of the victims were males, of which 114 (71%) were white and 46 (29%) black. The proportion of military victims who were male is slightly higher than for the civilian U.S. population (78%), but that finding may be attributed to the larger proportion of males in the military. The proportion of victims who were black, however, is significantly lower than for the civilian U.S. population (49%). This finding is probably due to several factors. First, many of the black-on-black homicides in the civilian sector arise from drug-related events, and there is a relative scarcity of drug-related killings in the military. Second, many

TABLE 6–4

ACTIVE DUTY AIR FORCE HOMICIDE VICTIMS (1981–1991) BY AGE/GENDER RELATIONSHIP BETWEEN OFFENDER AND VICTIM

Offender/Victim	Number
Adult Female vs Adult Female	2
Adult Female vs Adult Male	31
Adult Male vs Adult Female	32
Adult Male vs Adult Male	123
Juvenile Male vs Adult Male	2
Unknown	5
Total	195

TABLE 6–5

ACTIVE DUTY AIR FORCE HOMICIDE VICTIMS (1981–1991) BY MILITARY GRADE

Enlisted		Officer	
Grade	Number	Grade	Number
E–1	6	O–1	3
E–2	15	O–2	2
E–3	41	O–3	8
E–4	48		
E–5	40		
E–6	21		
E–7	9		
E–8	2		
Total enlisted	182 (93%)	Total officer	13 (8%)

of those most prone to violence either do not try to enter the military in the first place or are not retained if they are successful in getting in because the military is unwilling to retain young males who enter the service but subsequently demonstrate contempt for authority or a propensity for interpersonal violence.

Although military homicide victims were killed by a variety of means, firearms led the count. A total of 106 of the victims (54%) died from gunshot wounds. This method was followed by stabbing (34), blunt trauma (18), and motor vehicles (13). These four methods represented 171 (88%) of the total. The military findings are consistent with civilian homicides in which two-thirds of the black homicide victims (66.5%) were killed with firearms and a slightly lower proportion (59.8%) of white victims were killed by firearms. After handguns, cutting and piercing instruments were the next most frequently used weapons in each group so that taken together firearms and cutting instruments were the weapons used in almost 9 out of 10 civilian homicides among blacks and 8 out of 10 homicides among whites and persons of other races.[1]

The majority of the homicides involved a lone active duty victim killed by a single offender (152 or 78% of the cases). Twenty-one (11%) of the homicides were committed by two assailants. Homicides are, therefore, primarily an interpersonal event between two individuals; this finding is consistent with the civilian experience in which among black males age 15 and above, for instance, the predominant form was a killing (by handgun) precipitated by a verbal argument.

TABLE 6–6

ACTIVE DUTY AIR FORCE HOMICIDE VICTIMS (1981–1991) BY DAY OF WEEK

Day	Number	(%)
Monday	36	(19)
Tuesday	19	(10)
Wednesday	15	(8)
Thursday	19	(10)
Friday	24	(13)
Saturday	39	(20)
Sunday	40	(20)
Unknown	3	(1)
Total	195	(100)

TABLE 6–7

HOMICIDES BY ACTIVE DUTY AIR FORCE MEMBERS (1981–1991) BY STATUS OF THEIR VICTIMS

Victims	Number	(%)
Civilians	84*	(32)
Military Family Members	124	(48)
Other Active Duty Military Personnel	51	(20)
Total	259†	(100)

*Includes one military retiree
†243 military offenders killed a total of 259 victims

One might hypothesize that these kinds of violent episodes are more likely to occur on the weekend than during the week, and the data tend to support that assumption. As Table 6–6 indicates, Saturday and Sunday account for more homicides than would be expected by chance alone ($\chi^2 = 6.6$, $p < 0.02$).

Active Duty Offenders

Homicides are dynamic events involving a killer, a victim, and a context. Both the victim and the offender make their own unique contribution to the homicide, and the nature of the event determines whether the killing is a manslaughter, a murder, or justifiable homicide. Homicides are rarely random; perhaps the cases that come closest to a random relationship between the victim and the offender are vehicular manslaughters in which the driver at fault had no intention of killing anyone but did so during the improper or illegal operation of a motor vehicle. Most killings arise out of arguments, insults, or rivalries, and most of the time the victim is at least acquainted with his or her killer. This is equally true of military and civilian homicides.

During the same period that 195 active duty U.S. Air Force members were killed, 243 other air force members killed someone else. In 52 of these cases, one military member killed another. (49 of the cases overlap and involved air force members who killed other air force members; the other three offenders were from another branch of the armed forces.) The distribution of air force homicides by the status of the victim is reflected in Table 6–7.

Unlike the situation with air force victims, the largest proportion of offender cases did not involve murders, but they came close. As Table 6–8 reflects, the murders and manslaughters are almost evenly divided.

As in the case of active duty victims, killings by active duty members span the full range of homicidal behaviors, ranging from serial murders to vehicular homicides. The following examples illustrate some of these events:

Case Study 8

The offender, a 21-year-old single male E–4 was involved in a minor auto accident with a civilian. As their dispute escalated into a fight, the E–4 beat the civilian on the head with a baseball bat, killing him at the scene.

Case Study 9

The offender, a 31-year-old separated male E–6 was in the process of being divorced by his wife, who was leaving him for another man whom she was going to marry as soon as the divorce was final. After strangling her with her own panty hose, the E–6 wrote "hooker" on her chest with her lipstick. He then inserted the lipstick applicator up her rectum (the crime scene was "staged" to make it look as if a sex maniac had murdered her).

Case Study 10

The offender, a 22–year-old married female E–3 who was human immunodeficiency virus (HIV) positive, beat her 18-month-old son to death with a belt and an electrical cord (according to her, to "discipline" him). The child was found to have multiple bruises to the face, old wounds over his entire body, burns to the left knee, and a portion of his left ear was missing. The E-3 stated that the child was better off dead.

Case Study 11

A 26-year-old married black male E–4 was irritated at his 1-month-old son's crying. He shook the infant and punched him in the head, as a result of which the child died. Three years earlier, this same individual placed another infant in scalding water, inflicting such severe burns that the baby died.

The relationship between military killers and their victims is shown in Table 6–9. The proportion of homicides that involve military husbands killing their wives or children is especially noteworthy. Many of these husband versus wife homicides are consistent with the spousal homicide syndrome in which men claiming to be in love with their wives kill them for reasons related to sexual propriety (eg, the wife leaving the husband for a new partner, promiscuity, pathological jealousy, and catching the wife in an adulterous affair). Male sexual jealousy and proprietorship as motives are illustrated in the following examples:

Case Study 12

A 30-year-old married male E–7 got into a heated argument with his wife over his suspicions of her infidelity. After she admitted to having an affair, the E–7 grabbed a kitchen knife and stabbed her several times, killing her.

Case Study 13

A 24-year-old married male E–4 was sent to Saudi Arabia during Operation Desert Storm. While he was gone, his wife moved in with another man. When the E–4 returned and learned of her infidelity, he confronted her in the parking lot of a shopping center and shot her twice with a .357 pistol.

Case Study 14

A 26-year-old married male E–5 became despondent when his wife returned from a trip and told him that she

TABLE 6–8

HOMICIDES BY ACTIVE DUTY AIR FORCE MEMBERS (1981–1991) BY CATEGORY OF INCIDENT

Category			Number	(%)
Justifiable Homicide			3	(1)
Manslaughter			130	(50)
Vehicular		34		
Involuntary		47		
Voluntary		49		
Murder			126	(49)
Felony Murder		19		
Arson	2			
Burglary	3			
Rape	7			
Robbery	7			
Serial Murders		7		
Other Murders		85		
Murder-Suicides		15		
Total			259	(100)

wanted a divorce. He went to his room with the intention of killing himself, and as he was looking in his dresser for his pistol, he found some love letters written by his wife to another man. He located his 9mm pistol and shot her instead.

Fully 82% of the killings by military members took place between individuals who were known to one another, with almost 60% occurring between relatives or intimates. The majority of the killers (223 or 92%) were males, and 20 (8%) were females. This difference is a finding consistent with trends in the civilian world in which killing is also concentrated among young men (primarily in their late adolescence and early adulthood).

TABLE 6–9

HOMICIDES BY ACTIVE DUTY AIR FORCE MEMBERS (1981–1991) BY VICTIM-OFFENDER RELATIONSHIP

Victim-Offender Relationship		Number	(%)
Relatives		127	(49)
Wife vs Husband	2		
Husband vs Wife	45		
Father vs Son	31		
Father vs Stepson	8		
Father vs Daughter	20		
Father vs Stepdaughter	5		
Mother vs Daughter	6		
Mother vs Stepdaughter	1		
Mother vs Son	4		
Subject vs Other Relative	5		
Intimates		23	(9)
Ex-spouses	4		
Lovers	17		
Prostitutes	2		
Acquaintances		62	(24)
Coworkers	21		
Friend	15		
Sex-Related Triangle	9		
Caretaker vs Child	7		
Drug-Related	6		
Offender vs Med. Patient	2		
Roommate	2		
Military Member vs Stranger		44	(17)
Other		3	(1)
Total		259	(100)

In terms of race, the majority of killers (165 or 68%) were white, while 75 (or 31%) were black. The remaining 3 (1%) represented all other races. The proportion of homicides committed by blacks is double their representation in the Air Force as a whole, which is in the same direction as black homicide rates in the civilian world (where black homicide rates are approximately five times greater than white rates). Most of the black offenders in the military (58 or 75%) killed black victims; of the 19 nonblack victims killed by black offenders, 4 were their own family members, 8 were civilians, and 7 were other active duty military members.

The average age for the active duty killers was 26, which is almost identical to the average age of the military victims. As in the case of the military victims, the age is lower than the civilian average because of the age distribution of the active duty force. The average military member enlists at age 20, and because career military personnel are eligible for retirement at 20 years, the proportion of military members above age 40 diminishes rapidly.

The marital status of the military offenders is reflected in Table 6–10. The proportion of military members who killed their spouses or children mirrors the proportion of military members who are married. The question of whether the killing was related to their marital status, their military status, or neither is problematic but interesting.

Most of the homicides committed by active duty members occurred off the military reservation (209 or 81%). Of those that took place on base, 25 (or one-half the on-base total) involved the killing of a family member, and most of the rest (18) involved the killing of another military member. As in the case of the active duty victims, sex played a role in many of these deaths. Of the 259 homicides a total of

TABLE 6–10

HOMICIDES BY ACTIVE DUTY AIR FORCE MEMBERS (1981–1991) BY MARITAL STATUS OF THE OFFENDER

Status	Number	(%)
Married*	152	(63)
Single	71	(29)
Divorced	20	(8)
Total	243	(100)

*Includes 18 separated

52 (20%) were sex-related. Most of the sex-related cases (47) involved heterosexual events, and the remainder involved homosexual events.

More of the active duty killers used a firearm than any other weapon; however, firearms were not used in a majority of the killings. Slightly less than one-third of the military killers used a firearm, which produces a noteworthy anomaly: military homicide victims are most likely to be shot, but military homicide offenders are not likely to shoot their victims. This finding suggests that military members are more likely to kill with less premeditation and more under the pressure of circumstances as they develop at the time of the homicide. Table 6–11 presents the methods used in killings by active duty members.

Most homicides by military members were committed by males whose principal targets were females and juveniles, and most of their victims were intimates or family members. In contrast, for civilian offenders in state prisons, males were the principal target (70%), and few of the victims were intimates or dependents (24%). However, it is worth noting that in populations in which the homicide rate is relatively low, the proportion of cases that occur in the family is relatively high, and this relationship holds true for the military. The age/gender relationships among the killers and their victims are reflected in Table 6–12.

The homicides committed by active duty military members tended to occur on the weekends as was seen for victims of homicide ($\chi^2 = 5.4$, $p < 0.02$). As Table 6–13 indicates, Saturday was the maximum and Thursday the minimum day for homicides to occur by day of the week.

In summary, an analysis of homicides within the military yields some interesting findings. For one thing, military members are more likely to kill than to be killed. Active duty victims are most likely to be killed by someone to whom they are related or whom they know, and they are most likely to be shot. Military killers are most apt to kill family

TABLE 6–11

HOMICIDES BY ACTIVE DUTY AIR FORCE MEMBERS (1981–1991) BY METHOD

Method	Number	(%)
Firearm	75	(29)
Blunt Trauma	55	(21)
Automobile	34	(13)
Stabbing/Cutting	31	(12)
Shaken Infant	27	(10)
Asphyxiation	16	(6)
Gross Negligence	8	(3)
Multiple Methods	4	(2)
Other	9	(3)
Total	259	(100)

TABLE 6–12

HOMICIDES BY ACTIVE DUTY AIR FORCE MEMBERS (1981–1991) BY AGE/GENDER RELATIONS BETWEEN OFFENDER AND VICTIM*

Offender/Victim	Number
Adult Female vs Adult Female	2
Adult Female vs Adult Male	7
Adult Female vs Juvenile Female	7
Adult Female vs Juvenile Male	4
Adult Male vs Adult Female	83
Adult Male vs Adult Male	80
Adult Male vs Juvenile Female	28
Adult Male vs Juvenile Male	47
Unknown	1

*NOTE: Sixteen males killed more than one person; 15 of them killed two victims and one, a serial murderer, killed five. For purposes of this table each event is counted separately. Thus, even though 223 men killed 239 victims, the total number of "relationships" in this table totals 259.

TABLE 6–13

HOMICIDES BY ACTIVE DUTY AIR FORCE MEMBERS (1981–1991) BY DAY OF WEEK

Day	Number	(%)
Monday	35	(13)
Tuesday	42	(16)
Wednesday	28	(11)
Thursday	25	(10)
Friday	30	(12)
Saturday	53	(20)
Sunday	46	(18)
Total	259	(100)

members or other members of the military, but they are less likely to use a firearm in the commission of the crime. Murders within the military seem to conform in general to those within the civilian community except that fewer are drug-related. The status of being in the military depresses the overall likelihood of homicide. That may be due in part to personnel selection and retention procedures and may be related in part to the closely ordered nature of the military community. The bottom line, however, is inescapable: a person is safer in the military than in the civilian world, and this is especially so for black males.

Homicide Prevention

Although preventing homicides is a great deal more problematic than preventing suicides, there is still a great deal that can be done. For example, the most common homicide within military quarters is the killing of infants by their parents or adult caretakers. The victim is usually under 1 year of age and is either suffocated by the mother or dies as a result of being shaken by a male caretaker (the father, stepfather, or boyfriend of the child's mother).

In some cases, parental behavior is more violent. An unfortunate case occurred overseas. Both parents were active duty, juggling demanding careers with parenting. Severe marital conflict developed, and a newborn infant became the object of the father's frustration and anger. Responding to the infant's inconsolable crying one day, the father repeatedly dropped the child on its head. The infant sustained severe injury and went into respiratory arrest, and the panicked father took the child to the local military treatment facility. He initially adamantly denied suspicions of child abuse. Subsequent investigations and prosecution uncovered the truth.

Not surprisingly, these violent deaths are significantly under-represented in homicide counts because most are never prosecuted as murders or manslaughters, and this illustrates an important point. The criminal justice system measures outcomes in terms of legal definitions rather than the larger antecedent conditions that produce them. Lethal outcomes that are the product of frustration and a lack of impulse control often slip between the cracks of the system. The people who commit these acts are typically immature, inadequate, and impulsive (indeed, this triad is a common denominator in the majority of homicides regardless of the age of the victim). Because relatively few of these deaths are intended consequences, the targeted behavior should be assaults rather than killings. If assaultive behaviors can be reduced, the number of homicides will almost certainly diminish correspondingly.

The prevention of homicide is an unrealistic goal. The force of history clearly demonstrates that violence is part of the human condition. Currently, the best option is reduction of risk factors associated with aggression.[7] The prediction of violence is fraught with error, particularly long-range assessments. Clinicians can more accurately define acute dangerousness.

The legal duty of clinicians to warn victims of violence was addressed in the landmark case *Tarasoff v. Regents of Univ of Cal.*[8] Since then, the medical community has repeatedly examined the subject. The duty to warn must be tempered by clinical judgment. The clinician must carefully weigh the risk of disclosure versus potential harm to the public. Each instance must be approached in a flexible manner to ensure that a reasonable decision is reached. One possible clinical outcome could be the absence of a mental disorder. Threatening behavior in this context could be prosecuted under military law.

From a social perspective, violence can be minimized by controlling factors that promote or facilitate the expression of violence. Substance abuse is a prime example. In the military, random urine drug screens seeking illicit drug use have conspicuously reduced consumption. Alcohol remains uncontrolled, although the military policies for treatment and, where necessary, punishment are well described.[9]

Community psychiatry emphasizes prevention. The early detection and referral of emotional problems and family conflicts and identification of poor parenting skills may forestall a later crisis. In addition, command education and sensitivity to the emotional health of their subordinates are critical to prevention. Army policy, for example, mandates suicide prevention task force committees.[10] This multidisciplinary body is charged with the specific task of addressing suicide prevention at all command levels.

SUICIDE

Suicide is regarded as a major public health problem and has received considerable attention in recent years, especially in light of the growing number of suicides among young people.[11] Between

1970 and 1980, almost 300,000 people took their own lives, amounting to an estimate of one suicide every 20 minutes.[12] The military is not exempt from the problem; in fact, suicide ranks third as a leading cause of death among active duty military members (following accidents and deaths from natural causes).

There were three reasons why suicide within the military historically received relatively little attention. First, suicides were anomalies within the military community. Because the absolute number of active duty suicides is low to begin with and because their distribution across time and space further diminished their visibility, they were commonly regarded as rare events. Second, suicide was viewed as a psychiatric problem, and its management had therefore been placed outside the mainstream of command responsibility. Because mental health professionals were responsible for treating those who make suicide attempts or gestures as well as those referred for suicidal ideation, the mental health profession had "owned" the problem. Because they regard it as a psychiatric problem, the mental health community had been slow to see the relation between suicide and command responsibility. Finally, suicides had been viewed as an individual rather than collective problem; therefore, they have been seen as a problem without a solution because the death of the victim precluded any possibility of a more favorable outcome. There may even have been some general sense that someone who attempted or committed suicide could not be a great loss to the service. In short, suicides within the military have historically been viewed as an individual problem rooted in the pathology of the victim and therefore beyond the control of command authorities.

This historical attitude has changed and moderated since the end of the Vietnam conflict. In the U.S. Army, the change was driven from the top, by directive of the senior army leadership. AR 600–63[10] describes the military approach to suicide evaluation and prevention. AR 600–63 requires that every military installation assemble a suicide prevention task force committee. As a multidisciplinary body, this committee is authorized wide latitude in education and consultation. Some installations, for example, have installed a central suicide crisis telephone line. Others routinely write articles about various aspects of suicide in local military publications. Direct consultation to units is common. AR 600–63 also gives to the Chaplain Corps and the family life centers the responsibility for suicide prevention education to unit leaders and more recently, also to unit families. The chaplains usually welcome mental health assistance with this duty.

The typical small unit commander is sensitized to the emotional needs of his subordinates. At various times in their professional development, Army leaders are reminded of suicide. On some posts, command emphasis has given junior- and middle-level commanders the impression that a suicide among their subordinates could adversely affect their careers. Close liaison with military community mental health resources affords the commander the opportunity to obtain informal consultation. All units have access to these professionals. In addition, progressive substance abuse evaluation and treatment programs exist throughout the military. Substance abuse and family support programs are unique in that army regulations also define these services as command-sponsored priorities. The strains of military life as they adversely impact domestic relationships can be referred to family advocacy evaluation and treatment programs.

Despite the best efforts of these well-intentioned activities, suicide still occurs. Following any completed suicide, military regulations require a psychological autopsy. These indepth evaluations help isolate any correctable, and potentially aggravating, factors. Recommendations from the psychological autopsy may be useful in prevention.

In terms of specific numbers, since 1975, the U.S. Army has averaged 74 active duty suicides per year, and the U.S. Air Force has averaged 66 (their approximate crude rates are 12.5 and 11.5 per 100,000, respectively).[13–15] These rates compare favorably with the 1986 civilian rate of 12.8; however, the military population is not a random sample of the civilian population and, in fact, differs from it in several systematic ways. The military population is largely male, has a larger proportion of racial minorities, and has virtually no members below the age of 17 and relatively few above the age of 50.

To better understand the relation between army and civilian death rates, the army death rates were calculated for males and females and blacks and whites in 5-year age intervals for each mode of death.[16] The same calculations were done for civilians, breaking them down by race, sex, and 5–year age intervals, and the results were compared. Using a scale normalized to 100 for the case when the number of deaths observed in the Army is exactly equal to the number predicted from the civilian rates, the result is a standardized mortality ratio. This procedure is an indirect standardization and enables one to compare military deaths with civilian deaths. A number over 100 means that the death rate is higher than the comparable civilian group, and a score below 100 indicates a lower death rate.

The findings were startling: Total deaths in the Army occur at one-half the rate expected from comparable civilians, with suicide occurring at about two-thirds the civilian rate. In other words, with a standardized mortality ratio of 68.8 for suicides in 1986, there were 31% fewer suicides among active duty members in the Army than would have been expected by chance alone. Comparable calculations for the Air Force for 1985 revealed a standardized mortality ratio of 58, indicating that suicide among active duty Air Force members is only slightly more than one-half the rate of a comparable civilian population.

Why are the military suicide rates lower than would be expected? The answer may lie at least in part with the fact that the military population is not randomly selected from the larger civilian population. The military population differs from the civilian population on the basis of age, race, and sex and is a filtered population consisting of those who have been physically and emotionally screened and found fit for military service. Moreover, the military population tends to be better educated and healthier and is supported by command, medical, and mental health systems that place a major emphasis on wellness. Finally, all members of the military are subject to much closer supervision and assessment than their civilian counterparts. This means that a military member who shows signs of physical or emotional dysfunction is more likely to be identified as needing care early on and is also more likely to get it in the free (and mandatory) healthcare system of the military.

Suicide Risk Factors

The information that follows is based on an analysis of 850 air force suicides that took place over a 13-year period (1979 through 1991). For purposes of this chapter, *suicide* is operationally defined as the self-inflicted death of a person, based on the victim's wish to die and an understanding of the probable consequences of his action in furtherance of that goal.[17] This definition is based on the Operational Criteria for Classification of Suicide (Exhibit 6–1). This definition, therefore, excluded certain deaths even though they resulted from the victims' own actions (such as autoerotic fatalities, eating disorders, and overly successful suicide gestures). This definition may include deaths resulting from Russian roulette if the victim fully understood and accepted the consequences of the act even though it was an act of bravado.

One of the most important relations an individual has with the military is that of rank. One's rank determines income, status, and power. In the military, a person's rank can also have a powerful

EXHIBIT 6–1

OPERATIONAL CRITERIA FOR DETERMINING SUICIDE

Self-Inflicted: There is evidence that death was self-inflicted. This may be determined by pathologic (autopsy), toxicologic, investigatory, and psychologic evidence and by statements of the decedent or witnesses.

Intent: There is evidence (explicit and/or implicit) that at the time of injury, the decedent intended to kill himself/herself or wished to die and that the decedent understood the probable consequences of his/her actions.

1. Explicit verbal or nonverbal expression of intent to kill self.
2. Implicit or indirect evidence of intent to die, such as
   - preparations for death inappropriate to or unexpected in the context of the decedent's life,
   - expression of farewell or the desire to die or acknowledgment of impending death,
   - expression of hopelessness,
   - effort to procure or learn about means of death or rehearse fatal behavior,
   - precautions to avoid rescue,
   - evidence that decedent recognized high potential lethality of means of death,
   - previous suicide attempt,
   - previous suicide threat,
   - stressful events or significant losses (actual or threatened), or
   - serious depression or mental disorder.

Reprinted from: Centers for Disease Control. Operational criteria for determining suicide. *MMWR.* 1988;37(50):773–780.

influence on his self-perception and personal as well as professional expectations. People whose age, education, or experience are not in harmony with their rank may experience more stress than their contemporaries. In addition, loss of rank or failure to progress in grade can produce considerable anxiety and stress for the individual. In the case of officers and senior noncommissioned officers, feelings of personal or professional disgrace can exceed the individual's coping mechanisms, in some cases leading to a professional crisis. The following case study illustrates this point:

Case Study 15

A 40-year-old O–4 was expected to appear in federal court to answer to charges of ordering and receiving child pornography. He was unable to keep this information from his superiors and feared public disgrace and the loss of his military status. Instead of appearing in court, he shot himself in the head with a 9mm pistol.

Table 6–14 shows the distribution of suicide victims by their military grade. In terms of their distribution, the overwhelming majority of these deaths (751 or 88%) involved enlisted members. Within the enlisted category, 68% involved people in the grade of E–3, E–4, and E–5. All but one of the remaining 98 suicides (11%) were officers; the one exception was an U.S. Air Force Academy cadet. Over one-half the officer suicides (56%) were in the grades of O–3 and O–4.

TABLE 6–14

ACTIVE DUTY AIR FORCE SUICIDES (1979–1991) BY MILITARY GRADE

Enlisted	Number	(%)	Officer	Number	(%)
E–1	33	(4)	O–1	8	(8)
E–2	39	(5)	O–2	19	(19)
E–3	156	(21)	O–3	31	(32)
E–4	180	(24)	O–4	24	(24)
E–5	178	(24)	O–5	8	(8)
E–6	93	(12)	O–6	7	(7)
E–7	47	(6)	Cadet	1	(1)
E–8	21	(3)			
E–9	4	(~0)			
Total	751	(99)	Total	98	(99)

The civilian suicide rate has historically been higher for whites than for nonwhites, with white males consistently having the highest suicide rates of any race or sex category. The ratio of white to black male suicides is 1.6 to 1, making the suicide rate for white males 67% higher than it is for black males.[12,18] Twice as many civilian white females kill themselves as do civilian black females. The same pattern is seen in the U.S. Air Force: Of the 850 suicides committed by active duty air force members from 1979 through 1991, a total of 747 (or 88%) were by whites and 85 (10%) were by blacks. The remaining 17 suicides (2%) were by all other categories.

The overall ratio of white to black suicides in the U.S. Air Force was 8.3 to 1, a figure consistent with the proportion of whites to blacks in the AirForce as a whole. Thus, race by itself does not appear to be a risk factor in the distribution of military suicides. These figures do suggest, however, that black males in the military are significantly less likely to commit suicide than black civilians. It is likely that the cultural factors that inhibit suicide among blacks within the civilian sector carry over into the military. Examination of the 86 suicides by black military members failed to disclose any unique or distinctive features related to race. Of those who left suicide notes, none indicated a racial connection to their decision; indeed, the general circumstances surrounding their deaths were indistinguishable from those of any other group.

According to the CDC,[12] almost three-fourths of all suicide deaths between 1970 and 1980 involved males. The CDC also reported that the suicide rate increased among males while decreasing among females. This pattern continued through the 1980s, with males having an overall suicide rate of 18 compared with a female rate of 5.4 or a ratio of 3.3:1. Although three times more men commit suicide than women, women attempt suicide more frequently than men. The reason for this inverse relation between gender and suicide and suicide attempts is not clear. Some have speculated that women are more likely to use drugs and poisons to attempt suicide, whereas men are more likely to use firearms,[18,19] yet there is an excellent chance that more men intend to commit suicide than women.[20] Regardless of the reasons why, suicide is more

TABLE 6–15

ACTIVE DUTY AIR FORCE SUICIDES (1979–1991) BY RACE AND SEX

	Number	(%)
Males		
White	702	(82)
Black	76	(9)
Other	16	(2)
Females		
White	46	(5)
Black	9	(1)
Other	1	(~0)

prevalent among males than females, and this relation holds true for the military as well. During the 13-year period, 56 women took their lives, representing 7% of the active duty suicides. Because women represent approximately 12% of the active duty force, females in the air force are less likely to commit suicide than males. The overall distribution by race and sex is shown in Table 6–15.

Although there were a wide range of methods used, 85% of these suicides were accomplished by three methods: firearm (502 or 59%), hanging (122 or 14%), and auto exhaust (100 or 12%). The full distribution of air force suicides is listed in Table 6–16. In virtually all cases, the event combined a highly lethal method and a low probability of rescue.

TABLE 6–16

ACTIVE DUTY AIR FORCE SUICIDES (1979–1991) BY METHOD

Method	Number	(%)
Firearm	503	(59)
Hanging	122	(14)
Auto Exhaust	100	(12)
Drug Overdose	44	(5)
Leap/Fall	17	(2)
Asphyxiation	12	(1)
Automobile	9	(1)
Cutting	9	(1)
Drowning	8	(1)
Unknown	1	(~0)
Other	25	(3)
Total	850	(99)

The distribution of suicides by month for 1979 through 1991 has been remarkably consistent over time. There were an average of five suicides per month with no statistically significant differences over time among the months of the year ($F_{11,144}=1.07$, $p = 0.39$, ns). Although there is a widespread belief that suicides increase during the fall holidays (Thanksgiving and Christmas), no such relation was noted in the Air Force.

Similarly, for day of week for 1979 through 1991, there were no excess suicides on weekends compared with weekdays ($\chi^2 = .14$, $p > 0.7$, ns), with the total average number of suicides per day for Monday through Sunday being 12, 9, 8, 10, 8, 9, and 9, respectively.

Suicide Precipitants

The term *dyad* as used in this context refers to a person's intimate associations, usually husband-wife or boyfriend-girlfriend. In some cases, understanding the exact role of dyadic relationships is complicated because of multiple simultaneous dyadic relationships (for example, unhappily married individuals who are also having problems with their girlfriends). However, the relation between dyad problems and suicide is clear and unavoidable. As Vorkorper and Petty noted, "Most suicides are dyadic. Even if the events prior to suicide are in isolation, the tension between two people continues to exist in one person's head. Frequently the tension is in the person's social relations: husband-wife, parent-child, lover-lover, employee-employer, etc."[21(p177)]

Marital status by itself offers little in the way of insight into suicide because gross figures (or percentages) do not speak to the quality of the victims' relationships. Just as a good marriage can be one of the most positive influences in a person's life, a bad marriage can create intolerable stress. Much the same can be said about other intimate relationships (ie, boyfriend-girlfriend). Table 6–17 reflects the distribution of the suicides by marital status. Some insight may be obtained from the fact that of those victims who were married at the time of their death, 32% were separated from their spouses, and fully 87% were having serious marital problems, with infidelity and abusive relationships occurring with great frequency. Of those who were single, 62% were having serious problems in their intimate relationships, to include a majority in which the relationship had recently terminated.

Case Study 16

An 18-year-old single male E–4 with a history of financial- and job-related problems was arrested for petty larceny. His girlfriend was highly critical of his behavior and threatened to leave him. He told her that if she did, he would kill himself. After she told him she wanted to end their relationship he shot himself in the temple with a .32 revolver.

Case Study 17

A 27-year-old male E–5 was an alcohol abuser and had serious financial problems. He was unhappy with his assignment. He believed it was his destiny to commit suicide because both his father and uncle had taken their own lives. After making suicidal threats and two gestures, he was admitted for psychiatric observation. On release from the hospital, he learned that his wife had moved out and filed for divorce; he then shot himself in the head with a high-powered rifle.

Although many people assume "You have to be crazy to kill yourself," this assumption does not hold up on close examination. Very few of the victims (less than 2%) were psychotic. However, there were clear indications that at least 48% suffered from some kind of mental or emotional problem. The most frequently noted mental health problem was depression, which occurred in 40% of the cases. This is consistent with the observation that suicide and clinical depression are closely linked in civilian studies.[22] It has been reported that 90% of suicides occur in individuals with serious mental disorders (depression, schizophrenia) or substance abuse. Because the signs of depression (and many other emotional disorders) can be quickly and easily recognized, their presence offers an excellent potential opportunity for positive intervention. Moreover, treatment of depression has advanced in recent years through the development of powerful antidepressants.

TABLE 6–17

ACTIVE DUTY AIR FORCE SUICIDES (1979–1991) BY MARITAL STATUS

Category	Number	(%)
Married	462	(55)
(Separated)	(148)	
Single	298	(35)
Divorced	88	(10)
Widower*	2	—
Total	850	(100)

*Includes one individual who was a widower because he murdered his wife.

Case Study 18

A 40-year-old divorced male E–6 was chronically depressed over the consequences of his history of compulsive gambling and the financial problems that resulted. He was also an alcohol abuser. Because of his problems he was being forced to retire and became even more depressed over his uncertain future. He shot himself in the head with a .357 revolver.

Case Study 19

A 35-year-old married (but separated) female O–2 was depressed over her marital separation and the difficulty she was having with her children. She was reassigned to another hospital (she was a nurse) and did not feel close to the staff as she had at her previous assignment. She took her life by ingesting a lethal quantity of drugs.

Almost one-third of the victims were either under mental healthcare at the time of their deaths or had been recently. It is hard to interpret what this means. Not all patients want treatment and not all of them who are in treatment will cooperate with their providers. In some cases, the healthcare system may have failed to properly diagnose the severity of the problem; in other cases, it simply could not reach the victim, as shown in the following case studies:

Case Study 20

A 25-year-old single male E–3 was released from a military hospital where he had been treated for a suicide gesture. He made specific and direct comments about his intention of killing himself. After his release from the hospital, he went to a mountainous area where he shot himself in the head with a 9mm pistol.

Case Study 21

A 30-year-old married male E–6 had been suffering from chronic depression and developed a sleep disorder that persisted for several months. After telling his family that they would be better off without him, he was sent to a mental health center where he was treated for the sleep disorder and his suicidal ideation. In spite of their efforts, he shot himself in the head with a .357 revolver.

Of the U.S. Air Force suicide victims, 27% had been involved with either alcohol (17%) or drugs (10%). Approximately 6% abused both drugs and alcohol. Although substance abuse is a problem in its own right, it may also be regarded as a symptom of other, deeper problems. For some people, substance abuse may seem an effective means for coping with life's problems. For others, it is simply a means of escape. In reality, substance abuse only complicates a person's problems by preventing a more mature, effective approach to life's stresses. In addition, it complicates life by adding the negative issues associated with substance abuse to other problems. Although substance abuse is a risk factor in its own right, it should not necessarily be viewed as a cause of suicide.

Like depression, substance abuse is often visible to others. In many military cases, family, friends, and coworkers knew the individual had a problem with either alcohol or drugs; however, there were few indications that any of them sought care for the impaired individual. In other cases, they failed to do so until it was too late. In some instances, helping the victim hide a substance abuse problem represented a misguided attempt to protect the person from his or her own problems; in other cases, it represented indifference, as shown in the following case study:

Case Study 22

A 22-year-old single male E–4 was having difficulty adjusting to the military. He had a history of disciplinary problems. He complained about "not fitting in" and was a cocaine abuser. After his request for a day off was turned down, he connected a tube from the tail pipe of his car to the interior where he died of carbon monoxide poisoning.

Not surprisingly, nearly one-half of the military suicides had problems at work. In some cases, the individual brought his personal problems to work and, as a result, added his job to his other problems. In other cases, they took work problems home and added them to their dyad problems. Of those who were married, over 30% had both marital- and work-related problems. Of those who were single, over one-third had both relationship- and work-related problems. The combination of both dyad- and work-related problems is particularly stressful because it leaves the victim with virtually no safe emotional haven.

Approximately one-quarter of the military suicide victims were having financial problems at the time of their death. In some cases, the problem was the victim's spouse, whose spending was beyond the control of the victim. In other cases, the problem was the victim's own doing. Some of the victim-precipitated financial problems resulted from immaturity, whereas others were a form of acting out. Although financial problems do not appear to be a common precipitant of military suicides, when they do occur, they can be a clue to the individual's need for help. Military commanders are frequently contacted concerning subordinates' indebtedness or failure to honor financial obligations. Alert commanders often recognize this as being symptomatic of a broader pattern of ineffective coping behavior. As such, it has the potential for being another point of intervention that might collectively reduce the overall suicide rate within the military, as shown in the following case study:

Case Study 23

A 33-year-old recently divorced male E–6 was diagnosed as a hypochondriac. He was $25,000 in debt, and his security clearance was recently revoked. The loss of his clearance added to his depression, and he killed himself via automobile exhaust after leaving multiple notes.

A small number of U.S. Air Force victims (about 12%) were involved in difficulties with law enforcement agencies at the time of their death. About one-half of those were under investigation for a suspected criminal offense, and about one half were involved in some fashion with local law enforcement agencies. Being under investigation for a suspected criminal offense, especially if the crime involves moral turpitude, is extremely stressful. This is because the legal outcomes are difficult to anticipate, and many suspects expect the worst. Legal problems almost always negatively influence one's career as conviction in court is also grounds for administrative action by the military. Thus, military members facing serious legal problems must also worry about public disgrace and a very real threat to their military careers. For many, this is simply too much to endure, as shown in the following case studies:

Case Study 24

A 39-year-old married male O–3, formerly commander of the security police squadron, was convicted by a court martial for larceny. On the day that he was scheduled to be sentenced, he shot himself in the heart with a .38 revolver. He was found wearing his security police uniform.

Case Study 25

A 49-year-old married male O–4 was interviewed by military investigators because of an allegation that he had sodomized a 9-year-old male. The O–4 agreed to take a polygraph examination to resolve the issue, and the day before he was scheduled to take the polygraph, he shot himself in the head with a .32 pistol.

Case Study 26

A 29-year-old divorced male E–5 was under investigation for a narcotics charge and was scheduled to stand trial by court martial. While the trial was pending, he was involved in a hit-and-run accident. His blood alcohol level (0.24) was over double the legal minimum for driving while intoxicated (0.10). Following his arrest on the traffic charge, he shot himself in the head with a .38 revolver.

Suicide Communications

The actual act of killing oneself may only take a few minutes to carry out; however, suicide normally involves a great deal more than the fatal event. Impulsive suicides are rare (occurring in only 4% of the cases studied) and usually occur in a moment of great stress, as the following case studies demonstrate:

Case Study 27

A 26-year-old married male E–4 had been arguing with his pregnant wife. In a rage, he produced a pistol and threatened to kill himself. A third-party witness told him he was only joking and could not do it. The victim replied, "You don't think I can do it?" and then put the pistol to his head and pulled the trigger.

Case Study 28

A 25-year-old married male E–4 confronted his wife and her boyfriend. As they were arguing, he grabbed a 20 gauge shotgun, placed it under his chin, and pulled the trigger. He had been extremely unhappy over his marital and financial problems as well as his wife's infidelity, for which he had been receiving counseling.

Most active duty suicides are preceded by a period of personal difficulty for the victim. Although a small proportion of the suicides are impulsive (like the ones noted above), in most cases, the victim first comes on the idea of suicide as a solution to his problems and then gradually focuses on suicide as the only solution. As this process occurs, the victim comes to see life in increasingly constricted terms until his problems are seen as hopeless and suicide as the only way out. During the evolution of this process, the individual will typically drop many hints, both verbal and behavioral.

Of the 850 military suicides examined, 386 (45%) communicated their intention to commit suicide before they actually killed themselves. In some instances, these communications were clear, concise, and direct. In one case, for example, a 33-year-old E–5 who was having marital problems told his wife that if she divorced him, he would shoot himself. She told him that if he did, she would be grateful if he would at least go outside so he would not leave a mess in the house. He then went outside to a utility shed where he shot himself in the head with a .22 rifle. In many of these cases, the victims told a number of people of their plans, including coworkers and friends. In most instances, they ignored the victim and later said they "did not think that he would actually do it."

Sometimes the communication of suicidal intent was vague and only took on meaning after the victim's death. These communications often take the form of "good-bye" statements or messages. Sometimes the victim simply comments that he or she has nothing to live for. These vague comments are easy to dismiss precisely because they are so vague. Sometimes the victim is ignored because he makes suicidal comments too frequently or too explicitly, and those to whom they are made simply do not believe him. However, any suicidal statement should be taken seriously and acted on at once, as shown in the following case studies:

Case Study 29

A 35-year-old married (but separated) male E–6 had a history of work-related problems, financial difficulties, and marital strife. He had just been released from an alcohol rehabilitation program and attempted to reconcile with his wife. He repeatedly told her that if she left him, he would kill himself. She left him and he shot himself in the head with a .22 pistol.

Case Study 30

A 30-year-old married (but separated) male E–5 had a history of poor duty performance; his wife left him, filing for divorce, and he had a stormy relationship with his girlfriend whom he told he was going to kill himself. He subsequently hanged himself.

Case Study 31

A 27-year-old white male disliked his job and was having difficulty adjusting to the service. He was under treatment by mental health professionals for a previous suicide attempt. On the day of his death, he bought a high-powered rifle and left the note illustrated in Figure 6–1 in his barracks room. He was found in the area defined by the circle. He had shot himself in the middle of the forehead. Note the statement below the word *anger*: "Too much damage to go on!" This is characteristic of the kinds of hopelessness found in many suicides.

The military experience clearly indicates that suicide attempters are analytically distinct from completers. Most people who intend to kill themselves are successful in doing so, and most people who make unsuccessful attempts or gestures do not really wish to end their lives. Although there are exceptions in both categories, these generalizations have held true for the past 13 years.

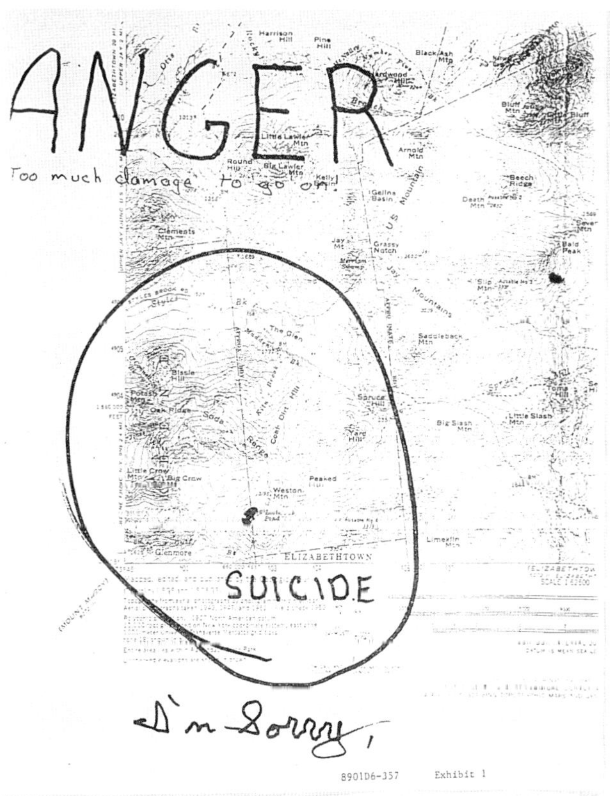

Fig. 6–1. Suicide note on map, with the word ANGER.

Suicide attempts are themselves a form of communication and can be best understood as a plea for help. Even when the attempt or gesture is manipulative in nature, it is still diagnostic of a problem of some kind. Of the 850 people who took their lives in this study, at least 13% had made a prior suicide attempt or gesture. These unsuccessful efforts often emerge as part of a larger pattern that, if ignored, can escalate into successful self-destruction, as the following case study illustrates:

Case Study 32

A 20-year-old single E–2 had been involved in a stormy relationship with his girlfriend. He would threaten suicide, and she would talk him out of it. During the course of this relationship, he lost a part-time job because he intentionally injured himself. At about this time, a close friend killed himself over a girl, after which the E–2 became obsessed with suicide. He talked about it constantly, played Russian roulette, and made several suicide gestures. His girlfriend got tired of his behavior and broke off their relationship. After she left him, he hanged himself.

Suicidal communications after the fact usually take the form of notes left at the death scene by the victim but may also include audio or video recordings. Of the 850 military suicide victims, 366 (43%) left a note. These notes take many forms. Some are angry; others are depressed and self-condemning and many simply take the form of a last will and testament. Over one-half of those who left suicide notes also communicated their intentions prior to taking their lives. The following are examples of some of the notes:

- "Call the police. I've killed myself in the Garage" (left by a 38-year-old married male O–3 who was a Reserve Officers' Training Corps (ROTC) instructor who was depressed over his marriage and stressed in his work. He hanged himself in his garage.)
- "To my beloved wife, This will be the last time we will talk! I want you to know I loved you so much! I kept asking myself why? I could come up with no answer! Don't worry about me now, I am at peace with GOD! Finally I thought I would be afraid to die and I am. God put me on earth & I was a FAILURE! I'm sure I can do his will much better in heaven. Please comfort

my mom. She will need you more than ever! I'm so sorry! I loved you more than life itself, if only you believed in me! I will be your holy spirit forever amen! I love you! XOXXOXO" (left by a 19-year-old male E–4 who had been married for 6 months when his wife left him, returning to live with her mother. She was extremely immature and dependent on her mother, who kept telling her that her husband was no good. Two days after she left him—at her mother's urging—he hanged himself, leaving this note on the back of their wedding picture)

- "I loved her so much. I'm so sorry but this is how its gotta be. I hate life. Life's done me wrong. Please God forgive me but I'm weak. My lifes finished." (A 20-year-old male E–3 had physical problems resulting from an earlier automobile accident. He was distraught over the recent death of a close friend and told his girlfriend he was going to kill himself. Shortly thereafter, she broke up with him. He shot himself in the head with a .38 revolver)

Suicide and Malingering

Certain institutional settings, such as the military and correctional facilities, are frequently confronted with malingered behavior. The goal of this conscious deception is to avoid unpleasant duty, work, or situations. Feigning illness or injury to avoid hazardous duty such as combat is particularly important. Such unchecked conduct can rapidly deplete necessary manpower requirements. This leaves the remaining units vulnerable.

The military has always been vigilant for shirkers. Included in the Uniform Code of Military Justice is the specific crime of malingering, Article 115, which, in part, states:

> Any person subject to this Chapter who for the purpose of avoiding work, duty, or service
> 1) feigns illness, physical disablement, mental lapse, or derangement; or
> 2) intentionally inflicts self-injury; shall be punishable as a court martial may direct.[4(§IVp68)]

The maximum punishment for malingering a self-inflicted injury in time of war includes a dishonorable discharge and confinement in prison for 10 years. Less serious malingering, such as feigning illness during peacetime, can be punished with a dishonorable discharge and confinement for 1 year.

The military crime of malingering does not discriminate mental disorder. An interesting conflict arises when suicide gestures are prosecuted. The military policy outlined in official regulations requires suicide be a command concern. Occasionally, however, repeated suicide gestures are punitively dealt with. At the unit level, frustrated commanders may respond to repeated suicide gestures with nonjudicial punishment or administrative separation from the service.

In only the rarest cases does a suicide attempt result in prosecution by court martial. This was the case in *U.S. v. Johnson*.[23] Johnson's legal case was complicated by the uncontroverted use of heroin. After his arrest for possession of the narcotic, Johnson fashioned a crude noose from an electrical cord and attempted to hang himself in the military police building. Johnson was hospitalized for a week following this attempt. Following discharge, Johnson purchased a quantity of heroin and injected a large amount. This near-fatal overdose represented a second serious suicide attempt. The gravity of this act was underscored by the accidental discovery of Johnson in a near-death condition. Prosecution and conviction were upheld by the U.S. Court of Military Appeal, the highest military court.

Assisted Suicide

In some rare cases, a suicide involves the participation of another person. These deaths raise difficult ethical, moral, and legal concerns. The military is not immune to such dilemmas.

In *U.S. v. Verraso*,[24] the accused soldier Verraso assisted in the suicide death of another soldier, Tamary Meza-Luna. Court records indicate that Verraso placed "the loop [of rope] around her [Meza-Luna's] neck leaving about three inches of slack between the rope and her neck." Verraso then left the area only to find out the next morning that Meza-Luna had indeed died. The relationship between these two people was complicated and had involved a prior joint suicide gesture. Verraso was convicted and received an 8-year prison term for her complicity.

Suicide Prevention

Some proportion (possibly as much as one-half) of active duty suicides may be preventable. Some individuals at high risk for suicide may exhibit signs that should alert coworkers. Military members work in units where their behavior is observable and where support is available. Because of this, the military is theoretically an ideal environment for suicide prevention. The problem in applying these resources is twofold: (1) getting first-echelon supervisors and coworkers to *recognize* the problem in the first place, and (2) getting them to *act* on it. With respect to the former, there are a number of hurdles to overcome. The overwhelming majority of active duty suicides involve people who are quite ordinary in most respects; however, their perceived problems are greater than their coping skills. As a result, they are likely to be depressed, and the symptoms of depression can serve as tripwires that indicate a need for remedial action. For example, many of them become distant and self-isolating. Their coworkers are likely to misread these signals and simply write them off as a jerks and reciprocate by ignoring them. Because they are essentially "normal" when they talk about suicide, their coworkers disregard them and assume they are either "kidding" or exaggerating how they feel.

Even if coworkers or immediate supervisors suspect a person might be at risk, many do not know what to do. Some of them ask the potential victim to promise not to do anything stupid; others ignore them because they feel uncomfortable about dealing with another person's personal problems. Some are unwilling to refer them to the mental health professionals because they think doing so will have a negative impact on their careers. Some simply do not know what to do and put off taking action until they are forced to do something.

This is ironic because military members are under almost constant surveillance by subordinates, peers, and supervisors. Any change in personality or overt behavior ought to be readily apparent and, when correctly interpreted as being symptomatic of a problem, should trigger an organizational response. Moreover, immediate coworkers are often aware of one another's problems, especially if those problems are serious. Thus, a coworker who knows a colleague is separated and in the process of getting a divorce, who is depressed at the prospect of losing custody of his children, and who has financial and substance abuse problems, should have good reason to suspect the victim is on seriously shaky grounds. When this is compounded by the victim making "good-bye" statements or even by talking about suicide, his colleagues need to recognize that the victim is in a serious emotional crisis and that suicide is a possible outcome. The following case studies illustrate this point:

Case Study 33

A 38-year-old E–5 had a history of marital problems. His wife told him she wanted a divorce. He had financial problems, and his performance at work was slipping. Shortly after going to mental healthcare for "stress," he shot himself in the head with a .22 rifle.

Case Study 34

A 40-year-old E–6 was separated from his wife. He had serious financial problems and had been arrested for driving while intoxicated. He complained about being overstressed at work and told several coworkers that he was thinking about killing himself. The coworkers told his first sergeant, and while the first sergeant was thinking about directing him to mental health, the E–6 shot himself in the chest with a shotgun.

Case Study 35

A 21-year-old E–2 was involved in a stressful relationship that was terminated by his girlfriend. He told her that if she left him, he would kill himself. She contacted his NCOIC (noncommissioned officer in charge), who took no action. The E–2 shot himself in the chest with a revolver.

Case Study 36

A 23–year-old E–4 was separated from his wife and had serious financial problems. He told several coworkers that he didn't think he could get "out of the hole he dug for himself." Three days before he was due to appear in court on a bad check charge, he shot himself in the right temple with a pistol.

All of the cases cited above (and none of them are unusual) share several common features. First, the victims were experiencing serious problems in their intimate relationships; second, each had colleagues who were well aware of the victim's problem; and finally, helping resources exist that could have addressed all of these problems but were not used.

Failure to prevent suicides generally occurs for one or more of the following reasons. First, the victim concealed the potential for suicide because of his problems, and coworkers were not aware of that possible outcome. In this connection, it is important to remember that a certain proportion of people at risk are going to kill themselves, and there is probably nothing that can be done to stop them. Second, some suicides are leadership failures. In this category, the signs and symptoms although clear were ignored. Most of the time when this happens, it is because others are afraid to "mess with another person's personal affairs" or because they do not know what to do or who to turn to for help. Finally, some suicides are mental health failures. A substantial minority of individuals at risk go to a mental health professional (either by referral or at their own initiative) and, for whatever reason, subsequently kill themselves.

The second problem in preventing suicides in the military involves how the system reacts to potential suicides when they are identified. The suicide "problem" is widely regarded as "belonging" to mental health. When people are identified as being at risk, they are likely to be sent to a mental health professional for evaluation and treatment. A good many mental health professionals believe that suicide is a psychiatric problem, and their evaluation protocols typically involve clinical interviews that look for psychiatric problems. If the person who has been referred is depressed but does not suffer from a psychosis or debilitating character or personality disorder, he may be able to talk his way out of treatment.

This is compounded by the fact that primary care providers in the military are typically young and at the entry phase of their careers. In a nutshell, many of them are easily misled by those whom they evaluate. If a person is sent to a mental health professional for suicidal ideation, all he needs to do is tell the provider he was feeling blue but now realizes the error in his thinking and is embarrassed at the stir his comments have set into motion. If the counselee shows the appropriate deference and talks a good game, he will be quickly released with the diagnosis of acute adjustment reaction and told to call back if he thinks doing so is necessary.

How then does one know if there is a suicide problem or if the number of suicides at a given military facility is "within normal limits?" It is the judgment of the first author that three suicides within any 12–month period constitutes a cluster and indicates the existence of a problem. When viewed as a tripwire, this figure can be used to initiate an examination of the context in which the suicides occurred to see if the problem is either a leadership or mental health professional failure.

Military communities interested in suicide prevention look for ways to keep people at risk from killing themselves. Suicide prevention programs may offer hot lines so people contemplating suicide can call someone who will listen to them or by putting out fact sheets or information bulletins on suicide. Although these approaches have value, they may not be the most effective way to prevent suicides. Based on the theme of failure seen in suicide notes, it might make more sense to offer programs to help people deal with failed relationships and financial, substance-abuse, and work-related problems. These people do not kill themselves because they want to die; they kill themselves because they cannot cope with their problems, and suicide is a vehicle for making the problems go away. Programs that deal with those kinds of problems may have the indirect consequence of reducing suicides.

CONCLUSION

Violent deaths are neither random nor mysterious events. They occur within specific contexts and can be understood in light of the overall events of which they are a part. They are difficult to prevent because they often represent circumstances largely created by people who then react badly to those circumstances. The prevention of violent deaths requires the identification of those at risk and intervention in ways that facilitate positive outcomes. The people in the best position to identify those at risk are the individual's coworkers and immediate supervisors; however, many of them do not know how to recognize risk factors or what to do even if they do recognize them. The military is in an ideal position to deal with this issue through its professional military education. By training supervisors to recognize the symptoms of those at risk and by encouraging them to make the appropriate referrals, it should be possible to offer the kinds of intervention that are likely to make the biggest difference.

In conclusion, homicide and suicide in the military have been less frequent than in civilian life. The circumstances of military and civilian deaths are similar with the preponderance of interpersonal conflict and the notable exception of the lack of drug-related murders within the military. We find no evidence that the lethal violence that is the mission of the military is reflected in the lives and deaths of active duty military personnel.

REFERENCES

1. Centers for Disease Control, US Department of Health and Human Services. *Homicide Surveillance*. Atlanta, Ga: USDHHS; 1986.

2. US Department of Justice. *Uniform Crime Reports for the United States, 1991*. Washington, DC: US Department of Justice; 1991.

3. US Department of Justice, Bureau of Justice Statistics. *Firearms and Crimes of Violence*. Washington, DC: US Department of Justice. February 1994.

4. *Manual for Courts-Martial, United States*. Washington, DC: GPO; 1984.

5. Daly M, Wilson M. *Homicide*. New York: Aldine DeGruyter; 1988.

6. Wolfgang ME. *Patterns in Criminal Homicide*. Philadelphia, Pa: University of Pennsylvania Press; 1958.

7. Moynihan DP. Defining deviancy down. *Am Scholar*. 1993;62(1):17–30.

8. *Tarasoff v. Regents of Univ of Cal*, [17 Cal.3d 425, 131 Cal Rptr. 14, 551 P.2d 334].

9. US Department of the Army. *Alcohol and Drug Abuse Prevention and Control Program*. Washington, DC: DA; 1988. Army Regulation 600–85.

10. US Department of the Army. *Army Health Promotion*. Washington, DC: DA; 1987. Army Regulation 600–63.

11. McGinnis MJ. Suicide in America—Moving up the public health agenda. *Suicide and Life-Threatening Behavior*. 1987;17(1):18–32.

12. Centers for Disease Control, US Department of Health and Human Services. *Suicide Surveillance, 1970–1980*. Atlanta, Ga: USDHHS; 1985.

13. Rothberg JM, Rock N, Jones FD. Suicide in US Army personnel, 1981–1982. *Milit Med*. 1984;149(10):537–541.

14. Rothberg JM, Jones FD. Suicide in the US Army: Epidemiological and periodic aspects. *Suicide and Life-Threatening Behavior*. 1987;17(2):119–132.

15. Rothberg JM, Ursano RJ, Holloway H. Suicide in the United States military. *Psychiatr Ann*. 1987;17:545–548.

16. Rothberg JM, Bartone PT, Holloway HC, Marlowe DH. Life and death in the US Army. *JAMA*. 1990;264:2241–2244.

17. Centers for Disease Control. Operational criteria for determining suicide. *MMWR*. 1988;37(50):773–780.

18. Monk M. Suicide. In: Last JM, ed. *Public Health and Preventive Medicine*. 12th ed. Norwalk, Conn: Appleton-Century-Crofts; 1986: 1385–1397.

19. McIntosh JL, Jewell BL. Sex differences in completed suicide. *Suicide and Life-Threatening Behavior*. 1986;16(1):18–32.

20. Rich CL, Ricketts JE, Fowler RC, Young D. Some differences between men and women who commit suicide. *Am J Psychiatry*. 1988;145(6):718–722.

21. Vorkorper CF, Petty CS. Suicide investigation. In: Curran WJ, McGarry LA, Petty CS, eds. *Modern Legal Medicine, Psychiatry and Forensic Science*. Philadelphia, Pa: F.A. Davis Company; 1980: 170–185.

22. Gelman D, et al. Depression. *Newsweek*. 1987;(May 4):48–57.

23. *US v. Johnson*, [26 MJ 415(CMA1988)].

24. *US v. Verraso*, [21 MJ 129(CMA1985)].

Chapter 7

ETHICAL ISSUES IN COMBAT PSYCHIATRY

EDMUND G. HOWE, M.D.*, AND FRANKLIN D. JONES, M.D., F.A.P.A.†

*Professor, Department of Psychiatry, and Director, Programs in Medical Ethics, Uniformed Services University of the Health Sciences, Bethesda, Maryland 20889–4799

†Colonel (ret), Medical Corps, U.S. Army; Clinical Professor, Uniformed Services University of the Health Sciences; Past President and Secretary and Current Honorary President of the Military Section, World Psychiatric Association

INTRODUCTION

Although some argue that combat itself is so highly unethical as to defy attempts to apply any ethical precepts, some cultures have had specific ethical principles for engaging in combat.[1,2] When cultures with divergent ethical standards have engaged in war, controversies have arisen. This was seen, for example, when European settlers came into conflict with Native Americans. Some tribes felt that the ultimate honor one could accord an enemy was to torture him to death so that he could display his courage.[3] Similarly, the Japanese outraged Americans by a "sneak attack" without a declaration of war on Pearl Harbor in 1941 with the Japanese position that this attack was a brilliant and ethical military maneuver, a position apparently endorsed by Israeli and Arab forces in some of their wars.[4,5] In subsequent wars, surprise initiation has become commonplace. Another example of divergent ethical positions occurred when American forces surrendered to the Japanese in the Philippine Islands. The samurai ethics of Bushido held surrender to be a heinous crime placing the perpetrator beneath contempt.[6] As a result, American prisoners of war were harshly treated and many perished.[7]

Starting with the medieval concept of chivalry, European ethics of combat were increasingly codified and formalized although there were many lapses.[8] In the American Civil War, General Sherman's slash-and-burn march through Georgia to isolate Confederate forces from supply support marked a major change in the American ethics of war because civilian populations became embroiled in what had been an occupation of professional military men.[2] In more modern times, one can see an extension of this concept in the fire bombing of Dresden,[9] the atomic bombing of Hiroshima and Nagasaki,[10] and the forced relocation of villagers in Vietnam.[11] The Nuremberg trials after World War II have shown, however, that there are definite limits to waging war on civilians.[12] Following his Vietnam service, the defense argued that First Lieutenant William Calley of the infamous My Lai massacre was no more guilty than pilots who bombed North Vietnam, killing thousands, because both were attempting to destroy the support infrastructure of the enemy.[13] The jury, composed almost entirely of combat veterans, did not agree, and Calley was convicted of over two dozen murders. In Calley's case, specific U.S. Army regulations were violated, and he was convicted not of ethical but of criminal offenses.

Psychiatry is not alone among the professions in having this sort of ethical dilemma when serving in the military, nor is the military the only institution in which it arises for psychiatrists. It is unavoidable that problems arise regarding conflicting loyalties and contradictory goals. Whether or not these are experienced as problems by the individual psychiatrist, or if they are so experienced, whether they are acknowledged, are important correlative issues and of special interest.

Finally, it needs to be emphasized that questions of professional ethics are not the sole prerogative of psychiatrists but also must be considered by other mental health disciplines and their noncommissioned officer and enlisted counterparts. In addition, it must not be forgotten that combat psychiatry is also practiced by general medical officers and physician assistants and, to some extent, by platoon medics and all other U.S. Army Medical Department clinicians on the battlefield.

ETHICS OF PSYCHIATRY IN WARFARE

Before the Vietnam conflict, military psychiatrists seemed confident that their goals and methods conformed to the values of both the military and the American people. These earlier military psychiatrists perceived that the rationale for America's military activities sufficiently satisfied the criteria for a "just" war and saw little role conflict or moral dilemma associated with encouraging the soldier-patient to return to combat regardless of residual psychiatric symptomatology.[14] However, in conjunction with the controversial Vietnam conflict, a frank and impassioned debate[14] erupted within psychiatry concerning the proper role for psychiatrists in time of war, especially military psychiatrists. Underlying this debate was the critical moral or ethical question for whom does the military psychiatrist work—the individual patient or the military organization? Novelists such as

Rosten (*Captain Newman, MD*)[15] and Heller (*Catch-22*)[16] have also addressed this issue, setting their stories in the context of World War II.

A military psychiatrist as a physician subscribes to the Hippocratic Oath and as an officer in uniform is governed by the Uniform Code of Military Justice and the oath sworn when commissioned. Conceptually, the potential conflict between these oaths reaches its most extreme point when the military psychiatrist must decide whether to conform to his soldier-patient's wish to be medically exempted from further exposure to the high-risk, high-stress combat environment or to satisfy the military's contrary expectation that he be returned to that environment even if he is in some emotional distress.

It is not new to observe[17] that psychiatric patients seen under combat conditions might themselves suffer with a conflict between self-protective motives and feelings of obligation to military comrades and goals. Likewise, psychiatrists who have not been sufficiently schooled in the goals and methods of military psychiatry have been noted[18] in previous wars to fail to understand the competing sides of the soldier's struggle to overcome his fear, to overly empathize with the soldier's self-protective side, and to overdiagnose psychiatric disturbance. What was new from the Vietnam period were the expressions of doubt as to what constitutes the ethical practice of psychiatry within the military—expressions that were vocalized primarily in the latter half of the war coinciding with the influx of civilian-trained psychiatrists into the services and with the increasing divisiveness among Americans regarding the war.[14]

By way of a literary example, in chapter 10, "Gentlemen, it works" of Glasser's fictionalized account[19(pp124–148)] of his experiences as an U.S. Army doctor assigned to an army evacuation hospital in Japan during the middle phase of the Vietnam conflict, he vividly portrays both sides by presenting an ersatz official stateside briefing on combat psychiatry's development, logic, and field methods (eg, brief, simple treatments provided near the soldier's unit and followed by rapid return to combat duty). The briefing was periodically interrupted by reflections of drafted psychiatrist Kohler regarding his own clinical experiences in Vietnam. Although initially skeptical of "the military machine with its emphasis on interpersonal rather than intrapersonal psychopathology,"[19(p140)] Kohler came gradually to appreciate the pragmatic value of the approaches used by military psychiatry to stem the psychological breakdown of stressed combat soldiers (and his patients expressed their appreciation). However, the piece ends with Kohler returning to his original worry that he could have been sending vulnerable soldiers back to face the risks of combat (echoing Livingston's 1969[20] concern): "It works. The men are not lost to the fight, and the terrifying stupidity of war is not allowed to go on crippling forever. At least, that's the official belief. But there is no medical or psychiatric follow-up on the boys after they've returned to duty. No one knows if they are the ones who die in the very next fire fight, who miss the wire stretched out across the tract, or gun down unarmed civilians. Apparently, the Army doesn't seem to want to find out."[19(p148)]

This chapter will examine the arguments that serve as justification for the policies, field principles, and techniques that compose the doctrine of combat psychiatric treatment. It also will examine a number of associated ethical questions surrounding military medicine and military service. The chapter will review challenges to the doctrine and provide an analysis of the effects of the competing value systems on military psychiatrists.

TREATMENT AND PREVENTION ISSUES

The Ethics of Military Medical Triage

The principles of medical triage[21(p182)] developed in disaster (mass casualty) situations for medical personnel were limited so that not all can be treated. In ordinary emergency situations, the most seriously ill would be treated first to save life and limb, but in military triage situations, the most seriously ill might be allowed to die so that limited medical resources can be devoted to salvaging the lives and limbs of the less seriously injured. In combat settings, this might be carried a step further in rendering care first to those most likely to carry out the combat mission, that is, the lightly wounded and combat stress casualties.

The military triage situation is "mission driven" and "resource scarce" and thus creates serious ethical dilemmas in terms of individual survival. Differing perspectives on impairment result in a conflict between putting the mission first versus the risk of increased morbidity. The principle of military medical triage[21] holds that individual soldiers' interests can be sacrificed when necessary either for the medical welfare of other soldiers or to further military goals. In practice, the need for such sacrifices may be rare. During the Vietnam conflict, for example, no efforts were spared to assist critically injured soldiers, and after evaluation, only those with the most severe head wounds were considered unsalvageable.[22(p156)]

The application of the military medical triage principle for the purpose of benefiting the military objective was exemplified during World War II in North Africa when penicillin was scarce in supply, but soldiers needed it. Some soldiers had been wounded in battle, and others had venereal disease. The available penicillin was given to the latter group because they could return to the front.[23,24,25(pp209–210)]

An application of the military medical triage principle being applied for the sake of other soldiers is reported by Hinds,[26] a British physician and medical historian. This situation occurred after an airplane on which he was traveling crashed in the desert. Eight men were badly injured and needed pain medication to survive the 120-mile journey to obtain care. Yet, there were but four doses of morphine. Hinds gave the limited morphine to those who had the best chance of survival.

Analogously, during combat, military physicians may have to decide which service persons' treatment should be given priority. More specifically, they may have to decide whether to give priority to treating soldiers so that they can return to the front or to saving the maximum number of lives. A relatively different emphasis between these two goals occurred, for example, during World War II. The German army placed greater priority on returning injured soldiers to the front, the United States, on sending injured soldiers to the rear for rehabilitation.[27]

Yet, triage and different degrees of risk-taking by certain groups is less than fully analogous. When triage takes place, no group is singled out on the basis of some preexisting characteristic that subjects some to a greater risk of morbidity or death.

The Right To Refuse Treatment

Many civil rights are lost or abridged when one joins the military, including the right to refuse legal orders even if they may result in one's death. Often decried[28,29] in medical circles is the loss of medical confidentiality although regulations[28,30,31,32] limit access to medical records to those with a need to know. Paradoxically, while this pillar of medical practice is pushed aside, the right to refuse medical treatment is preserved except in emergency situations in which the patient may lose life or limb.

The military has occasionally been subjected to the same difficult situation encountered in civilian jurisdictions when an involuntarily detained patient meets detention or commitment criteria but has the right to refuse treatment. A military member may be ordered into a psychiatric facility for evaluation by his commander; however, this situation does not give physicians the right to treat involuntarily. With psychotic mental patients, this situation may result in lengthy hospitalization until spontaneous improvement allows nonhospital disposition or persuasion or deterioration to the point of danger to life or limb allows hospital treatment. Such a case described by Beighley and Brown[33] resulted in 5 weeks' delay in treating a psychotic manic-depressive patient.

The military does have a procedure by which a member who refuses treatment may be eliminated from the military. This lengthy procedure involves review by the applicable surgeon general. In 1973, the second author, in his capacity as chief of psychiatric services at a major army medical center, encountered a case in which the procedure took one-half a year and was still unsatisfactory because the military member did not get appropriate care after being discharged.

Military Physicians Treating Combat Fatigue

The handling of psychiatric breakdown during the stress of combat was generally considered to be a command issue until the introduction of psychiatrists into the Russian medical support structure during the Russo-Japanese War.[34] Previously, such combat breakdown was attributed to physical causes (such as "soldier's heart" in the U.S. Civil War) or moral weakness (cowardice).[35] Management tended to be medical (rest and medications) or coercive (court martial or death). Russian psychiatrists[34] offered an alternative by labeling such stress casualties as "insane," "neurasthenic," or otherwise not responsible. As recently as World War II, America's General Patton[36] frankly considered combat stress casualties to be cowards.

Gradually, the medical view held sway because this approach appeared more humane and pragmatically resulted in a greater salvaging of casualties who could return to combat or combat support duties. The battalion surgeon and the psychiatrist shared some of the commander's responsibility for sending men back into combat where they might die. Because of inherent ethical dilemmas, this situation can become an uncomfortable role for physicians.

One justification is expounded by Jones[37] who cites numerous examples that illustrate that when military psychiatrists treat combat stress casualties on the basis of principles such as proximity and expectancy, not only the military but also, over the long-run, these service persons also benefit. That is, if they are returned to the front after a few days, they have appeared to experience no subsequent psychological morbidity greater than their untreated fellow soldiers.

Thus, in this situation, the conflict cannot be fairly characterized as the military's interests versus soldiers' interests. Rather, to some extent, the military and service persons' interests are in agreement. If the combatant dies after returning to duty, this may not be the case; but, this outcome may be justified on other grounds. Further, if military psychiatrists actively tried to protect combatants with combat fatigue from reentering combat, they would violate the soldiers' prior expectations and break an implicit promise to them. Furthermore, some other, less-experienced and presumably less-skilled individual would have to assume the risks from which the combat stress casualty had been removed.

Combat stress casualties seek medical handling and rarely overtly ask to be removed from combat. If they should ask to be removed from combat and if the ethical principle of respect for their autonomy were prioritized, this would require military physicians to permit their request, even though they might at that time be psychologically impaired. The consequence of granting their request might be subsequent morbidity from feelings of guilt and low self-esteem, and furthermore, they might be subject to court martial. Desertion in the face of the enemy is a capital offense. Even if a combatant showed manifestations of combat fatigue, this is not usually sufficient to justify medical evacuation beyond first or second echelon levels. Ethically, it may be that the stressed soldier should retain decision-making capacity because he is still competent to decide what he wants. For comparison, in civilian settings, physicians may not be justified in overriding their patients' desire to refuse a life saving operation even when the patient is depressed.

Even if such patients are considered to retain competence, however, military psychiatrists would have some justification, when unsure, to err by treating them as if they primarily had combat fatigue and, once recovered, would want to return to duty. This usually is the case,[38,39] and psychiatrists lack the means of determining when it is not. Moreover, treating most combatants with combat fatigue so that they can return to duty is necessary for the welfare of the unit and the military combat mission. The soldier's return to duty also, in at least a majority of instances,[38] is necessary to prevent numerous others who also feel afraid during combat from following suit. Just as they may have to sacrifice their lives, if necessary, for the combat effort, those who show symptoms of combat fatigue, to some degree, may have to sacrifice their autonomy. To this extent, the benefit to the military *is* opposed to the interests of the soldier with combat fatigue.

The incident regarding combat fatigue cited often in the ethical literature[40–42,43(pp261–262)] is a press report of an air force sergeant who had flown many combat missions in Vietnam and subsequently asked to be relieved from further combat duty. Air force psychiatrists assessed his condition, diagnosed it as a stress reaction, treated him for combat stress with psychotropic medication and psychotherapy, and returned him to duty.[42]

Veatch reports that Newman, a physician, argued, however, that the psychiatrists who treated this sergeant created an "iatrogenic psychosis."[42(p246)] Newman was asserting, of course, that this soldier's request to be removed from combat was "genuine," and therefore, he should not have been treated for combat fatigue. As just discussed, however, there is sufficient justification for military physicians to treat service persons for combat fatigue even when their request to be removed from duty is in part genuine. Namely, military psychiatrists lack the means of distinguishing combat fatigue from "genuine" requests, the military will benefit, and to the degree combat fatigue exists, the service person will benefit if he survives combat. Service persons also have agreed implicitly, even when conscripted because they could refuse conscription and face penalties, when entering the military to give their lives, if necessary, much less their autonomy, for the combat mission. They also expect the military to do what they can to protect them.

It could be asserted, in agreement with Newman's[42] claim, that any soldier entering combat willingly is irrational. Lifton[44] contends, for example, that service persons sometimes initially seek out combat experience enthusiastically because of "male bravado." Lifton gained this impression from the not unbiased comments of "rap groups" of antiwar veterans, and his description of their attempts to understand their earlier motivation for entering combat is noteworthy: "They probed unsparingly the source and fears beneath their male bravado in enthusiastically (in many cases) 'joining up' and even seeking out the war."[44(p807)]

Lifton's observations, although involving only one small group of disaffected veterans, might be generalizable to others. That is, surely most Americans would prefer not to risk their lives in combat, although there have been societies in which this was the standard for males. For this reason, practices such as those that follow are designed to enhance service persons' "willingness" to take this risk. For example, a historical principle illustrated by Frederick the Great, and reaffirmed by army senior commanders often as late as World War I, is that the common soldier must fear his officer more than the enemy. General Wolfe in 1755 exemplified this practice. Wolfe informed his troops that "A soldier that quits his rank or offers to flag, is instantly to be put to death by the officer or Sergeant in the rear of that platoon: a soldier does not deserve to live who will not fight for his king and country."[45(p69)] A second example would be the threatened use of courts-martial.

It must be reiterated that combat fatigue casualties rarely claim that they wish to escape combat. In fact, they are more likely to evince a desire to return to combat but cannot do so due to their symptoms. Thus, their initial psychiatric symptoms temporarily speak for them; that is, requesting an honorable exit from combat.

As noted, Newman[42] states that when military psychiatrists "treat" soldiers so that they again become willing to enter combat, they create "iatrogenic psychosis." This assertion is stated in another way by Lifton. Referring to military chaplains and psychiatrists, Lifton states "We can . . . speak of the existence of a 'counterfeit universe' in which pervasive spiritually reinforced inner corruption becomes the price of survival."[44(p808)]

The answer to Newman and Lifton's claim, however, is suggested by the last part of General Wolfe's statement, just quoted. That is, although few persons would *want* to risk their lives for their country, the vast majority would choose to do so despite their fear of death because they are willing to fight for their country. In suppressing this fear, however, they are exceptionally subject to combat fatigue, but they are better able to overcome this fear if their commanders, fellow service persons, and military psychiatrists, among others, exert pressure on them to do so. Such soldiers' decisions to reenter battle, fundamentally, however, are autonomous because they can refuse to give up their symptoms or can refuse combat and take the consequences.

Newman[42] questioned military psychiatrists' ability to assess combat fatigue accurately. He stated, "It is virtually impossible to refute a psychiatric diagnosis and the harder one tries, the more the attempt is viewed as additional confirmation of the severity of the 'mental illness.'"[42(p246)] Newman argued that military psychiatrists lack objectivity. However, all physicians—like military physicians—are at risk of having their objectivity distorted by the conditions under which they practice. Before the Civil War, for instance, when slaves ran away, they were sometimes given the diagnosis of drapetomania.[40] In the former Soviet Union, the mere expression of dissidence could raise the suspicion of schizophrenia.[46] Daniels,[47] a sociologist, has cited an example she considered particularly illustrative of military physicians' institutional bias. She asked a military physician his response to sending soldiers to possible death. This doctor corrected her and told her that he was returning them only to "arduous duty."[47(p4)]

Bok[48] argued more generally that professional groups such as physicians and military personnel become increasingly insensitive because of the frequent crises occurring in their work. Insensitivity is not the same as bias but would be conducive to it. If Bok's assertion is correct, military psychiatrists, as other military physicians, would be doubly susceptible to acquiring bias. Jones'[49] argument that soldiers suffering combat fatigue should be given the message that they are "just tired" and "will recover when rested" is consistent with this possibility. This assumption, pragmatically, is true. Yet, the phrase "just tired" can be construed as carrying within it the presupposition that if service persons were not just tired, they would want to return to duty. As discussed, this may not be the case. To the degree, then, that military physicians using this phrase have lost sight of the fact that it is not normal to want to risk being killed, they may appear biased. In fact, military psychiatrists are well aware of the nuances of these phrases. The phrase *just tired* saves the soldier from the self-doubt and self-guilt that he is a coward.

The possibility of clinical bias would superficially seem to be supported by Jones'[49] report that military personnel were willing during World War I to consciously delay service persons' diagnosis for the sake of military needs. Military aidmen were instructed to "tag" casualties of combat fatigue as "not yet diagnosed."[49] This was necessary because poorly trained, nonphysician personnel had been tagging patients as "war neurosis" or "gas neurosis." By the time physicians saw them later and noted the transient nature of the problem, soldiers had latched onto the incorrect diagnosis as a ticket out of combat. This practice, thus, does not represent deception, which ethically may be seen as a greater wrong than coercion and pragmatically, if discovered by service persons, could have significant adverse consequences on military physician-patient trust. Rather than being deceptive, this measure postponed the diagnostic labeling until specialists could render it and prevent unfortunate labeling from adversely affecting treatment. In World War II, better trained personnel tagged such soldiers correctly as "combat fatigue," a transient disorder.[38]

Observing French and British treatment of combat stress reactions before U.S. entry into World War I, Salmon[50] abjured aversive techniques used by French and German physicians, such as the application of faradic current to ostensibly "paralyzed" muscles. In a report to the Austrian military after World War I, Freud[51] noted that coercive electrical procedures were ineffective, usually producing only temporary results. Salmon[50] relied on persuasion, which on the surface may appear to be a less dramatic and weaker approach. In a situation of strained resources, persuasion may appear to be a luxury that takes time and resources; however, when policies were well-established toward the end of World War II and after the first few months in the Korean conflict, most soldiers could be returned to combat after a few nights' rest.[49] The system became quite efficient. Ethically, of course, it is much easier to justify persuasion than coercion in treatment.

The Use of Drugs to Prevent and Treat Combat Fatigue

Different kinds of ethical problems are raised by the ways in which military psychiatrists could attempt to prevent or treat combat fatigue. Military psychiatrists could, for example, give drugs to reduce fear,[52] and drugs have been given to those who have experienced combat fatigue to help them return to battle.

While few psychiatrists would contend that psychological treatments of combat stress disorders are unethical, Holloway[53] has argued that pharmacological interventions to treat or prevent such disorders may be unethical. From ancient times, soldiers have utilized pharmacological agents to enhance combat motivation. The most utilized drug has been alcohol, an effective and readily available anxiolytic that unfortunately impairs motor performance. Vikings of the first millennium often fought after being intoxicated on mead (beer made from honey), and during the middle ages, armies often went into battle intoxicated. As late as World War II, Japanese troops sometimes prepared themselves for final, desperate banzai charges with saki. A medieval Moslem sect gave the word "assassin" to the English language because of its members' use of hashish (they were called "hashishim") before they were sent to kill their leader's critics. Like alcohol, cannabis can seriously impair combat performance, and it is unclear whether the hashishim were still "stoned" as they committed the assassinations or just convinced that they had experienced, briefly, the paradise that was to be their eternal reward.[52]

During World War II, using a newly discovered technique in which psychiatric casualties were sedated with barbiturates given intravenously and then were asked to recall traumatic battle scenes (abreaction), Grinker and Spiegel[54] were able to return some otherwise unreachable cases to effective service. This technique may still have some applicability in treatment resistant chronic post-traumatic stress disorder cases. It was quickly learned that this procedure was rarely necessary when casualties were given early forward treatment with rest and expectation. In Italy during World War II, Glass[38,55] found that the traditional treatment principles were adequate, and when he became Pacific consultant during the Korean conflict, he emphasized them and discouraged pharmacological interventions.

The Vietnam conflict was the first time U.S. forces had true anxiolytic and neuroleptic drugs.[56] Most widely used were the major tranquilizers chlorpromazine (Thorazine) and prochlorperazine (Compazine), medications that also decrease neurological ability to respond to threat. They slow troops down, decrease motor skills, and result in greater risk of injury from clumsy behavior and decreased alertness. Anxiolytics, primarily chlordiazepoxide (Librium) and diazepam (Valium), were also used in Vietnam to treat less severe psychiatric casualties and for alcohol detoxification.

A sometimes unintentional treatment of psychiatric symptoms occurred in Vietnam when soldiers would complain to battalion surgeons of the physiological components of anxiety (such as diarrhea) and would be given prochlorperazine (Compazine), a standard but powerful antiemetic, antidiarrheal drug that is also a major tranquilizer. Because such medicated soldiers were typically returned to their units, ethical issues can be raised. By impairing motor skills, these drugs may have increased the soldiers' risks in combat. Should the physician inform troops of the consequences of the medications they are taking, and should the soldier be involved in the decision?

Following the disastrous results of a "medical" (inhospital sedation on a medical ward) approach to psychiatric casualties in the 1973 Arab-Israeli War, the Israelis banned hypnosis and medications, having read the U.S. literature and consulted with Walter Reed Army Institute of Research personnel.[57] In the 1982 Lebanon War, however, a few depressed patients were treated with antidepressants.

If drugs are used to render soldiers less fearful before combat, Gabriel[58] has expressed concern that these drugs also could render service persons less emotionally able to appreciate the consequences of their actions. As a result, they might be willing to carry out otherwise unacceptable acts. Whether or not this speculation has a basis in fact is unknown. Yet, persons using alcohol clearly become less inhibited and show more aggressive behavior. Whether drugs such as buspirone would have a similar disinhibiting effect during combat is unknown; however, most persons given buspirone become less aggressive. Other, as yet unknown, drugs might be used in the future to prevent combat fatigue in a beneficial manner. However, they might also increase the soldier's tendency to carry out overly aggressive acts during combat as suggested by Gabriel.[58]

Holloway[53] has speculated that the use of chlorpromazine (Thorazine) and similar medications in Vietnam rendered some soldiers more susceptible to subsequent psychological morbidity, that is, chronic post-traumatic stress disorder. He further speculated that these drugs (and possibly illegal drugs such as heroin) prevented service persons from having the capacity to "process" what they were feeling so that neither then nor later could they have the same capacity to express or "abreact" their emotional responses. There are no studies to confirm or deny this hypothesis.

DIAGNOSTIC ISSUES

Combat Refusal as a Form of Combat Stress Casualty

Although some military psychology writers[59] are inclined to lump combat stress casualties with genuine combat refusal cases (conscientious objectors), one must be careful to distinguish them to avoid the misuse of psychiatry as exemplified by the former Soviet treatment of dissidents.

Handling those who refuse combat while evidencing combat stress symptoms as stress casualties is beneficial because the soldier avoids being prosecuted for a capital offense, and after appropriate treatment, the military retains a soldier who is capable of further service.

At the other end of the spectrum are soldiers refusing to leave combat when impaired. An Israeli physician served with an infantry commander who became increasingly reckless of his own safety and was finally killed on a combat mission. In retrospect, the physician felt that the commander was suffering from increasing anxiety and degradation of performance ("old sergeant syndrome") but chose death rather than admit to a psychiatric breakdown. The Israeli physician felt that he might have erred in not medically evacuating the commander, but the grounds for doing so would have been difficult to establish.[60]

Conscientious Objectors

The U.S. military has recognized that certain religious creeds forbid aspects of military service. Army Regulation 600–43, *Conscientious Objection*,[61] recognizes two kinds: (1) 1–0, which precludes any military involvement, and (2) 1–A–0, which allows one to serve in uniform but not to engage in combat. The military has generally held that an individual's scruples against combat must be based on religious affiliation to qualify for conscientious objector status. Furthermore, if the objection is to a particular war because one believes it to be illegal or unjust, this is not considered justification for conscientious objector status.

The military has been disinclined to grant conscientious objector status to service members who declare conscientious objector convictions after entry to active duty, particularly if their conversion occurred after receiving orders to a combat zone or if it followed lengthy education or training and the service member is scheduled to put that training into action. Such a person may be viewed as using conscientious objector status as a ruse to evade obligated duty.

Case Study

About 1 year after completing a military psychiatric residency, Captain MC stationed in the United States declared himself a conscientious objector who could not wear the military uniform. Captain MC had been an exemplary psychiatrist in his military-affiliated residency and, during his senior year, had been selected as chief resident. Background information revealed that his decision to enter psychiatry had been influenced by his mother's chronic mental illness. After completing residency, he had attended meetings with the Society of Friends (Quakers) and had gradually identified with their creed of nonviolence. He was in no danger of being assigned to the combat zone (South Vietnam), but he became convinced that he could not contribute to the war effort. After lengthy administrative evaluations, his conversion was accepted as genuine, and he was separated a few months earlier than he would have been had he served out his obligation.

Comment: While one could speculate on the identity crisis faced by one reared in this psychiatrist's circumstances, those who know him well could not doubt the genuineness of his convictions or the validity of his conversion as a Quaker. It is military policy to obtain evaluations by chaplains, psychiatrists, and commanders to validate the genuineness of the alleged conscientious objector status and to ensure that this religious conviction is not secondary to a mental illness.

Individual Service Persons Taking Exceptional Risks

War is replete with examples of individual gallantry and heroism. We honor such valor with medals, memorials, and national holidays, and their sacrifices have become an enduring aspect of our national heritage. However, equity may be violated if individual service persons are permitted repeatedly to take exceptional risks. During his tour as a division psychiatrist during the Vietnam conflict, the second author saw one man who volunteered initially to be a "tunnel rat." If he had continued to volunteer for this unusually hazardous duty, the risk he would have been taking would have become increasingly disproportionate to the risks taken by others. At some point, this risk might become unjust. This soldier, however, subsequently declined this role and allowed others to volunteer for this particularly dangerous mission.

Service persons might, of course, volunteer to take exceptional risks for several reasons. Some may enjoy engaging in highly risky behavior. Others may volunteer for altruistic reasons, but in some cases, this altruism may reflect hidden guilt and an unconscious need to be punished.

Those who can repeatedly carry out dangerous missions may have exceptional capacities for withstanding this stress, and the military's utilizing their strengths may enhance the combat mission. Helicopter pilots, for example, may carry out risky missions because of physiological or psychological characteristics.[62] Yet, if service persons take disproportionate risks, equity is violated, and their repeatedly taking these risks at some point could be forbidden.

The principle of respecting service persons' autonomy may be opposed to the principle of equity. That is, the service person who enjoys high risks or has exceptional capacity to function under stress might, like the service person volunteering to be a tunnel rat, freely volunteer. The assumption that a person's freedom to take risks should sometimes be limited so that he does not take on an unfair burden is commonplace. In civilian settings, for instance, a limitation is placed on the kinds of research for which subjects can volunteer.[12] Even if researchers themselves volunteer, a human use committee may disapprove the research on the ground that it is unduly dangerous. For a similar rationale, some limit should exist when service persons repeatedly volunteer for dangerous duty even if their motivation seems genuinely altruistic.

The service person in combat differs considerably from the subject of research. Potentially, a service person's bravery could save his unit and, using the example of World War II, conceivably thousands of lives. This, theoretically, could also be the case with research, as, for example, in research that could provide a cure for acquired immunodeficiency syndrome (AIDS). It is more likely, however, that allowing a service person to take exorbitant risks will be justified because of the great number of lives saved. At the very least, then, a service person should be permitted to take repeated dangerous risks only when attempts to enlist other volunteers (capable of performing the duty) for the same hazardous duty have been unsuccessful.

The military recognizes the need to share the risks of hazardous duty and, in the past, has initiated limited tours of combat duty and fixed numbers of combat aviation missions. In addition to serving the principle of equity, this policy enhances morale.[62]

COMMAND ISSUES

Practices After Nuclear Attack

Fatally irradiated troops pose pragmatic and ethical issues. Such troops cannot always be readily identified and require enormous medical expenditures in personnel and other costs to treat. For example, a few might be saved by bone marrow transplants. On the other hand, many of these troops are not debilitated in the early stages after exposure. In a combat setting, the most rational approach might be to consider them fatalities, consider euthanasia for the most debilitated, and utilize the nondebilitated for high-risk missions. If euthanasia is not available, mere palliative procedures could consume medical resources needed elsewhere.

Exceptional circumstances obviously could exist after nuclear attack. Jones[63] raised several questions such as whether service persons fatally exposed to radiation should be sacrificed for the "greater good" by having them carry out high-risk delaying actions, kamikaze attacks, or operations in contaminated areas. Further, closely related questions are whether service persons should be sent back to irradiated areas when their degree of previous exposure is unknown, and whether if they are sent back, they should be told beforehand that their additional exposure may be fatal.

The last question is particularly complex because service persons who know that they could be exposed to fatal doses of radiation might refuse to return to the front. Under normal circumstances, as previously stated, it would be ethically permissible to ask service persons to make sacrifices to benefit their unit. The question Jones[63] raised involves primarily this issue: Is there any reason after nuclear attack that an exception to the usual ethical priorities should be made?

The answer is possibly yes. Although it is ethically permissible in most instances to withhold specific information from service persons so that they can carry out combat duties more effectively, after nuclear attack, the consequences may be so devastating to service persons that the priority should shift to truth telling to preserve what dignity remains.

Soldiers' dignity could be furthered, for example, by their commanders' choosing not to "use" them primarily as "means" to the units' end by sending them to certain death as would be the case if sending them on kamikaze attacks. Alternatively, because the use of weaponry had "progressed" to the point of nuclear attack, it might be argued that more than ever, all-out attempts to win the conflict would be justified, and permitting service persons under these conditions to give their lives for their country would enhance their dignity.

After nuclear attack, then, combat actions that are carried on might best be construed as falling into either of two categories, noncritical versus critical means to achieve victory. In the former instance, to preserve service persons' dignity, they might not be sent back to the front because it could be anticipated that this would probably mean their dying. At the very least, they should be told the truth regarding this likely consequence of their returning to battle.

When further engagement by irradiated soldiers is critical on the other hand, the usual justification for permitting soldiers to sacrifice their lives will remain—despite the assault to human dignity likely to result after nuclear attack. In this circumstance, respecting service persons' dignity maximally might require allowing them to give their lives in, for example, any of the three ways Jones has described.[63] Further, it may be that respecting soldiers' dignity in this situation also might mean *not* telling them that their reentering irradiated areas would or could mean their deaths. Withholding this knowledge could be justified in this instance if this were necessary to enable these service persons to continue to fight effectively.

Ethically, the justification for giving priority to the combat mission—like allowing service persons who have been fatally injured to die—would be based on the principle of equity. That is, all soldiers risk death during combat. Soldiers who happen to have been injured should not necessarily be protected from this risk. As with soldiers who are healthy, they, too, may be required to sacrifice their lives so that the combat mission can be accomplished.

Sacrifices During Combat

It is sometimes necessary for commanders to allow some soldiers to lose their lives knowingly for the greater interest of other soldiers and the mission. Jones[49] referred to such a possible instance in the first case he discussed involving a soldier who was pinned down by enemy fire. Jones notes that in this instance that the soldiers felt that there may have been a need to sacrifice some troops for the sake of the mission.[49] Jones described this same necessity, implicitly, when he stated that during the U.S. Civil War, commanders sometimes felt that it was desirable to "blood" the troops (expose them to wounded and dead fellow soldiers) to increase their effectiveness in later battles.[64] In addition, risky training exercises sometimes result in deaths, for example in parachute jumps.

The principle underlying commanders' practices in these anecdotes is the same as the principle underlying military medical triage. Namely, as stated, it is sometimes necessary to sacrifice some service persons' lives to achieve victory, if this sacrifice is necessary or seems necessary. Again, there is little question regarding the ultimate justification of this principle. The significant ethical questions involve the limits that should exist on allowing such sacrifices.

Impaired Commanders

When a physician becomes aware that a commander is obviously impaired, he can and should request that the commander be relieved. In neuropsychiatric conditions, however, the impairment may be subtle. General George Patton's belief[36] that he was the reincarnation of great warriors of the past, while possibly pathological, did not apparently impair him as a commander. One of the authors became aware that one of his high-ranking commanders suffered from amyotrophic lateral sclerosis, a degenerative disease of motor neurons. The author did not see evidence that this impaired the commander's judgment. It is not the prerogative of the physician to rule on incompetent (as opposed to impaired) commanders.

Improper or Illegal Commands

Illegal orders come in many guises and may be far from dramatic. When he was a division psychiatrist during the Vietnam conflict, the second author observed a high-ranking commander of limited combat experience (he had been a transportation officer) who ordered physicians to take sick call outside during the rainy season. The commander reportedly believed that soldiers going on sick call were largely malingering. Fortunately, the physicians simply ignored the order rather than challenging it. Another example occurred when a commander ordered his battalion surgeon to read openly excerpts from the medical records of a troubled, mentally ill soldier who was related to a World War II military hero. The second author in his position as division psychiatrist objected; however, his objection was ignored by higher medical personnel.

A dilemma exists when military physicians believe that the probable sacrifice of soldiers' lives lacks sufficient justification. The question that then arises is what action, if any, should military physicians take to protect soldiers from what physicians see as unnecessary or exorbitant risks. Military physicians who believe that they should follow orders unquestioningly in all circumstances follow what is often referred to as a "role-specific" ethic.[39] According to this ethic, military physicians would obey the orders of their superiors as long as they are legal and would delegate all decision-making authority to their superiors.

Alternatively, military physicians could believe that ethically they may assess independently the situations in which sacrifices are called for to see if they are reasonable. Military physicians who took this position might conclude that there are some occasions in which they should take action on service persons' behalf. Hopkins and colleagues[65] expressed this latter view, for example, during World War II when the U.S. Army was sending many soldiers with malaria and dysentery back to the front in Southeast Asia. Hopkins et al stated that he considered it a "disgrace upon the Army Medical Department that ranking medical officers had not insisted upon the total evacuation of the 2nd and 3rd Battalions of 5307 after Nphum Ga"[65(p371)] and added:

> If pressure from high ranking field officers can be applied to Army Generals and Evacuation Hospitals as well as to medical officers in general to such an extent (regarding their) prerogative of protecting the health of the fighting men and guaranteeing that men unfit for combat are kept out of combat, then those hospitals as well as the medical officers are robbed of sacred duties and rights to which their medical knowledge and service entitles them.[65(pp379–380)]

Physicians in the military are unlikely, however, to have knowledge comparable with that of their superiors regarding the overall strategy of command decisions. Therefore, when a military physician independently assesses command policy, he risks being short-sighted in determining his ethical obligations. Hopkins and coworkers,[65(p372)] for example, in the instance just described, may have been unaware of several important factors.

A similar question regarding the obligation of military physicians to take action also may occur in situations that do not involve risks to their own troops but to "innocent" civilians. The option of speaking out or refusing to carry out orders is available to line officers and all other service persons, of course, as well as military physicians. In the case of line officers, however, the argument that they should not act because they lack information would tend to be weaker.

Jones[66] cited the example of Colonel Eli Geva who refused to lead his troops into Beirut because he objected to the killing of civilians and felt that the military objectives did not justify the losses of his soldiers. Jones indicated also that Geva was criticized for showing too much concern for civilians. Military physicians refusing to obey orders for the sake of either their troops or civilians might be subject to the same complaint.

Yet, Jones[66] also commented in speaking of Geva's refusal that the decision subsequently was made to launch a "more discriminating attack" designed to reduce these casualties. It would seem plausible that Geva's refusal may have had some effect on saving civilians' lives. Even if it did not, however, his or military physicians' refusal to obey an order may be justified on so-called deontological grounds alone; that is, that "some actions are right (or wrong) for reasons beyond their consequences."[67(p36)] During World War II, for example, Nazi physicians' protesting may have accomplished no consequential benefit; they may even have lost their lives as a result of refusing some orders. Yet, because they would have been respecting another human being's dignity, their refusal would have been justified. Similarly, Geva's refusing to carry out an order he considered immoral might be justified solely on the ground that by his refusal, he was avoiding implicitly sanctioning an act he considered immoral. This would be true regardless of the consequences.

Thus, although some soldiers' lives must be sacrificed for the benefit of other service persons and/or for military goals, military physicians may be justified ethically in refusing to carry out orders that they consider immoral. Ideally, of course, mechanisms should exist within the military to prevent the need for disobeying an order from ever arising, and physicians or other service persons should never find themselves in a situation of having to decide whether to protest. Field Marshall Carver[45] reported that during World War II, between the Normandy invasion and the end of the war, as an armored brigade commander, he had to remove many officers for the sake of their units and themselves. He pointed out that all of these officers had been highly decorated and respected men with more battle experience than himself and that none of their subordinates gave him a clue that he should act as he did because they were too loyal.

Despite attempts by the military, such as the inspector general system, adequate checks may not exist, particularly because of the hierarchical ranking in the military. Although the indications that a military physician should refuse an order or should act to protect service persons or civilians are likely to be unclear, nonetheless, they may exist.

Atrocities

Every significant war has witnessed atrocities against civilians or enemy soldiers. Most militaries attempt to prevent or punish such atrocities either from moral precepts or because they recognize that atrocities impair the morale of the perpetrators and may inadvertently spur greater resistance by the enemy. The 1990 to 1991 atrocities imputed to Iraqi forces in Kuwait earned United Nations condemnation and strengthened a multinational coalition to intervene against Iraq.[68] During the My Lai atrocity in Vietnam, at least one U.S. soldier became a casualty when he shot himself in the leg rather than participate.[69]

Military psychiatrists during combat may witness or suspect acts that are illegal or whose legal status is uncertain. Jones[66] suggested that atrocities are particularly likely, for example, in low-intensity guerrilla warfare in which terrorism tends to brutalize both sides.

Several examples can be cited from the past. Gault[70] refers, for example, to enemy prisoners in Vietnam who were thrown out of helicopters if they refused to provide information. This atrocity apparently was intended as a lesson to other prisoners indicating what would happen to them if they also failed to give information. Other more equivocal examples include captured enemies being given less than optimal care before being interrogated,[71] women being interrogated while they were breast feeding,[72(p455)] children being asked to incriminate their parents,[72(p456)] and prisoners being turned over to other parties when it was anticipated that the other parties would mistreat them.[73(p402)]

Military physicians, like all service persons, have obligations under international agreements to treat enemy prisoners of war with decency. Military physicians not only have additional obligations to actively intervene to prevent atrocities as a result of their implicit promise made when they became physicians to not harm patients, but also they have the legal obligation of all service members to try to prevent such atrocities and to report any that have occurred. A military physician's medical role should give him a stronger obligation to speak out against or oppose atrocities than other service persons. The obligation arguably exists even when speaking out might pose some danger to the physician. Implicitly, when becoming a physician, one accepts a degree of self-sacrifice. The American Medical Association[74] has taken the position that all physicians, for example, should be willing to treat patients with AIDS despite the risk that they could give themselves a fatal needlestick. The example given about Nazi physicians further supports these assertions. Rosebury stated that "It is a matter of record that the majority of [German] physicians practiced ethically during the Holocaust except for not protesting."[75(p517)]

Reasonable ethical arguments support two limitations to military physicians' obligation to oppose atrocities: (1) instances in which mistreatment of enemy service persons could produce information that would save a unit or even the nation and (2) instances in which physicians' or their families' lives would be endangered. The first limitation is based on utilitarian values. It assumes that harm to one is outweighed by harm to multiple others. Yet, it is usually, if not always, uncertain that atrocities will be the only means of avoiding harm to others, and the use of atrocities to prevent such harm might contradict the ends for which the war is fought. As Supreme Court Justice Douglas stated, in another context, "It would indeed be ironic if, in the name of national defense, we would sanction the subversion of . . . those liberties . . . which [make] the defense of the nation worthwhile. . . ."[76(p264)]

As already stated, physicians made an implicit promise when entering the medical profession to work for the good of others even when this involves some degree of self-sacrifice, and they agreed when joining the military to uphold the U.S. constitution, which through treaties supports international law. If, then, military physicians' or their families' lives would not be endangered, at least when their opposing an atrocity would be beneficial, they have a prima facie obligation to act. Thus, if they do not act immediately, they would have a strong obligation to do so at the first opportunity that presents itself at which this degree of sacrifice would not be necessary.

A potential risk of this position—that military physicians need not act when their own or their families' lives are at stake—is that physicians could acquire justification for never acting and show the same kind of inaction shown by Nazi physicians. It hardly seems possible, however, that military physicians would *never* acquire an opportunity to be sufficiently protected from repercussions against themselves and their families to act against atrocities. Thus, as opposed to holding military physicians, or others for that matter, to an heroic standard implausible to achieve, this standard might justifiably be lowered.

SUMMARY AND CONCLUSION

Ethical issues abound in military psychiatry as in military medicine in general, but few issues are specifically limited to psychiatry. Those limited to psychiatry generally relate to the psychiatrist's unique role in treating combat stress casualties and in ruling out mental illness as a cause of proscribed behavior (for example, homosexuality, criminal behavior, alleged conscientious objector status, and so forth).

Despite its reputation for rigidity and conservatism, the military has generally reflected the prevailing American ethos and has sometimes led the way in reforms. This was demonstrated when the military was the first large governmental organization to be desegregated and when it pioneered in developing drug and alcohol rehabilitation programs around the concepts of amnesty and confidentiality. Nevertheless, psychiatrists, who have their own reputation for strong individualism, will always find a substantial number of individuals who will not feel at ease in an organization that sometimes views individuals as replaceable parts in a large machine. Their struggles with ethical issues will invariably reflect not only the issues themselves but also the individual biases of the psychiatrist in conformity and confrontation.

REFERENCES

1. Dabaghian J. *Mirror of Man: Readings in Sociology and Literature.* Boston: Little, Brown; 1970: 482–489.
2. Durant W, Durant A. History and war. In: Durant W, ed. *The Lessons of History.* New York: Simon and Schuster; 1968: 81–86.
3. Erikson EH. Hunters across the prairie. In: *Childhood and Society.* 2nd ed. New York: Norton; 1963: 114–165.
4. Williams MH. 1941. In: *US Army in World War II: Special Studies: Chronology—1941–1945.* Office of the Chief of Military History, US Army. Washington, DC: GPO; 1960: 3–10.
5. Carver M. Arab-Israeli wars. In: *War Since 1945.* New York: Putnam's Sons; 1981: 234–272.
6. Benedict R. *The Chrysanthemum and the Sword.* Boston: Houghton Mifflin; 1946.
7. Nardini JE. Survival factors in American POW's of the Japanese. *Am J Psychiatry.* 1952;109:241–248.
8. Durant W. Feudalism and chivalry. In: *The Age of Faith.* New York: Simon and Schuster; 1950: 572–579.
9. Vonnegut K. *Slaughterhouse 5.* London: Cape; 1970.
10. Hersey J. *Hiroshima.* New York: Modern Library; 1946.
11. Carver M. *War Since 1945.* New York: Putnam's Sons; 1981:179.
12. *The Nuremberg Code. Trials of War Criminals Before the Nuremberg Military Tribunals.* Washington, DC: GPO; 1948.
13. Jones FD. Personal Observation, 1971.
14. Camp NM. The Vietnam war and the ethics of combat psychiatry. *Am J Psychiatry.* 1993;150:1000–1010.
15. Rosten LC. *Captain Newman, M.D.* New York: Harper; 1962.
16. Heller J. *Catch-22.* London: Cape; 1962.
17. Zabriske EG, Rhein JHW, Strecker EA, Leopold S, Raynor MW, Steckel HA. Division, corps, and army neuropsychiatric consultants. In: P Bailey, FE Williams, PA Komora, TW Salmon, N Fenton, eds. *The Medical Department of the United States Army in the World War.* Vol X. *Neuropsychiatry.* Washington, DC: GPO; 1929: 303–324.
18. Glass AJ. Psychotherapy in the combat zone. *Am J Psychiatry.* 1954;110(10):725–731.
19. Glasser RJ. *365 Days.* New York: Braziller; 1971.
20. Livingston GS. Letter from a Vietnam veteran. *Saturday Review.* 1969;(September 20):22–23.
21. US Department of Defense. Sorting of casualties. In: Bowen T, Bellamy RF, eds. *The Emergency War Surgery NATO Handbook.* 2nd revision. Washington, DC: GPO; 1988.
22. US Department of Defense. *Emergency War Surgery.* 1st revised ed. Washington, DC: GPO; 1975.
23. Winslow G. The concept of triage in modern medicine. In: *Triage and Justice: The Ethics of Rational Life-Saving Medical Resources.* Berkeley: University of California Press; 1982: 1–11.
24. Beecher HK. Scarce resources and medical advancement. In: Freund PA, ed. *Experimentation with Human Subjects.* New York: George Braziller; 1969: 66–104.

25. Beecher HK. *Research and the Individual/Human Studies.* Boston: Little, Brown & Co.; 1970.

26. Hinds SW. Triage in medicine. A personal history. In: Lucas GR, Jr., ed. *Triage in Medicine and Society.* Houston: Institute of Religion and Human Development; 1975: 6–22.

27. Bellamy R. Contrasts in combat casualty care. *Milit Med.* 1985;150:405–410.

28. Howe EG. Special problems for military psychiatrists. In: Simon RI, ed. *Review of Clinical Psychiatry and the Law.* Vol 2. Washington, DC: American Psychiatric Press; 1991: 306–324.

29. Auster SL. Confidentiality in military medicine. *Milit Med.* 1985;150(7):341–346.

30. Knoll DD. The physician-patient privilege, article 31, and the military doctor. *Milit Med.* 1971;136(7)640–643.

31. Ruben HL. Confidentiality and privileged communications: The plight of the military physician. *Milit Med.* 1973;138(4):211–213.

32. US Department of the Army. Confidentiality of medical information. In: *Medical Record and Quality Assurance Administration.* Washington, DC: DA; 1982. Army Regulation 40–66.

33. Beighley PS, Brown GR. Case report: Medication refusal by psychiatric inpatients in the military. *Milit Med.* 1992;157(1):47–49.

34. Richards RL. Mental and nervous disorders in the Russo-Japanese War. *Milit Surgeon.* 1910;26(2):177–193.

35. Deutsch A. Military psychiatry: The Civil War, 1861–1865. In: *One Hundred Years of American Psychiatry: 1844–1944.* New York: Columbia University Press, 1944. 367–384.

36. Essame H. *Patton: A Study in Command.* New York: Scribner; 1974.

37. Jones FD. Section A: Combat stress casualties. In: Jones FD, Sparacino LR, Wilcox VL, Rothberg JM, eds. *War Psychiatry.* Part 1. In: *Textbook of Military Medicine.* Washington, DC: Office of The Surgeon General, US Department of the Army and Borden Institute; in press: chapters 1 through 5.

38. Glass AJ. Lessons learned. In: *Neuropsychiatry in World War II.* Vol 2. In: Mullens WS, Glass AJ, eds. *Overseas Theaters.* Washington, DC: GPO; 1973. GPO Stock No. 0832–00047, 989–1027.

39. Howe EG. Ethical issues regarding mixed agency of military physicians. *Soc Sci Med.* 1986;23(8):803–815.

40. Engelhardt HT. Fear of flying: The psychiatrist's role in war. *Hastings Center Report.* 1976;6:21.

41. Friedson E. Commentary on: In the service of the state: The psychiatrist as double agent. *Hastings Center Report.* 1978;8(special suppl):3–6.

42. Veatch RM. The psychiatrist's role in war. In: *Case Studies in Medical Ethics.* Cambridge, Mass: Harvard University Press; 1977: 245–251.

43. Brody H. *Ethical Decisions in Medicine.* Boston: Little, Brown & Co.; 1976.

44. Lifton RJ. Advocacy and corruption in the healing professions. *Conn Med.* 1975;39:803–813.

45. Carver L. Morale in battle—The medical and the military. *J R Soc Med.* 1989;82:67–71.

46. Reich W. The case of General Grigorenko. *Encounter.* 1980;54:9–24.

47. Daniels AK. In the service of the state: The psychiatrist as double agent. *Hastings Center Report.* 1978;8(special suppl):3–6.

48. Bok S. *Lying/Moral Choice in Public and Private Life*. New York: Vintage Books; 1976.

49. Jones FD. Psychiatric lessons of war. In: Jones FD, Sparacino LR, Wilcox VL, Rothberg JM, eds. *War Psychiatry*. Part 1. In: *Textbook of Military Medicine*. Washington, DC: Office of The Surgeon General, US Department of the Army and Borden Institute; in press: chapter 1.

50. Salmon TW. *The Care and Treatment of Mental Disease and War Neuroses ("Shell Shock") in the British Army*. New York: The War Work Committee of the National Committee for Mental Hygiene; 1917.

51. Freud S. The war neuroses (1919). In: *An Infantile Neurosis and Other Works (1917–1919)*. Vol 17. In: Strachey J, ed. *Standard Edition of the Complete Psychological Works of Sigmund Freud*. London: Hogarth Press; 1955: 205–215.

52. Jones FD. Sanctioned use of drugs in combat. In: Pichot P, Berner P, Wolf R, Thau K, eds. *Psychiatry: The State of the Art*. Vol 6. New York: Plenum; 1985: 489–494.

53. Holloway HC, et al. Vietnam psychiatry revisited. Presented at the American Psychiatric Association Annual Meeting; 19 May 1982; Toronto, Ontario, Canada.

54. Grinker RR, Spiegel JP. *Men Under Stress*. Philadelphia: Blakiston; 1945.

55. Glass AJ. Psychiatry in the Korean campaign (installment I). *US Armed Forces Med J*. 1953;4:1387–1401.

56. Jones FD, Johnson AW. Medical and psychiatric treatment policy and practice in Vietnam. *J Soc Issues*. 1975;31(4):49–65.

57. Shabtai N. Personal Communication, 1983.

58. Gabriel RH. *No More Heroes: Madness & Psychiatry in War*. New York: Hill and Wang; 1987.

59. Kormos HR. The nature of combat stress. In: Figley CR, ed. *Stress Disorders Among Vietnam Veterans*. New York: Brunner/Mazel; 1978: 3–22.

60. Harris P. Personal Communication, 1983.

61. US Department of the Army. *Conscientious Objection*. Washington, DC: DA; 1987. Army Regulation 600–43.

62. Jones D. Air Force combat psychiatry. In: Jones FD, Sparacino LR, Wilcox VL, Rothberg JM, eds. *War Psychiatry*. Part 1. In: *Textbook of Military Medicine*. Washington, DC: Office of The Surgeon General, US Department of the Army and Borden Institute; in press: chapter 8.

63. Jones FD. Neuropsychiatric casualties of chemical, biological, and radiological warfare. In: Jones FD, Sparacino LR, Wilcox VL, Rothberg JM, eds. *War Psychiatry*. Part 1. In: *Textbook of Military Medicine*. Washington, DC: Office of The Surgeon General, US Department of the Army and Borden Institute; in press: chapter 4.

64. Jones FD. Traditional warfare combat stress casualties. In: Jones FD, Sparacino LR, Wilcox VL, Rothberg JM, eds. *War Psychiatry*. Part 1. In: *Textbook of Military Medicine*. Washington, DC: Office of The Surgeon General, US Department of the Army and Borden Institute; in press: chapter 2.

65. Hopkins JET, Stelling HG, Voorhees TS. The marauders and the microbes: A record of righteous indignation. In: Stone JH, ed. *Crisis Fleeting*. Washington, DC: Office of The Surgeon General, Department of the Army, 1969: 293–396.

66. Jones FD. Nostalgia. In: Jones FD, Sparacino LR, Wilcox VL, Rothberg JM, eds. *War Psychiatry*. Part 1. In: *Textbook of Military Medicine*. Washington, DC: Office of The Surgeon General, US Department of the Army and Borden Institute; in press: chapter 3.

67. Beauchamp TL, Childress JF. *Principles of Biomedical Ethics*. 3rd ed. New York: Oxford University Press; 1989.

68. Murphy C. U.S. says Iraq stepping up campaign of executions and torture in Kuwait. *Washington Post*. February 24, 1991; 114(81):A–1, A–22.

69. US Department of the Army. *The My Lai Massacre and Its Cover-up: Beyond the Reach of the Law?: The Peers Commission Report*. New York: Free Press; 1976.

70. Gault B. Some remarks on slaughter. *Am J Psychiatry*. 1971;128:450–454.

71. Testimony and questioning of Donald Duncan. In: Duffett J, ed. *Against the Crime of Silence/Proceedings of the International War Crimes Tribunal*. New York: Simon and Schuster; 1968: 463–464.

72. Testimony and questioning of Peter Martinsen. In: Duffett J, ed. *Against the Crime of Silence/Proceedings of the International War Crimes Tribunal*. New York: Simon and Schuster; 1968: 425–457.

73. Solange BA. Juridical report on the treatment of war prisoners and civilians. In: Duffett J, ed. *Against the Crime of Silence/Proceedings of the International War Crimes Tribunal*. New York: Simon and Schuster; 1968:392–402.

74. American Medical Association. Denial of care. *Digest of HIV/AIDS Policy*. Chicago, Ill: American Medical Association; 1994: 9.

75. Rosebury T. Medical ethics of biological warfare. *Perspect Biol Med*. 1963;6:511–523.

76. *US v. Robel*, 386 U.S. 258, 1967.

Chapter 8

ETHICAL CHALLENGES FOR THE PSYCHIATRIST DURING THE VIETNAM CONFLICT

NORMAN M. CAMP, M.D.*

*Colonel, (ret), Medical Corps, U.S. Army; Associate Clinical Professor, Medical College of Virginia, Virginia Commonwealth University, Richmond, Virginia 23298–0710

INTRODUCTION

Psychiatrists who serve in the military function in the ethical shadow of an enormous and strict hierarchy, the central organizing principle of which is the subordination of individual values to those of the organization—presumably for the benefit of society.

There have been various attempts to examine and reconcile potential loyalty conflicts for the military psychiatrist, which may be similar to those faced by psychiatrists who work for other organizations. However, little specific attention has been paid to the exquisite and absolute contradiction of values that may affect military psychiatrists when they serve in a combat theater. As came to light during the Vietnam conflict, whereas combat psychiatrists' clinical decisions can have far-reaching consequences, they may face organizational expectations, codified in the military treatment doctrine, that they function in ways which are perceived, at least by others, if not by themselves, as violating the most basic ethical tenets of psychiatry serving the welfare of the individual. To understand how this value clash can arise, one must understand certain fundamental distinctions between psychiatric reactions to combat and similar civilian casualties.

The treatment of combat psychiatry casualties differs from the treatment of similar casualties in civilian settings because the soldier-patient faces not only the extraordinarily stressful combat but also the arousal of his own moral conflict.[1,2] Even if the soldier is reluctant, he has a duty on recovering to risk further sacrifices, perhaps to the point of giving his life. The military psychiatrist is similarly in a unique position. Also a soldier and also subject to the authority and hierarchical values of the military, the psychiatrist is obligated to aid his patient in fulfilling this duty—even if the psychiatrist is reluctant. More specifically, because the combat psychiatrist's foremost military responsibility is that of stemming the flow of individuals who manifest a psychological incapacity or reluctance to soldier,[3] he may be obligated to deny a psychologically traumatized soldier's expectation of medical exemption from further exposure to combat (or from a court martial) to conform to the military's expectation that the soldier be returned to that environment if he can function, regardless of whether he has persisting psychiatric symptoms or is opposed to returning.[4]

Before the Vietnam era, the potential for conflict between military and civilian value systems when psychiatrists in military service treated combat casualties was rarely mentioned in the psychiatric literature;[5] however, it was often implied.[6–8] For example, Peterson and Chambers[6] acknowledge the discomfort their colleagues experienced in satisfying military priorities during the Korean conflict:

> It is easy to evacuate a soldier from combat and difficult to do the reverse. It is easier to say, "this man should never have been drafted," than to help him adjust to his duties. It is easier to send a frightened young soldier, who reminds one of one's self or one's own son, to the rear than to return him to combat duty. . . . One's own feelings of guilt over returning another to combat duty, make it difficult for the psychiatrist to function effectively and without anxiety.[6(p253)]

Nevertheless, in World War I, World War II, and the Korean conflict, thousands of psychiatrists, typically mobilized civilians, performed their professional duties with a sustained allegiance to the military objectives and accepted that their clinical goals, techniques, and values would be altered by expediency associated with fighting those wars.[9,10] Important in this regard is the huge impact of World War II on the course of American psychiatry. At one point (June 1944), 26% of the members of the American Psychiatric Association (APA) were in military uniform.[11] Following the war, many who had served became the leaders of American psychiatry.[10] In their experience, the combat psychiatry doctrine—a treatment regimen that utilizes basic physical and psychologically supportive treatments, deemphasizes patienthood, and encourages rapid resumption of duty function—seemed validated through its effectiveness in treating large numbers of soldiers, and their influence on psychiatric thinking in America was revolutionary.[12] The development of civilian applications of social and behavioral therapeutic strategies[13,14] and the modalities of brief psychotherapy[15] and crisis psychotherapy[10] were natural extensions of the doctrine.

The implementation of the traditional combat psychiatry doctrine in the Vietnam conflict, however, came to be severely criticized, primarily on ethical grounds. As will be described, the new opponents of military psychiatry, including some who served as psychiatrists in Vietnam, argued that the doctrine's treatment goals and methods violated psychiatry's humanitarian principles by neglecting the needs of the soldier in order to wage an unjust war. After the United States withdrew its forces from Southeast Asia, however, these issues were mostly forgotten[10] as were many related societal controversies associated with the conflict.

TRADITIONAL VIEWS OF COMBAT PSYCHIATRY

When Fear Overshadows Combat Motivation

A review of selected aspects of combat psychiatry is pertinent to understanding its potential value conflicts. It has only been within the era of the modern battlefield, essentially beginning with World War I, that acute, disabling psychiatric reactions to the stress of combat have arisen in numbers sufficient to constitute a military medical problem.[16–18] Throughout the 20th century, weapons have become increasingly destructive and their delivery systems more precise; consequently the stress levels sustained by troops, as measured by the proportion of nonfatal combat casualties that are psychiatric, have risen proportionally. Furthermore, because disabling psychological and behavioral reactions to the stress of modern combat have at times arisen in sufficient numbers to alter the course of military engagements, the U.S. military has come to value highly the services of its psychiatrists and allied medical department personnel.

Clinical Presentations of Combat Stress Reactions

The psychiatric symptoms associated with combat stress may range in severity from hyperalertness, irritability, difficulty concentrating, and insomnia, to gross and disabling disturbances in affect, thinking, and behavior.[19] Collectively, they have been labeled with uniquely military names such as shell-shock, war neurosis, and combat fatigue (or exhaustion).[20] More lately they have been referred to as battle stress (or shock) casualties and combat stress reactions.

Behavior disturbances as a reaction to combat stress include such obviously avoidant behaviors as combat refusal, malingering, self-inflicted wounds, and desertion, as well as less direct ones such as alcohol and drug misuse; neglect of healthcare, weapons, or equipment; indiscipline; short-timers syndrome; and combat atrocities.[21,22] Of special importance to military objectives, both psychiatric and behavioral reactions can spread by suggestion and reach epidemic proportions (eg, as with the incidents of group gas hysteria in World War I[23] and the heroin problem in the latter years in Vietnam[24]). Consequently, soldiers with combat stress reactions may jeopardize other soldiers, reduce a unit's combat effectiveness, and affect the outcome of a combat situation. Although suggesting there is more homogeneity than experience dictates, for discussion purposes, the collection of combat-generated conditions will be referred to generally as combat stress reactions.

Diagnosis and Pathogenesis

The clinical presentations of combat stress reaction cases have at times conformed to various specific *Diagnostic and Statistical Manual of Mental Disorders* (3rd ed., revised, DSM III–R)[25] diagnostic categories.[10] However, presenting symptoms tend to be diffuse and variable with particular patterns influenced by the combat situation and "ecology."[26] In fact, because of their typically protean nature and apparent reversibility when managed according to the doctrine,[19] military psychiatrists have concluded that the combat stress reaction is essentially the battlefield equivalent of the acute reaction[27] or catastrophic reaction[28] to stress. The soldier with a combat stress reaction is considered to have suffered a reversible, if profound, regression as a consequence of having had his psychological defenses, as well as his combat motivation,[6] overwhelmed by the rigors, dangers, losses, and horrors of the combat situation.[29] Although combat stress reactions do not meet the criteria for post-traumatic stress disorder (PTSD) and do not generally evolve into diagnosable PTSD,[30] without effective treatment, chronic debilitating forms will develop.[28]

From World War I, when combat stress reactions were determined to be psychiatric rather than neurologic disorders, it was concluded that they were caused by the combination of combat intensity or duration and individual predisposition[7] (often with insinuations of cowardice[8]). More recently, this etiologic dialectic, often referred to as "every man has his breaking point," has been expanded to encompass a more complex biopsychosocial model.[31–33]

Such a model suggests that a variety of individual and social risk factors can interact with a variety of combat stresses to undermine a soldier's combat adaptation. The preventive activities of military psychiatrists have typically utilized their understanding of these factors to influence military policies and planning regarding screening, indoctrination and training, physical conditioning, morale and leadership, social supports, and combat conditions and tactics.[22,34,35] Personality factors are posited to have relatively less etiologic importance in combat stress reactions[36,37] but to be of increasing importance in cases arising in low-intensity combat[38] as well as influence recovery.[39] However, as Erikson's[31] analysis of a specimen combat stress reaction case from World War II suggests, a theory of intrapsychic conflict may be especially useful in explaining breakdown and recovery at the level of the individual soldier.

In conclusion, combat stress reactions are considered by military psychiatry to represent a normal reaction to an abnormal circumstance at least in their acute stages. Although not the primary etiology, the combat stress reaction commonly expresses the soldier's "refusal to fight"[40(p11)] and thus represents a situation in which his fear overshadows his combat motivation.[41]

The Use of Psychoactive Drugs

Through the ages, the extreme physical and emotional demands of combat naturally led warring states to experiment with various psychoactive substances to limit excitement and fear and reduce exhaustion and dysfunction among its warriors.[16] In the American wars before the Vietnam conflict, the use of medications in the treatment of psychiatric casualties was generally limited to sedatives, primarily barbiturates.[42] The addition of recently discovered neuroleptics and anxiolytics in the Vietnam theater represented a powerful new tool to the armamentarium of combat psychiatrists. The numerous reports from those serving in South Vietnam[43–46] and the prescription prevalence study conducted there by Datel and Johnson[47] indicate the widespread, enthusiastic use by military psychiatrists and other military physicians of these newer psychoactive medications in the treatment of combat-related psychiatric symptoms. However, the effects of these drugs on soldiers and their combat performance have never been studied. Current doctrine discourages the use of all but the short-acting sedatives and anxiolytics,[22] and those are to be used only when reassurance, strong suggestion, and behavioral methods have been tried without sufficient effect. However, psychiatric and medical units in a combat theater are still equipped with a wide range of psychoactive medicines.

The Critical Nature of Expectancy

The goal of traditional U.S. Army combat psychiatrists has been to fulfill the U.S. Army Medical Department's mission of contributing to the achievement of the combat objective (the motto of the U.S. Army Medical Corps is "To Conserve Fighting Strength"[48]). Over the course of World War I, World War II, and the Korean conflict, combat psychiatrists empirically derived a set of clinical principles that appeared to restore quickly the affected soldier's critical physical and psychological functions so that he could return to his military unit and comrades and resume the fight.[18] These principles have become condensed in the mnemonic PIES: proximity, immediacy, expectancy, and simplicity.[13] These principles refer to elementary physical (ie, rest, replenishment, and psychoactive medication in selected instances) and psychosocial treatments (ie, assisted anamnesis, reassurance, and encouragement) that are applied as rapidly as possible and as close to the soldier's unit and the fighting as the tactical and clinical situations permit.

Especially central to this review are the ethical implications surrounding expectancy. *Expectancy* refers to an overarching clinical attitude that has been recognized since World War I to be essential in restoring soldiers and returning them to duty.[7] The treatment team's collective attitude of expectancy shapes the various physical, psychological, and environmental interventions to bolster the patient's self-confidence as a soldier and discourage self-protective feelings and invalidism (eg, to reduce the secondary gain wish for medical exemption from further combat).[6,8] As will be illustrated in a later section of this chapter, the soldier is managed more as a soldier and less as a patient. While hospitalized, he is regarded as if his symptoms represent simply a temporary, normal reaction to stress and fatigue. He is encouraged to believe that after a brief period of rest and recuperation and with the psychiatric team's assistance in ventilating his traumatic combat experience, he can and will recover quickly, rejoin his comrades, resume his military job, and regain his self-respect. Shaw describes this exhortative approach:

> Reinforcement is given to the soldier's softly heard voice of conscience, which urges him to stay with his buddies, not to be a coward, and to fulfill his soldierly duty. Encouragement is given to patriotic motivation, pride in the self and the unit, and to all aspects of one's determination to go through with one's commitment.[32(p131)]

Current U.S. Army doctrine[49–54] divides the dysfunctional combat stress behaviors into battle fatigue and misconduct stress behavior. Battle fatigue covers all subtypes and syndromes that are treated according to PIES[13] and the four Rs: reassure, rest, replenish, and restore confidence. Misconduct stress behavior refers to conditions that are judged to be willful violations of unit regulations, the Uniformed Code of Military Justice, or the law of land warfare and are presumed to respond better to disciplinary action.

The doctrine recognizes that there may be gray areas at the minor end of the misconduct spectrum where command can choose to treat the misbehaving soldier for battle fatigue and return him to duty. However, it states unequivocally that "once serious misconduct has occurred, it must be punished to prevent further erosion of discipline. Combat stress, even with heroic combat performance, cannot justify criminal misconduct."[53(¶2–9d)]

VIETNAM PSYCHIATRY: FROM CONFIDENCE TO DISMAY

Unanticipated Challenges in Vietnam

Over the 8 years of conflict in Southeast Asia (1965 to 1973), an estimated 135 U.S. Army psychiatrists, as well as smaller numbers of U.S. Navy and U.S. Air Force psychiatrists, were sent to provide care for the almost 3 million American men and women who served there. During the first few years following the insertion of American ground forces into South Vietnam, troop morale remained high, and few Americans opposed the conflict. Rates for psychiatric admissions and evacuations remained well below those seen in earlier wars.[55] Psychiatric observers remarked on the apparent effectiveness of the combat psychiatry doctrine[56,57] and the value of newly discovered neuroleptic and anxiolytic drugs in the treatment of a broad range of psychiatric symptoms among combat-exposed troops.[43,46,47,58]

Then, from 1968 until all U.S. troops were withdrawn in 1973, antiwar and antimilitary sentiment accelerated in the United States and among U.S. troops in Vietnam. Collectively, the spectacular increase in the Vietnam theater rates of disciplinary actions and of psychiatric disorders, including heroin dependency,[59] indicated that a very large proportion of U.S. troops were unable or unwilling to accept the risks of combat, acknowledge military authority, or tolerate the hardships of an assignment in Vietnam. The resultant challenge to the assigned military psychiatrists was unprecedented.[60]

Shifting Professional Attitudes Toward the Conflict

As increasing numbers of Americans denounced the conflict in Southeast Asia, military psychiatry and its doctrine came under attack.[61] Criticism came both from psychiatrists and other physicians who had served in Vietnam as well as from those who had not served there. Lifton,[62] a psychiatrist with experience with military populations, veterans, and survivors of extreme military and civilian stress, is a prominent example of the latter. In his opinion, the military psychiatrists in Vietnam were "technicist" professionals who had colluded with an "absurd and evil organization."[62(p808)] Later, he equated them with German physicians who worked for the Nazis in their death camps.[63]

Spragg[64] and Boman,[21] two Australian military psychiatrists, drew on their experiences with Australian troops who fought in Vietnam and were also very critical of the U.S. combat psychiatry doctrine. Boman referred to the published accounts by American military psychiatrists as "hair raising reading."[21(p111)]

Mental health organizations also reacted strongly to the conflict's increasing unpopularity. In March 1971, 67% of APA members responding to a poll indicated that they wanted the U.S. government to terminate all military activity in Vietnam.[65] This poll was followed by APA Board of Trustees' passing of official resolutions that condemned the conflict and argued for an American withdrawal.[66] In July 1972, the American Psychological Association joined seven other mental health associations in the following public statement, "we find it morally repugnant for any government to exact such heavy costs in human suffering for the sake of abstract conceptions of national pride or honor."[67(p1)] In raising questions about the morality of the U.S. military intervention in Vietnam, these organizations increased the ethical dilemmas for psychiatrists, psychologists, and social workers in uniform, yet they neglected to provide their colleagues with the guidance for addressing these dilemmas.

The debate between psychiatrists Bloch and Maier illustrates the shift in professional attitudes from the more sanguine early conflict period to the late conflict enmity. In 1969, Bloch[43] wrote an article describing the psychiatric goals and methods used at the 935th U.S. Army Medical (Psychiatric) Detachment in 1967 to 1968 in Vietnam. A civilian-trained psychiatrist in uniform, Bloch confidently explained how his team adapted the U.S. Army's traditional doctrine for the treatment of combat casualties to fit the unique features of the low-intensity, counter-insurgency combat theater of Vietnam. He also highlighted the value of previously unavailable psychoactive medications, primarily chlorpromazine, in the treatment of seriously combat-disabled soldiers.

Maier, a psychiatrist who treated psychiatric casualties from Vietnam while he served with the U.S. Army in Japan in 1965 to 1967, reacted in a letter to the editor[68] that was intensely critical of the ethics and practices of military psychiatrists in Vietnam. He concluded, "By acting to 'conserve the fighting strength' in this war of boundless immorality, [the military psychiatrist] partakes of the passive complicity that is the mark of guilt in our time. . . . Whatever else Army psychiatry may be, I see neither moral nor scientific justification for the dignity of its definition as clinical psychiatry."[68(p1039)]

Bloch[69] replied that in his experience in Vietnam, soldiers who struggled with concerns regarding the morality of the conflict typically were driven by pre-Vietnam psychological conflicts. He also defended the goals and methods of military psychiatry in Vietnam, "If reality is that America's youth are now fighting, then they deserve the best psychiatric care that can be afforded them. Such care neither oversimplifies issues nor encumbers and compromises the evaluation or treatment setting by intrusion of the psychiatrists' moral judgments and emotions."[69(p1040)]

Livingston, a West Point graduate who volunteered to serve in Vietnam, was not a psychiatrist at the time he served as a medical officer there in 1968. However, his account[70,71] of the moral outrage he developed from serving in the conflict (" . . . one of the most antilife enterprises of our time"[70(p272)]) is noteworthy because of his specific condemnation of the combat psychiatry doctrine. He remarked:

> I was confronted with several cases of 'combat neurosis' who told me that they saw nothing in what they were doing that justified the risks they were being asked to take. In effect, they had seen enough of death to know that they preferred life.
>
> What was I to do with deviant behavior like that? They were given a brief respite and returned to their units; the fighting strength was conserved. How many were later killed I do not know, nor do I wish to.[70(pp268–269)]

Compared with the more confident accounts by psychiatrists who served in the first half of the conflict,[43,46,58,72–74] ones who went during the second half, such as Camp (as quoted in Ingraham and Manning),[18] Char,[75] Colbach,[45] Fisher,[76] Joseph,[77] and Ratner,[78] exhibited more frustration and cynicism. Collectively, they give the impression that conventional military psychiatric structures and doctrine were inadequate to address the burgeoning psychiatric and behavioral problems of the later years of the Vietnam conflict.

The anguish described by Colbach, also a civilian-trained psychiatrist, suggests the moral uncertainty of those who served in the second half of the conflict. Shortly after Colbach's service in Vietnam (1968 to 1969), Colbach and Parrish published an overview of U.S. Army mental health activities since the conflict began that included a justification for the combat psychiatry doctrine there: "If one soldier is relieved of this duty, another will have to replace him. And the soldier replaced by another will have to live a long time with the realization that he was so 'sick,' so weak, that someone else had to take over for him when the chips were really down."[79(p341)]

Fifteen years later, Colbach[45] wrote a personally and professionally wrenching retrospection on his role and activities in Vietnam, which evidently haunted him long after his return. Throughout his narrative, there are expressions of conflict and regret. For example, he believed that his anger at being sent to Vietnam interfered with his empathy for his soldier-patients: ". . . in many ways I was a failure in actually reaching out to those fellows and touching them and alleviating their suffering"[45(p265)] Like Bloch, Colbach was resigned to being the "guardian of reality."[45(p265)] However, this position seemed to give him little relief from his role-linked guilt: "I tried to help my patients learn that lesson [that all of life is a struggle], not to quit but to go on. Probably a few of them did learn that, if they survived."[45(p265)]

Ultimately, Colbach found an ethical position he hoped would bring him peace of mind: "Whether the Vietnam conflict fits these criteria [of a just war] or not is really beyond me to say. I did accept it as a just war when I agreed to serve in it. . . . I then had to accept that my obligation to my individual patient was far superseded by my obligation to the military and, eventually, to my country."[45(p265)]

A Survey of Psychiatrists Who Served in Vietnam

The results of a 1983 survey by Camp and Carney[80,81] of 115 psychiatrists (of an estimated total of 135) who served with the U.S. Army in Vietnam appear to verify that Colbach's struggle was not unique. When respondents were asked to include personal reactions to the professional challenges they faced there, a large proportion, especially among those who served in the second half of the conflict, emphasized that they still felt quite strongly—typically, embittered—about the conflict and their role in it. For example, one psychiatrist noted, "I have yet to find the peace of mind that would allow [me] to watch any of the Vietnam conflict movies, or talk about the war without threat of loss of control."[81(p28)] Many indicated that they had felt overwhelmed, betrayed, and blamed—overwhelmed by a raging drug epidemic, eruptions of racial animosities, and outbreaks of violence; betrayed by the army because of their poor preparation and support in the theater; and blamed by their stateside colleagues and countrymen for doing the job they were required to do.

The following quotes (collected during Camp and Carney's research[80,81] but not previously published), all from individuals who received their psychiatric training in civilian programs and who served in the second half of the conflict, illustrate the confusion that many acknowledged:

> I soon adapted by realizing I could only be of use by cooperating with the military in most ways. To have tried to be another Ghandi would have been pointless and would have deprived those few I could help with my expertise.

> As my year in Vietnam passed my ethical dilemma increased some, but I was hired by the Army, not the specific patient. The second fact was that I knew if I wanted to try to do something for a specific person, I knew someone else would have to come to Vietnam to take his place.

> . . . I accepted my assignment as an obligation despite my conviction as early as 1964 that our involvement was stupid, would fail, would be a disastrous waste of wealth, power, and lives, and was unjustified politically, historically, and morally. . . . I did not feel strong ethical conflict over my role in the Army in Vietnam. . . . The therapeutic technique of psychiatry is inimical to the military cast of mind and would probably undermine morale and exacerbate disciplinary problems with many soldiers.

On the other hand, some study participants denied feeling ethical strain in Vietnam, while others indicated that they intentionally shielded patients. For example, a psychiatrist who served with one of the specialized psychiatric units responded, "What [ethical] dilemma—I evac'd them all to Japan!"

Role Dilemmas for All Psychiatrists During the Conflict

A number of Vietnam-era authors explored the functional and ethical dilemmas inherent in military psychiatry that are indirectly linked to the combat theater role.[82–90] Many suggested that psychiatrists serving in the military had invariably abandoned or corrupted their medical ethics. For example, Daniels referred to the military psychiatrist as a "captive professional."[84(p255)] Friedman saw him as ". . . the overseer of a system of social control which is distinctly nonmedical in its character."[87(p122)] Locke[88] contended that psychiatrists who serve with the military are systematically persuaded to dehumanize the soldier, prosecute the war, and betray their individualist values. Barr and Zunin[86] took the criticism of military psychiatrists a step farther and recommended that their designation be changed from medical officer to "psychiatric military officer" in order to warn drafted psychiatrists and soldiers of the replacement of their medical ethics by those of the institution.

Concern for these ethical dilemmas was not confined to the psychiatrists serving with the military services during the Vietnam conflict. A number of civilian psychiatrists indicated that they were deeply troubled by conducting evaluations of young draft-eligible men with symptoms that apparently arose in response to the threat of being drafted.[91–97] Several were overtly suspicious of the allegiances of military psychiatrists. For example, Kirshner[96] suggested that military psychiatrists were antitherapeutic when they evaluated and treated dissenting soldiers because of countertransference obstacles based on the psychiatrist's unresolved identity issues. Ollendorff and Adams defined the military-oriented "establishment" psychiatrist as one who is corrupt and who "declares as fit everybody who is not dead."[95(p89)]

In Support of Military Psychiatry

There were a few publications in the latter half of the conflict and afterward that sought to justify the role, doctrine, and methods used by military psychiatrists in Vietnam. Generally, these publications were by career military psychiatrists, such as Arthur,[10] Brown,[61] Gibbs,[98] Hays,[99] Parrish,[100] and Johnson,[101] and were more restrained than those of critics.

One exception is found in the review by Bey and Chapman;[41] Bey is a civilian-trained psychiatrist who served with a combat division in Vietnam (1969 to 1970). They unapologetically argue that the "vast differences" between military and civilian psychiatry are necessary to support wartime mobilization, and the military psychiatrist's first priority must be the predominance of collective goals and values over those of the individual.

Lingering Criticism of the Treatment Doctrine Since Vietnam

As the numbers of veterans reporting post-Vietnam psychiatric symptoms and adjustment difficulties grew in the years following the cessation of hostilities in Southeast Asia, criticism of the doctrine of combat psychiatry resurfaced in the form of speculations that it had generated these delayed casualties for the sake of questionable military goals.[62,102–105] For example, Abse comments:

> Such [PTSD] patients in my experience have not received early effective treatment with emphasis on cathartic psychotherapy. On the contrary, they received, while in Vietnam, treatment which emphasized massive psychotropic medication, followed by crowding out with sundry recreational activities any focus on their essentially traumatic and pathogenic experiences. Such temporary suppressive treatment invited the reinforcement of dissociation though it may have worked for the while, while the soldier was in active service overseas.[103(p20)]

However, no correlation has been found between proximate combat-generated psychiatric difficulties in Vietnam and psychiatric problems in readjustment to stateside life.[106]

ETHICAL DILEMMAS IN THE TREATMENT OF COMBAT STRESS REACTIONS

The Military Psychiatrist as a "Double Agent"

Before an attempt to analyze the ethical conflicts associated with the treatment of combat reaction cases can be made, the military psychiatrist's "double agent" status must be underscored.[107] For physicians, being a double agent refers to professional situations that involve responsibilities to a patient that may contradict fiduciary ones (a contractual arrangement based on trust). More specific to the military psychiatrist, the double agent conflict follows from the fact that because they work for the military, their professional responsibilities typically include both patient-centered, therapeutic decisions and organization-centered, administrative decisions.[108] Furthermore, because there is considerable professional disagreement about mental health norms,[109] balancing loyalties can become more difficult for psychiatrists than for other types of military physicians. In addition to being affected by the values of the military organization, their clinical decisions may also reflect their personal ideology,[85,90] training, and experience,[81] as well as changing social contexts.[45]

Effective Treatment May Not Be Ethical Treatment

In November, 1967, Specialist 4th Class (Sp4) Frank Gentili (case material disguised), a 20-year-old infantryman who had been assigned in Vietnam for 5 months, was transported by helicopter to a U.S. Army evacuation hospital along with other combat casualties. On his arrival, he was observed to be mute, grunting incomprehensibly, and posturing. He was quite disorganized and could not communicate with his examiners. He was easily startled by noises and walked with a slow, shuffling gait. When he sat in a chair, he rocked with his eyes closed and occasionally mumbled "Mama." The results of his physical examination were otherwise normal.

On the psychiatric unit, Sp4 Gentili was given a shower, reassurance, and was "put to sleep" with chlorpromazine (dose not available). When he awoke 18 hours later he seemed alert, coherent, and rational. He was issued a fresh uniform and received instructions about the quasi-military ward routine. The staff told him that he was recovering from overexposure to combat and that he could expect to be returned to his military unit soon. In the group therapy meeting, Sp4 Gentili emotionally told how he had been serving as a fire team leader when six of his friends were killed and mutilated by enemy fire and described how he had become agitated and began screaming while loading their bodies into a helicopter. He talked of his revulsion at the killing and his regret that he had "gone to pieces." He felt torn because he always sought to be "good" and wanted to be a good soldier, but that it just was not his "make-up" to kill. He declared that he could not return to the field. The record notes that the psychiatric staff responded to Sp4 Gentili's feelings "with reality-testing and ego support of his duty and mission." That night he was informed that he would be returning to his unit the following day, and he was again given chlorpromazine.

Because of his rapid improvement and lack of a past psychiatric history, Sp4 Gentili was discharged back to his unit with the diagnosis of "combat exhaustion." It was also recommended that he be reexamined by his division psychiatrist if his symptoms recurred.

Except for the addition of chlorpromazine, this soldier would have been managed similarly by military psychiatrists during the latter phases of World War I, in World War II, or in the Korean conflict, and probably with the same rapid return to duty.[43] In those wars, the military doctrine's effectiveness in fulfilling its treatment goal was unambiguous.[18] However, just as legality is not a sure test of morality, neither is treatment effectiveness. The challenges to the military treatment doctrine from the Vietnam conflict era raised questions centered around how loyal military psychiatrists were to the welfare of their soldier-patients in the process. Using the case of Sp4 Gentili, a closer look at the criticisms, such as that of Livingston,[70] suggests two confounded questions: (1) Was his treatment and disposition by military psychiatrists unethical because it primarily served, as some believed, the prosecution of an immoral war? (2) Was his treatment and disposition unethical because it served military expediency at the expense of his interests or welfare?

The answer to the first question is logically straightforward. Any professional activity by military psychiatrists that contributes to an immoral or unjust war would be immoral and unethical. However, in reality such a judgment on the morality of a war remains inconclusive with respect to Vietnam.[110] Many share the view that the Vietnam conflict was categorically immoral.[2,111] In addition, specific combat activities, such as atrocities, may be readily distinguishable as immoral. Others would justify the U.S. intervention in Vietnam on the basis of the principles of international law established after World War II by the military tribunal at Nuremberg.[112] Furthermore, a link between particular immoral combat activities and the specific clinical activities of military psychiatrists may be very difficult to establish.

The Challenge of Distinguishing Harm and Benefit

The second and more general question regarding the psychiatrist's obligation to the soldier is also complicated and has implications for the use of the military treatment doctrine in any war. Because of his double agent position, the combat psychiatrist faces an array of competing values and influences and, therefore, is responsible for the effects of his treatments in terms of the balance of harm and benefit.[113]

The Question of Harm to the Soldier

Is it likely that Sp4 Gentili was harmed by the combat psychiatry treatment approach because it put him in unreasonable jeopardy in subsequent combat? If he was only partially treated, or if he was still under the sedating effect of chlorpromazine, or because of his already demonstrated susceptibility, his vulnerability in combat may have been greatly increased.[114]

As was mentioned previously, the question of the effects of the neuroleptic and anxiolytic drugs on the performance (or vulnerability) of combat soldiers who served in Vietnam has not been studied. A study by Palinkas and Coben[115] did, however, suggest that, at least for some diagnostic groups, returning soldiers to combat exposure after psychiatric hospitalization may have increased their risks. According to these authors' review of the records for all U.S. Marines deployed in Vietnam throughout the conflict (N = 78,756), psychiatric hospitalization was significantly associated with an increased risk of becoming subsequently wounded among those diagnosed with social maladjustment, psychosomatic conditions, "nervous and debility [sic]," transient situational disturbance, and acute situational maladjustment. However, the 243 Marines listed specifically as having combat fatigue were not shown to be at greater risk.

The Question of Benefit to the Soldier

Is it likely that Sp4 Gentili benefitted by being treated according to the combat psychiatry doctrine? Psychiatric morbidity in prior wars was greatly reduced among soldiers affected with combat stress reaction who were treated and managed according to the traditional doctrine[57] because it apparently (1) reinforced the soldiers psychological defenses against subsequent breakdown in combat and (2) opposed the fixation of his symptoms into a "self-protective disabling neurotic compromise."[7(p731)] It was the impression of the earlier military psychiatrists that through suppressive and repressive clinical means, they could strengthen the affected combat soldier's investment in his combat comrades, leaders, and objectives, as well as reinforce his confidence in his own capabilities, thereby reestablishing his primary psychological resistance against further combat-induced disorganization:

> [To adapt to combat the soldier must] fuse his personal identity with the new group identity, to form deep emotional relationships with his buddies and with his leader, in sharing boredom, hardship, sacrifice and danger with them, and whether by compromise or illusion, to become oriented with them toward the destructive goals which he understands to be necessary for the common good.[19(p365)]

Deeper, longer, or more complicated treatments, and especially those occurring far from the soldier's original unit and in more comfortable surroundings, were found as far back as World War I to favor the development of chronic psychiatric disability.[116] Glass commented on the disadvantage of using uncovering therapies:

> Indeed, any therapy, including usual interview methods, that sought to uncover basic emotional conflicts or attempted to relate current behavior and symptoms with past personality patterns seemingly provided patients with logical reasons for their combat failure. The insights obtained by even such mild depth therapy readily convinced the patient, and often his therapist, that the limit of combat endurance had been reached as proved by vulnerable personality traits.[7(p727)]

The Question of Coercive Treatment and Its Benefit to Society

Was Sp4 Gentili's treatment unethical because his combat stress reaction represented the combat refusal of a dissident or because it is normal not to want to return? By labeling him with the exclusively military diagnosis combat exhaustion, disregarding his opposition to further combat, and imposing the military doctrine's treatment regimen, were his military psychiatrists blaming the victim?[84] Some writers have even referred to the soldier's new willingness to enter combat after such coercive treatment as an iatrogenic psychosis.[1,62]

The matter of informed consent or refusal is especially critical when psychiatrists are representing the interests of other parties in addition to those of their patients.[117] In Sp4 Gentili's presenting condition of near catatonia, he was not competent to understand an adequate consent process and there can be little doubt about the rightfulness of treating him as the military psychiatrists deemed necessary. However, on the following day, his regression and decompensation had largely resolved, and the situation became quite different. He was treated with more chlorpromazine and behavioral strategies, including exhortation of the duty side of his conflict to sway him from his expressed (at least initially) opposition to killing, and he was rapidly returned to more combat duty. No matter what efforts the treatment team might have expended to obtain Sp4 Gentili's consent, the existence of a powerful negative incentive, that is, the threat of a court martial, eliminated the possibility of informed consent or refusal. Because these clinical techniques were imposed on an individual who was sufficiently competent and rational to cooperate with a consent process, Sp4 Gentili's treatment was technically coercive by definition and violated a "moral rule" (against causing pain and depriving freedom).[113]

There may, however, be overriding moral justification for coercive treatment when it is felt to serve the best interests of the patient (so called paternalistic treatment[113]), but in civilian settings, the paternalism exception to the moral rule does not apply to rational, competent adults. However, because the rights of those in active military service have historically been abridged by law, these boundaries are less certain.[2] In fact, there are numerous military regulations and policies that shape the practice of psychiatry to represent the preeminence of institutional goals and values over those of the individual.[41,118] Besides the absence of a right to informed consent or refusal with regard to hospitalization or psychiatric treatment, there are also limitations in the service member's rights to privileged communication[22] and to psychiatric due process.[119]

There also may be overriding moral justification for coercive treatment when the treatment is deemed necessary for the welfare of others (so called utilitarian value). Was there sufficient benefit to society to justify treating Sp4 Gentili according to the combat psychiatry doctrine? That is, in overriding his autonomous choice and quickly returning him to fight again in spite of some additional risk to him, was his treatment team serving a superseding value representing the welfare of the American people? As a soldier, was he obligated to unconditionally sacrifice his self-interest for the common good?

Some individuals would argue that a treatment approach that justifies the sacrifice of the interests of the individual soldier in the service of society may simply coincide with the military's value of teamwork and combat efficiency in some situations. The military's values can diverge from those of society, as many believe was the case in Vietnam. In practice, it is unrealistic to believe that the combat psychiatrist can distinguish at any given time whether the military treatment doctrine serves essential public welfare or only conforms to military objectives, political goals, or a war's popularity. Furthermore, this uncertainty may compound the already difficult task of determining clinically whether a soldier who is opposed to returning to combat is suffering from a mental disorder or expressing a rational refusal.[109] Brill's comment from World War II illustrates the influence of the seeming utilitarian values on clinical judgment: "It was difficult to define exactly how much of such patients' ineffectiveness was due to illness and how much to lack of desire to do their part."[120(p242)]

DISCUSSION

The Ethical Foundation of Traditional Military Psychiatry

How can we understand the emergence of such strenuous opposition to the combat psychiatry doctrine in Vietnam and the subsequent weakening of the professional credibility of military psychiatry during the Vietnam conflict era? Evidently, under the conditions of more "popular" wars—World War I, World War II, and the Korean conflict—psychiatrists serving in the military apparently experienced little ethical strain, even though they required reorientation from civilian values.[8] The traditional military treatment doctrine rested on a foundation of mutually reinforcing ethical positions that seemed sufficiently humanitarian to provide military psychiatrists with the moral context for their clinical interventions. These earlier combat psychiatrists believed that not only were they conforming to the expectations and values of the military, but even more important, there was congruence between what was perceived to be best for the soldier and best for society. It was felt that the doctrine not only contributed to America's defense but also represented the most effective, scientifically based regimen for protecting soldiers from further combat traumatization and from chronic psychiatric disability. Thus, it seemed apparent that the psychiatrist who failed to understand both sides of the soldier's struggle to overcome his fear and his own moral dilemma could overly empathize with the soldier's self-protective tendencies and "overdiagnose" and "overevacuate" such soldiers, inadvertently increase psychiatric morbidity, and risk negatively affecting the military situation.[4]

Furthermore, these early psychiatrists had confidence in the morality of their treatment goals and methods because of supportive positions taken by organized psychiatry.[9] They believed that their professional activities were consistent with the ethical principles of their profession.

Psychiatry's Ethical Ambiguity Concerning Vietnam

The Vietnam conflict provides a vastly different picture. Evidently, the alignment of justifying moral principles for combat psychiatry's doctrine that had held throughout the earlier wars was precariously balanced. As the conflict in Vietnam dragged on and the numbers of casualties reached an intolerable level for the American public, doubts arose about what constituted the ethical practice of military psychiatry. Such doubts also coincided with the rising social consciousness in the late 1960s and early 1970s and the increased proportion of civilian-trained psychiatrists assigned to the military in Vietnam.[81] Many military psychiatrists who served in the second half of the Vietnam conflict felt inclined to identify with the dissent of the vast numbers of soldiers who were—for the first time in the modern history of American warfare—themselves opposed to the nation's political and military objectives. These replacement psychiatrists became concerned that the military treatment doctrine was not humanitarian and might only serve authoritarian and political ends (ie, violating *primum non nocere*). They questioned the treatment regimen that would induce soldiers to believe that further exposure to combat was in their best interests and evidently worried that they could "expect" soldiers to risk their lives or their mental stability without moral justification.

In spite of their attempts to find the balance between harm and benefit, military psychiatrists in Vietnam functioned in the dark. Although they knew of the successful implementation of the military treatment doctrine in past wars, they had no reliable information about whether their patients might face unacceptable risks because of its use in Vietnam. Nor could they comprehend whether the doctrine truly served public welfare. Even if the conflict met the standard for a just war by international law, its morality for the psychiatrist in Vietnam, just as for the soldier or citizen, may have been far more subjectively determined.[2]

The Military Psychiatrist as Scapegoat

The ethical burden for Vietnam's combat psychiatrists was magnified because they struggled with these issues alone. Psychiatry failed to recognize their dilemma, provide them with ethical sanctions, or monitor the institutional regulations, policies, and treatment doctrine that affected the practice of military psychiatry. Furthermore, the tendency for critics such as Lifton[62] to equate the questions about the institutional abuse of psychiatry with those regarding the conduct of the individual psychiatrist greatly added to the combat psychiatrists' role confusion. A more realistic consideration would acknowledge the impossible contradiction of military and professional obligations under those circumstances. In the words of Boman, "The role of the military psychiatrist in a conflict like Vietnam encompasses so many ambiguities and moral dilemmas that one would not be surprised at his lapsing into almost a state of frozen ambivalence"[21(p124)] London[121(pp249–250)] went further by challenging the new "moralistic 'right think'" of those who would fault military psychiatrists for not actively opposing the military in Vietnam, "... it is unseemly, if not immoral, to retrospectively condemn the doctors of last decade's war for doing what then looked like their duty. . . ."[121(p250)]

Section three of the APA's principles of medical ethics with annotations especially applicable to psychiatry[117] speaks of the psychiatrist's obligation to provide the best possible care within the constraints of the system while striving to change those conditions that are not in the best interests of the patient. However, it is unclear what could have been done differently by military psychiatrists during the Vietnam era. Opposition to military regulations and policies by individual professionals appears self-defeating if one considers the examples of social worker Meshad,[122] general medical officer Livingston,[71] psychiatrist Locke,[88] and the well-publicized court martial in 1967 of dermatologist H. Levy, as commented on by Veatch.[123]

CONCLUSION

Although this chapter seeks to understand the negative impact of the Vietnam conflict on the psychiatrists who served there and the degradation of the prestige of military psychiatry, perhaps it contributes little more than to express lamentations following a failed war. If the United States had achieved its military and political goals in Southeast Asia, would concerns about a doctrine that urges soldiers to return to the fight be taken seriously? It certainly seems self-evident that as the country loses its will to make sacrifices for the sake of fighting a war, soldiers will quickly become demoralized, and the psychiatrists sent to support them will struggle as well.

Still, it has been amply documented how the Vietnam conflict's unpopularity and the collective sense of its wrongfulness affected America's combatants; however, far too little has been said regarding the impact of these aspects on healthcare providers such as psychiatrists and allied medical personnel. This chapter's inclusion of the personal reactions from the Vietnam era—testimony that is typically absent from the analyses of moral philosophers and bioethicists—seeks to recognize the agony of the psychiatrists (and others) who wrestled with the Vietnam conflict's moral and ethical questions.

The moral dilemma for combat psychiatrists in Vietnam was no greater than that for the soldier or military leaders. Furthermore, their service there was clearly less physically hazardous. Nevertheless, might psychiatry and the nation owe some measure of gratitude and acknowledgment to these men and women in consideration of their impossible task and the personal sacrifices they sustained in performing the duties that their country asked of them?

Regarding the more general questions surrounding the implementation of the traditional combat psychiatry treatment doctrine, in the more than two decades since American troops were withdrawn from Vietnam, there has been regrettably little interest in resolving challenges that arose during the conflict regarding its ethical justification. In the wars before Vietnam, this doctrine had proved to be highly effective for treating individuals with combat stress reactions and returning them to duty. Furthermore, it was uncontroversial and later successfully adapted for use with civilian populations. As this review of the doctrine's rationale and ethical quandaries suggests, combat psychiatrists are influenced by powerful, potentially competing value systems but cannot always appreciate some of the most important factors that affect the balance of harm and benefit associated with their treatment decisions.

Surely, it can be said that psychiatry as a profession buried its bitter Vietnam memories after the conflict and that they have yet to be assimilated. Yet critical moral and ethical questions regarding the loyalties of combat psychiatrists remain. Rather than replacing the wrenching memories of the Vietnam conflict and the associated decadent and divisive epoch with amnesia, psychiatry and its military representatives should seek consensus regarding the unique collection of ethical dilemmas that can surround the delivery of psychiatric care under combat conditions. More specifically, future research and study should be devoted to the establishment of fundamental ethical standards and formalized professional guidelines for the treatment of military casualties. Otherwise, there remains, as there was during the Vietnam conflict, a greater burden of conscience borne by each psychiatrist who serves.

REFERENCES

1. Veatch RM. The psychiatrist's role in war. In: Veatch RM, ed. *Case Studies in Medical Ethics*. Cambridge, Mass: Harvard University Press; 1977: 245–251.
2. Walzer M. *Just and Unjust Wars: A Moral Argument with Historical Illustrations*. New York: Basic Books; 1977.
3. US Department of the Army. *Neuropsychiatry and Mental Health*. Washington, DC: DA; 1984. Army Regulation 40–216.
4. Johnson AW, Jr. Combat psychiatry: Part I. A historical review. *Med Bull U.S. Army Europe*. 1969;25:305–308.
5. Maskin M. Something about a soldier. *Psychiatry*. 1946;9:189–195.
6. Peterson DB, Chambers RE. Restatement of combat psychiatry. *Am J Psychiatry*. 1952;109:249–254.
7. Glass AJ. Psychotherapy in the combat zone. *Am J Psychiatry*. 1954;110:725–731.
8. Glass AJ. Lessons learned. In: *Overseas Theaters*. Vol 2. In: Glass AJ, ed. *Neuropsychiatry in World War II*. Washington, DC: GPO; 1973: 989–1027. GPO Stock No. 0832–00047.
9. Glass AJ. Army psychiatry before World War II. In: *Zone of the Interior*. Vol 1. In: Glass, AJ. Bernucci RJ, eds. *Neuropsychiatry in World War II*. Washington, DC: GPO; 1966: 3–23.
10. Arthur RJ. Reflections on military psychiatry. *Am J Psychiatry*. 1978;135:2–7.
11. Farrell MJ, Berlien IC. Professional personnel. In: *Zone of the Interior*. Vol 1. In: Glass, AJ. Bernucci RJ, eds. *Neuropsychiatry in World War II*. Washington, DC: GPO; 1966: 41–51.
12. Grob GN. Origins of DSM–I: A study in appearance and reality. *Am J Psychiatry*. 1991;148:421–431.
13. Artiss KL. Human behavior under stress—From combat to social psychiatry. *Milit Med*. 1963;128:1011–1015.

14. Glass AJ. Military psychiatry and changing systems of mental health care. *J Psychiatr Res.* 1971;8:499–512.

15. Budman SH, Gurman AS. *Theory and Practice of Brief Therapy.* New York: Guilford Press; 1988.

16. Gabriel RA. *No More Heroes: Madness & Psychiatry in War.* Westport, Conn: Greenwood Press; 1987.

17. Keegan J. *The Face of Battle: A Study of Agincourt, Waterloo and the Somme.* New York: Penguin Books; 1978.

18. Ingraham L, Manning F. American military psychiatry. In: Gabriel RA, ed. *Military Psychiatry: A Comparative Perspective.* Westport, Conn: Greenwood Press; 1986: 25–65.

19. Bartemeier LH, Kubie LS, Menninger KA, Romano J, Whitehorn JC. Combat exhaustion. *J Nerv Ment Dis.* 1946;104:358–389.

20. Glass AJ. Introduction. In: Bourne PG, ed. *The Psychology and Physiology of Stress: With Reference to Special Studies of the Viet Nam War.* New York: Academic Press; 1969: xiii-xxx.

21. Boman B. The Vietnam veteran ten years on. *Aust N Z J Psychiatry.* 1982;16:107–127.

22. Ursano RJ, Holloway, HC. Military psychiatry. In: Kaplan I, Sadock BJ, eds. *Comprehensive Textbook of Psychiatry IV.* Baltimore: Williams and Wilkins; 1985: 1900–1909.

23. Bailey P, Williams FE, Komora PO. In: *Neuropsychiatry in the United States.* Vol 10. In: *The Medical Department of the United States Army in the World War.* Washington, DC: GPO; 1929.

24. Robins LN, Helzer JE, Davis DH. Narcotic use in Southeast Asia and afterward. *Arch Gen Psychiatry.* 1975;32:955–961.

25. American Psychiatric Association. *Diagnostic and Statistical Manual of Mental Disorders.* 3rd ed. Revised. Washington, DC: American Psychiatric Association; 1987.

26. Jones FD. Future directions of military psychiatry. In: Gabriel RA, ed. *Military Psychiatry: A Comparative Perspective.* Westport, Conn: Greenwood Press; 1986: 181–204.

27. World Health Organization. *Mental Disorders: Glossary and Guide to Their Classification in Accordance with the Ninth Revision of the International Classification of Diseases.* Geneva, Switzerland: World Health Organization; 1978.

28. Rahe RH. Acute versus chronic psychological reactions to combat. *Milit Med.* 1988;153:365–371.

29. Shaw JA. Unmasking the illusion of safety. *Bull Menninger Clin.* 1987;51:49–63.

30. Blank AS, Jr. The longitudinal course of Posttraumatic Stress Disorder. In: Davidson JRT, Foa EB, eds. *Posttraumatic Stress Disorder: DSM–IV and Beyond.* Washington, DC: American Psychiatric Press; 1992.

31. Erikson E. Relevance and relativity in the case history. In: Erickson E, ed. *Childhood and Society.* New York: WW Norton; 1950: 23–47.

32. Shaw JA. Psychodynamic considerations in the adaptation to combat. In: Belenky G, ed. *Contemporary Studies in Combat Psychiatry.* Westport, Conn: Greenwood Press; 1987: 117–132.

33. Horowitz MJ. Posttraumatic stress disorder. In: *Treatments of Psychiatric Disorders: A Task Force Report of the American Psychiatric Association.* Washington, DC: American Psychiatric Association; 1989: 2065–2082.

34. Marlowe D. The human dimension of battle and combat breakdown. In: Gabriel RA, ed. *Military Psychiatry: A Comparative Perspective.* Westport, Conn: Greenwood Press; 1986: 7–24.

35. Belenky GL. Varieties of reaction and adaption to combat experience. *Bull Menninger Clin.* 1987;51:64–79.

36. Glass AJ. Observations upon the epidemiology of mental illness in troops during warfare. In: *Symposium on Preventive and Social Psychiatry.* Washington, DC: Walter Reed Army Institute of Research; 15–17 April 1958: 185–198.

37. Noy S. Stress and personality as factors in the causation and prognosis of combat reaction. In: Belenky G, ed. *Contemporary Studies in Combat Psychiatry.* Westport, Conn: Greenwood Press; 1987: 22–29.

38. Tischler GL. Patterns of psychiatric attrition and of behavior in a combat zone. In: Bourne PG, ed. *The Psychology and Physiology of Stress: With Reference to Special Studies of the Viet Nam War.* New York: Academic Press; 1969: 19–44.

39. Strange RE. Combat fatigue versus pseudo-combat fatigue in Vietnam. *Milit Med.* 1968;133:823–826.

40. Kormos HR. The nature of combat stress. In: Figley CR, ed. *Stress Disorders Among Vietnam Veterans.* New York: Brunner/Mazel; 1978: 3–22.

41. Bey DR, Chapman RE. Psychiatry—the right way, the wrong way, and the military way. *Bull Menninger Clin.* 1974;38:343–354.

42. Grinker RP, Spiegel JP. *Men Under Stress.* New York: McGraw-Hill; 1963.

43. Bloch HS. Army clinical psychiatry in the combat zone—1967–1968. *Am J Psychiatry.* 1969;126:289–298.

44. Bloch HS. Brief sleep treatment with chlorpromazine. *Compr Psychiatry.* 1970;11:346–355.

45. Colbach EM. Ethical issues in combat psychiatry. *Milit Med.* 1985;150:256–265.

46. Strange RE, Arthur RJ. Hospital ship psychiatry in a war zone. *Am J Psychiatry.* 1967;124:281–268.

47. Datel WE, Johnson AW, Jr. *Psychotropic Prescription Medication in Vietnam.* Alexandria, Va: Defense Technical Information Center: 1981. Document AD A 097–610.

48. Office of the Adjutant General. *Coat-of-Arms for Medical Field Service School.* Washington, DC: War Department; 1921: 424.5 Coats of Arms. Memorandum.

49. US Department of the Army. *Management of Stress in Army Operations.* Washington DC: DA; 1986. Field Manual 26–2.

50. US Department of the Army. *Health Service Support in a Theater of Operations.* Washington DC: DA; 1991. Field Manual 8–10.

51. US Department of the Army. *Brigade Division Surgeons' Handbook—Tactics, Techniques, and Procedures.* Washington DC: DA; 1991. Field Manual 8–10–5.

52. US Department of the Army. *Planning for Health Service Support.* Washington DC: DA; 1994. Field Manual 8–55.

53. US Department of the Army. *Leader's Manual for Combat Stress Control.* Washington DC. DA, In press, 1994. Field Manual 22–51.

54. US Department of the Army. *Combat Stress Control in a Theater of Operations.* Washington DC: DA; In press, 1994. Field Manual 8–51.

55. Allerton WS. Army psychiatry in Vietnam. In: Bourne PG, ed. *The Psychology and Physiology of Stress: With Reference to Special Studies of the Viet Nam War.* New York: Academic Press; 1969: 1–17.

56. Bourne PG. Military psychiatry and the Vietnam experience. *Am J Psychiatry*. 1970;127:481–488.

57. Baker SL., Jr. Traumatic war disorders. In: Kaplan HI, Freedman AM, Sadock BJ, eds. *Comprehensive Textbook of Psychiatry III*. Baltimore, Md: Williams and Wilkins; 1980: 1829–1842.

58. Motis G, Neal RD. Freud in the boonies: II. The 4th Infantry Division psychiatric field program at work in a sustained combat situation. *U.S. Army Vietnam Med Bull*. 1968;(January/February):27–30.

59. Camp NC, Stretch RH, Marshall WC. *Stress, Strain, and Vietnam: An Annotated Bibliography of Two Decades of Psychiatric and Social Sciences Literature Reflecting the Effect of the War on the American Soldier*. Westport Conn: Greenwood Press; 1988. Figures 1 and 2.

60. Jones FD, Johnson AW, Jr. Medical and psychiatric treatment policy and practice in Vietnam. *J Soc Issues*. 1975;31:49–65.

61. Brown DE. The military: A valuable arena for research and innovation. *Am J Psychiatry*. 1970;127:511–512.

62. Lifton RJ. Advocacy and corruption in the healing professions. *Conn Med*. 1975;39:803–813.

63. Lifton RJ. *The Nazi Doctors: Medical Killing and the Psychology of Genocide*. New York: Basic Books; 1976.

64. Spragg GS. Psychiatry in the Australian military forces. *Med J Aust*. 1972;1:745–751.

65. APA members hit meeting disruptions in opinion poll results. *Psychiatr News*. 1971;(March 3):1.

66. Tarjan G. Highlights of the 124th annual meeting. *Am J Psychiatry*. 1971;128:137–140.

67. Psychologists, MH groups attack Vietnam war. *Psychiatr News*. 1972;(July 5):1.

68. Maier T. The Army psychiatrist: An adjunct to the system of social control. *Am J Psychiatry*. 1970;126:1039. Letter.

69. Bloch HS. Dr. Bloch replies. *Am J Psychiatry*. 1970;126:1039–1040. Letter.

70. Livingston GS. Medicine in the military. In: Visscher M, ed. *Perspectives in Medical Ethics*. Buffalo, NY: Prometheus Books; 1972: 266–274.

71. Livingston GS. Letter from a Vietnam veteran. *Saturday Rev*. 1969;(September 20):22–23.

72. Conte LR. A neuropsychiatry team in Vietnam 1966–1967: An overview. In: Parker RS, ed. *The Emotional Stress of War, Violence and Peace*. Pittsburgh, Penn: Stanwix House; 1972: 163–168.

73. Jones FD. Experiences of a division psychiatrist in Vietnam. *Milit Med*. 1967;132:1003–1008.

74. Motis G. Freud in the boonies: A preliminary report on the psychiatric field program in the 4th Infantry Division. *U.S. Army Vietnam Med Bull*. 1967;(September/October):5–8.

75. Char J. Drug abuse in Vietnam. *Am J Psychiatry*. 1972;129:463–465.

76. Fisher HW. Vietnam psychiatry: Portrait of anarchy. *Minn Med*. 1972;55:1165–1167.

77. Joseph BS. Lessons on heroin abuse from treating users in Vietnam. *Hosp Community Psychiatry*. 1974;25:742–744.

78. Ratner RA. Drugs and despair in Vietnam. *U Chicago Mag*. 1972;64:15–23.

79. Colbach EM, Parrish MD. Army mental health activities in Vietnam: 1965–1970. *Bull Menninger Clin*. 1970;31:333–342.

80. Camp NM, Carney CM. U.S. Army psychiatry in Vietnam: Preliminary findings of a survey: I. Background and method. *Bull Menninger Clin*. 1987;51:6–18.

81. Camp NM, Carney CM. U.S. Army psychiatry in Vietnam: Preliminary findings of a survey: II. Results and discussion. *Bull Menninger Clin*. 1987;51:19–37.

82. Clausen RE, Daniels AK. Role conflicts and their ideological resolution in military psychiatric practice. *Am J Psychiatry*. 1966;123:280–287.

83. Dubey J. Military psychiatrist as social engineer. *Am J Psychiatry*. 1967;124:52–58.

84. Daniels AK. The captive professional: Bureaucratic limitations in the practice of military psychiatry. *J Health Soc Behav*. 1969;10:255–265.

85. Sullivan PR. Influence of personal values on psychiatric judgement. *J Nerv Ment Dis*. 1971;152:193–198.

86. Barr NI, Zunin LM. Clarification of the psychiatrist's dilemma while in military service. *Am J Orthopsychiatry*. 1971;41:672–674.

87. Friedman HJ. Military psychiatry: Limitations of the current preventive approach. *Arch Gen Psychiatry*. 1972;26:118–123.

88. Locke K. Notes on the adjustment of a psychiatrist to the military. *Psych Op*. 1972;9:17–21.

89. Perlman MS. Basic problems of military psychiatry: Delayed reaction in Vietnam veterans. *Int J Offender Ther Compar Criminol*. 1975;19:129–138.

90. Weitzel WD. A psychiatrist in a bureaucracy: The unsettling compromises. *Hosp Community Psychiatry*. 1976;29:644–647.

91. Frank IM, Hoedemaker FS. The civilian psychiatrist and the draft. *Am J Psychiatry*. 1970;127:497–502.

92. Liberman RP, Sonnenberg SM, Stern MS, with Brown DE, Jr. Psychiatric evaluations for young men facing the draft. *Am J Psychiatry*. 1971;128:147–152.

93. Moskowitz JA. On drafting the psychiatric "draft" letter. *Am J Psychiatry*. 1971;128:69–72.

94. Roemer PA. The psychiatrist and the draft evader. *Am J Psychiatry*. 1971;127:1236–1237. Letter.

95. Ollendorff RH, Adams PL. Psychiatry and the draft. *Am J Orthopsychiatry*. 1971;41:85–90.

96. Kirshner LA. Countertransference issues in the treatment of the military dissenter. *Am J Orthopsychiatry*. 1973;43:654–659.

97. Robitscher J. *The Powers of Psychiatry*. Boston: Houghton Mifflin; 1980.

98. Gibbs JJ. Military psychiatry: Reflections and projections. *Psych Op*. 1973;10:20–23.

99. Hays FW. Lest we forget. *Milit Med*. 1977;142:263–267.

100. Parrish MD. A veteran of three wars looks at psychiatry in the military. *Psych Op*. 1972;9:6–11.

101. Johnson AW. Jr. Combat psychiatry: Part II. The U.S. Army in Vietnam. *Med Bull U.S. Army Europe*. 1969;25:335–339.

102. Shatan CF. How do we turn off the guilt? *Human Behav*. 1973;2:56–61.

103. Abse DW. Brief historical overview of the concept of war neurosis and of associated treatment methods. In: Schwartz HJ, ed. *Psychotherapy of the Combat Veteran.* New York: Spectrum Publications; 1984: 1–22.

104. DeFazio VJ. Psychoanalytic psychotherapy and the Vietnam veteran. In: Schwartz HJ, ed. *Psychotherapy of the Combat Veteran.* New York: Spectrum Publications; 1984: 23–46.

105. Kolb LC. Post-traumatic stress disorders in Vietnam veterans. *N Engl J Med.* 1986;314:461–642. Editorial.

106. Research Triangle Institute. *National Vietnam Veterans Readjustment Study.* Research Triangle Park, NC: Research Triangle Institute; 1988.

107. Hastings Center Report. *In the Service of the State: The Psychiatrist as Double Agent: Special Supplement.* Washington, DC: The Hastings Center Institute of Society, Ethics and the Life Sciences; 1978.

108. Lomas HD, Berman JD. Diagnosing for administrative purposes: Some ethical problems. *Soc Sci Med.* 1983;17:241–244.

109. Sider RC. Mental health norms and ethical practice. *Psychiatric Annals.* 1983;13:302–309.

110. Butterfield F. The new Vietnam scholarship. *NY Times Mag.* 1983;(February):26–35, 45–47, 52–58.

111. Falk RA, Kolko G, Lifton RJ, eds. *Crimes of War.* New York: Random House; 1971.

112. Ferencz BB. War crimes law and the Vietnam war. *Am U Law Rev.* 1968;17:403–423.

113. Group for the Advancement of Psychiatry. *A Casebook in Psychiatric Ethics.* New York: Brunner-Mazel; 1990.

114. Brass A. Medicine over there. *JAMA.* 1970;213:1473–1475.

115. Palinkas LA, Coben P. Psychiatric disorders among United States Marines wounded in action in Vietnam. *J Nerv Ment Dis.* 1987;175:291–300.

116. Jones FD, Hales RE. Military combat psychiatry: A historical review. *Psychiatric Annals.* 1987;17:525–527.

117. American Psychiatric Association. *Principles of Medical Ethics with Annotations Especially Applicable to Psychiatry.* Washington, DC: American Psychiatric Association; 1985.

118. Bitzer R. Caught in the middle: Mentally disabled Vietnam veterans and the Veterans Administration. In: Figley CR, Leventman S, eds. *Strangers at Home: Vietnam Veterans Since the War.* New York: Praeger; 1980: 305–323.

119. Grant WH, Resnick PJ. Right of active duty military personnel to refuse psychiatric treatment. *Behav Sci Law.* 1989;7:339–354.

120. Brill NQ. Hospitalization and disposition. In: Glass AJ, Bernucci RJ, eds. *Medical Department, United States Army, Neuropsychiatry in World War II (Vol I, Zone of the Interior).* Washington, DC: GPO; 1966: 195–253.

121. London P. Quoted by: Veatch RM. The psychiatrist's role in war. In: Veatch RM, ed. *Case Studies in Medical Ethics.* Cambridge, Mass: Harvard University Press; 1977: 245–251.

122. Meshad S. *Captain For Dark Mornings: A True Story.* Plaza Del Rey, Calif: Creative Image Associates; 1982.

123. Levy H. Cited by: Veatch RM. Soldier, physician and moral man. In: Veatch RM, ed. *Case Studies in Medical Ethics.* Cambridge, Mass: Harvard University Press; 1977: 61–64.

Chapter 9

PSYCHIATRIC CONSULTATION TO COMMAND

JAMES E. MCCARROLL, Ph.D., M.P.H.,* JOHN J. JACCARD, M.D.,† AND ALAN Q. RADKE, M.D., M.P.H.‡

*Colonel, Medical Service Corps, U.S. Army; Department of Military Psychiatry, Walter Reed Army Institute of Research, Washington, D.C. 20307–5100

†Lieutenant Colonel, Medical Corps, U.S. Army; Chief, Psychiatry Consultation-Liaison Service Department of Psychiatry, Walter Reed Army Medical Center, Washington, D.C. 20307–5001

‡Medical Director, Willmar Regional Treatment Center, Willmar, Minnesota 56201–1128

INTRODUCTION

Command consultation in the field of military medicine is the process of providing expert mental health advice to commanders on matters affecting the mental health and performance of military personnel, usually in the context of their military organization. The term *unit consultation* is a synonym that emphasizes the unit-based focus of command consultation rather than the focus on the individual. Command consultation normally occurs on the request of the commander or another person in the chain of command who has detected the potential for or existence of a problem that could be helped by mental health consultation. While this topic is presented from a psychiatric perspective, many of the principles presented here can be applied to consultation by physicians in other branches of medicine. The same principles and methods of consultation are practiced by the other disciplines in the mental health or combat stress control team: social work officers, clinical psychologists, psychiatric nurses, occupational therapists, and their noncommissioned officer counterparts.

We begin with a brief review of the origins and development of command consultation in the military. The balance of the chapter is devoted to highlighting the major steps involved in performing the consultation, ethical considerations, and risks to the consultant. We have provided many examples of previous consultations and included the experiences of senior consultants to illustrate these points.

ORIGIN AND HISTORY OF PSYCHIATRIC COMMAND CONSULTATION

Psychiatric consultation in the U.S. Army began in World War I, based on the experiences of British psychiatrists as reported by Salmon.[1] A psychiatric consultant was assigned to each corps and division. Army psychiatric consultation continued to grow, learning from the experiences of World War II[2,3] and the Korean conflict.[4] As the understanding evolved of how the stresses of military service and combat affected soldiers, the approaches of psychiatrists and other mental health professionals also evolved.

The Attempt to Screen for Psychiatric Vulnerability

Before and during the early part of World War II, psychiatrists followed the theories of psychoneurosis that were prominent at that time. These theories held that the personality was vulnerable, and breakdown occurred as a result of exposure to extreme stress.[5] They believed that psychiatric disorders did not occur in normal persons, but in weaklings or those with emotional instability that predisposed them to emotional breakdown and psychiatric illness, illness that required evacuation.[6] It was also thought that psychiatrists could screen out such conditions in advance.[7] Short interviews with psychiatrists and nonpsychiatric physicians were set up at induction stations to examine recruits for the presence of or potential for psychoneurotic illness. This screening proved to be a failure and was one of the great lessons learned in World War II psychiatry. Menninger noted that "From the point of view of manpower, we must frankly face the fact that although they were poor risks, many unstable individuals could and did make excellent records. Many men who were rejected as questionable prospects might have been good soldiers under favorable circumstances."[8(p289)]

Effective screening would have required examiners to accurately judge the degree of resistance a soldier could marshall against stress. The strengths of the emotional supports provided by social forces operating in the army were underestimated, and there was no way to measure the capacity of the soldier to identify with his unit and to obtain strength from such a social process. The resiliency of the soldier and the capacity to regain equilibrium under stress was not anticipated.

Forward Management of Psychiatric Casualties

On the war front, there was a clear need for the forward management of psychiatric casualties; major manpower losses occurred where such efforts were not made. Forsaking the practice of World War I, psychiatrists were not assigned to U.S. Army divisions until November 1943. The principles of combat psychiatry required that psychiatric casualties be treated close to their units, as soon as possible, and with the expectation that they would soon return to duty. These ideas were later conceptualized by Artiss[9] as proximity, immediacy, and expectancy, abbreviated to the acronym PIE by others. As it was put by Colonel William C. Porter, "Treat them within the sound of the artillery."[10(p350)] The implementation of these principles resulted in the return to duty of the majority of psychiatric casualties following very brief treatment and rest. It was very difficult to obtain reliable figures on the numbers of troops returned to duty, but the estimate was that after 1943, psychiatrists returned 70 to 80% of psychiatric battle casualties to duty who were thereafter indistinguishable from their soldier comrades.[8]

Whether psychiatrists could predict behavior, especially in combat, was another matter. Fortunately, some kept notes on what they did and wrote about their experiences. Several rich anecdotes were provided by Plesset[11] based on his forced "experiment" with soldiers who would most likely have been screened out by both the psychiatrist and the commander:

> It is not always possible in the army to dispose of men who appear to be undesirable. Furthermore, it is, and has been, one of the functions of the division psychiatrist to salvage and to encourage the retention of men rather than to increase the loss of manpower. For these reasons and others, there were remaining in my division after the gang plank was raised, 138 men who during training had presented sufficient adjustment difficulty to necessitate psychiatric attention. Most were the chronic complainers who were referred by their unit surgeons. They represented an assortment of neuroses and so-called constitutional psychopathic states. It was with some apprehension that I viewed their future adjustment to combat, and in order to salvage some satisfaction through the virtue of prophetic powers, I labelled the records of 25 of these as especially poor risks. I anticipated seeing most of the group of 138 in the first few days of combat or perhaps even earlier, for these were the "known" problems.
>
> Case History: Soldier aged 28—married with two children—first seen June 1944, at which time he had more than 3 years' service. Family history revealed that his parents had been separated for 16 years, and that his mother had been in a state mental hospital for 4 years. Work history indicated intermittent and variable employment. Soldier completed the 7th grade at the age of 16. He complained of headaches, dizzy spells, nervousness. He said that he felt "all tore up" and that he had periods when he remembered nothing he did for a whole day. During the interview, he was tense and fearful. He had four courts martial for A.W.O.L. He was labelled as a poor risk for combat. During combat he served in an infantry battalion and received the Bronze Star Medal for heroism. At termination of the war he was still on duty.
>
> At the end of 30 days of combat, only one of the entire group had been evacuated for "exhaustion" (army terminology in medical units forward of evacuation hospitals for psychoneurosis or other psychogenic disorders). No other had been evacuated for any reason—137 were still on duty. . . . During the first month, one had been decorated with a Bronze Star for bravery. After 60 days of combat—3 had been admitted to the Division Clearing Station for "exhaustion," 134 remained on duty. In the subsequent 3 months of combat there were no other admissions from this group for "exhaustion." Eighteen had been evacuated or transferred for other reasons (2 had been killed in action, 1 was a battle casualty, 7 were non-battle casualties and 8 were transferred for various reasons). At the termination of the war there were 120 remaining on duty. Nine had received a Purple Heart for wounds; eight had received a Bronze Star Medal for heroic or meritorious service.[11(p88)]

Army policy regarding combat psychiatry did not change until the spring of 1944, from screening to conservation of manpower,[7] and the psychiatrist's role changed from disposition of personnel to advice on how to use marginal personnel. Psychiatrists then began to function in a true preventive fashion advising on training, personnel, morale, and discipline, and lecturing on mental health and human relations. War Department Circular 48 in February 1944[7(p400)] specified the commander as responsible for developing the mental health of trainees and officially designated psychiatrists to give mental hygiene lectures to officers and enlisted men at all training camps.

Development of Preventive Psychiatry and the Consultative Approach to Mental Health Problems

Based on their findings from combat, psychiatrists felt that they had proved that social-environmental circumstances were overriding determinants of behavior, and the basis was set for wider application of preventive and consultative psychiatric services. Rioch[6] wrote that during World War II, psychiatric concepts of prevention and treatment underwent pronounced changes, almost reversals, and Appel[7] wrote that prevention began where screening left off. The preventive measure that Rioch[6] considered most important was the understanding of human relationships. The greatest defense against breakdown in combat, which can be considered a form of acute situational stress, was the development and reinforcement of group cohesiveness. One of the major lessons learned in World War II was that psychiatric disability correlated positively with external stress and was not limited to so-called intrapsychic determinants, as had been predicted.

While many psychiatrists were occupied with screening, others had been assigned to training camps. Consultation services by psychiatrists were seen with suspicion by higher level commanders who thought that consideration for the adjustment of the individual soldier was mollycoddling and would weaken the fighting man. They thought that the existence of such clinics would give official recognition to maladjustment and that lectures about mental hygiene would give soldiers the tools to malinger. These fears proved to be unfounded because 80% of maladjusted soldiers were returned to their units to complete their training, and the others were expeditiously removed.[10]

After World War II and before the consultative approach was taken, trainees with adjustment problems were treated as patients in outpatient clinics. These clinics were overwhelmed by disgruntled soldiers. Extensive psychiatric and psychological examinations did not predict future performance. Information derived from observations of work and study of the actual nature of the soldier's relations with persons in his unit were more valid predictors of performance than were extensive psychiatric and psychologic examinations. In doing traditional psychiatric examinations of trainee adjustment problems, U.S. Army mental health professionals overemphasized pathology and overpredicted failure of adjustment.[12] Psychiatrists assigned to training centers organized mental hygiene consultation centers to apply what they considered to be preventive psychiatry concepts to the stresses of basic training. During World War II, mental hygiene consultation centers were established but, after the war, were abandoned. After the Korean conflict, 35 were again established.[13] These facilities were located separately from the hospital, both geographically and administratively, and were attached to the training center headquarters. For this reason, and others, they became identified with the viewpoint of the troop commanders instead of the hospital.[7] Psychiatrists frequently observed the behavior of the troops on duty and participated in training with them, thus learning important aspects of camp life. Cases of maladjustment in training were treated by attempting to increase the soldier's affiliation with his unit and to make his adjustment to the military a positive occurrence in his life.[14] Efforts were centered on prevention: primary, secondary, and tertiary.[4,15] When treatment was performed, it was done in a milieu, mostly by technicians with the psychiatrist as supervisor.[13]

Cruvant[16] commented that the intelligent line officer is the military psychiatrist's first bulwark of offense and defense for early prevention, recognition, and prompt elimination of the psychiatrically unfit. One of the major goals of early preventive psychiatry was education of the line officers about the functions of psychiatrists. Cruvant wrote about the need for a close relationship between the line and training officers, a need that remains unchanged today. This relationship was called laborious ". . . when the psychiatrist exists as a remote, unapproachable entity within the cloistered halls of the station hospital."[16(p42)] War Department Field Manual 8–10, June 1946,[7(p410)] noted that the majority of the factors that determine the mental health of troops fall in the province of command, that staff psychiatrists and commanders would maintain close liaison, and that the psychiatrist would monitor the mental health of the command and conduct a continuous education program by formal lecture and informal discussion to instruct enlisted people and officers in mental health. He was also advised to closely monitor such matters as training schedules, leave policies, disciplinary procedures, and the need and opportunity for rest and recreation. The three areas that most affected the mental health of the men were morale, leadership, and personnel policies. The idea that psychiatric knowledge could be helpful in these areas was new to army leadership.

True primary preventive psychiatry occurred late in World War II when psychiatric advice was applied to large numbers of men. For example, psychiatrists in the Fifth Army recommended that infantry replacements be sent forward in groups who had trained together rather than as individuals.[7] Other preventive measures that were recommended were discussed by Appel and Beebe:[17] providing incentives and rewards for infantrymen, establishing a length of combat tour policy, increasing the meaning of the importance of tactical objectives for soldiers, and communicating to the soldier the reasons for fighting the war. They also noted that for preventive psychiatry to be successful, it had to demonstrate that environmental changes can contribute to the mental health of the population. Its ultimate success depended on whether stress factors could be identified that were both important causes of psychiatric disorders and subject to modification or control.

The efforts of the World War II and Korean conflict era consultative and preventive psychiatry programs were judged to be successful although evaluations of the effectiveness of the preventive psychiatry programs were difficult to obtain. Menninger[18] noted that preventive efforts during World War II were an outstanding achievement, but that no statistics were available. He concluded that the education of line and medical officers and their advice to command on mental health and morale undoubtedly accounted for a tremendous saving of manpower.

In 1960, the Group for the Advancement of Psychiatry prepared a report[19] to summarize the programs of preventive psychiatry in the armed services, to evaluate their effectiveness, to derive operational concepts, and to indicate possible applications of the principles to nonmilitary settings. The group found that there had been a decrease in the hospitalization of identifiable psychiatric disorders both in war and peace; there had been a continuing decline in medical separations for psychiatric illness; there had been no corresponding increase in loss of manpower through administrative channels or through medical separation for nonpsychotic illness when corresponding periods of time were involved; and there had been a decrease in the number and rate of disciplinary confinements. The group concluded that although the data were not as complete as might have been desired, they did indicate a significant trend showing that a loss of manpower from psychiatric disorders had been prevented. The group noted that the data could not support the idea that emotional difficulties had been prevented, but rather that ineffectiveness had definitely been reduced through the early recognition and prompt outpatient treatment of emotional difficulties during adjustment situations, combat, and noncombat.

CURRENT MODELS OF COMMAND CONSULTATION

Training

Command consultation is not a subspecialty of any mental health discipline, but is a set of skills that begin in training and increase as the individual gains experience. The same consultation skills that are used in command consultation are used in other areas of psychiatry. For example, similar skills are used by a child psychiatrist consulting to a school, in community psychiatry consulting to community agencies, and in the hospital consulting to other physicians. In hospital-based training programs, one model that seems particularly useful is that of liaison training in medical and surgical consultation, often based in consultation-liaison psychiatry training.[20] This area of training and practice is multidisciplinary and involves many of the same medical and behavioral sciences disciplines, for example, psychology and social work, that consult to commanders.

There are no firmly established training models of command consultation training, but we note one example of what was reported as an effective training program. In one psychiatric residency, command consultation training was provided over a 1 year period, consisting of consultation to a unit in the field on a weekly basis.[21] A biweekly seminar on consultation by an experienced consultant was also held in the hospital. A recent article by psychiatrists at Letterman Army Medical Center describes a similar program.[22] A good base of literature in the command consultation field is severely lacking. Most of the writings tend to be oriented around consultation in different settings such as in combat,[23] in training environments,[24] or in esoteric settings such as a refugee camp.[25] Other authors have stressed technical points such as the development of roles for the various professions in consultation,[26] the necessity of having high-level command support for consultation to be maximally effective,[27] unit group consultation,[28] and the allocation of resources to consultation.[29]

Development of a high level of skill in consultation seems best taught in an apprenticeship model in which a senior psychiatrist takes a resident or junior staff member with him on a consultation visit and teaches the particulars of the case.

On a local level, the primary basis on which a good consultative relationship between the mental health professional and the commander is often established is by the good clinical work of the would-be consultant. The consultant who gains credibility through his clinical work is then likely to be sought for future work. The assistance of the mental health professional is made known to the higher levels of command, and he soon has a reputation as being helpful and competent or not useful.

There are many types of problems for which mental health consultation is sought, from the adjustment problems of recruits at a training center to questions of the conduct and judgment of high-level officers. The knowledge, skills, and attitudes of the consultant will change with experience, and the approach will vary depending on the type of consultation. It is difficult to anticipate all the types of consultation that could occur, but the following seem to be the major categories.

Problem-Oriented Consultation with Local Unit

A psychiatrist is called on to consult with a unit with which he has a history but does not maintain a close relationship. Accidents involving military personnel, for example, provide a scenario in which a consultant can provide assistance to a unit, as well as form a relationship with a commander.[30,31] A common example of this type of consultation is the army division psychiatrist who consults to units in the division. Another example is the air force psychiatrist who consults to the flight surgeon. Flight surgeons often call on the psychiatrist for assistance with cases, particularly pilots about whom there is some question about their fitness to fly.[32]

The need for consultation in a combat environment is given by Kurtz,[33] who described his observations as a commander in Vietnam with a nonpsychiatrist physician who helped his unit. The education of other physicians by psychiatrists to do consultative work is one of the most important tasks of the psychiatric consultant:

> My best experience with doctors was in Vietnam when I was a battery commander. The battalion surgeons were young captains. As far as treating wounds went, they hardly ever got into that process because the evacuation system was so efficient. No matter where we were, even when I was wounded, the brigade aid station was usually the first stop, if any, before reaching a surgical hospital. They [the battalion doctors] didn't serve a real medical purpose in combat; they weren't there doing open heart surgery on the battlefield, but they were there, and did a great job, along with the chaplains, with keeping the lid on things in terms of human emotions. They had just enough training, enough general knowledge of psychiatry and psychology to where they were able to handle things. If a kid was under stress, they were able to identify that and they were able to create little situations to alleviate that stress. I think they took very good care of commanders, and I think they knew to keep anybody healthy, they kept the commanders healthy. So they were able to take care of a commander who was getting tense to the point of almost becoming dysfunctional. They, in their own way, put their arms around company commanders who were getting stressed out. Almost all of what they were doing was keeping us functional.

Kurtz[33] also noted some problems that could be of interest to a battalion commander. These consultations were not performed, but were needed:

> I would say, "I'm trying to raise standards in my battalion and it's going to cause stress. Advise me, what do I do. How do I package the program? What kind of stress can I anticipate? How do I deal with it?" Or, "We are going into a night training cycle. What do you know about sleep deprivation? Can you watch my outfit work for awhile and tell me who is sleeping and who is not. Why are things going wrong? Why are staffs up 24 hours? Give me some background, what happens when we don't get enough sleep?"[33]

Problem-Oriented Consultation with Remote Unit

This type of consultation is sometimes called a "one-shot consultation" because the consultant or consulting team will go to a site, perform the consultation, return home, and be unlikely to see the recipients of the consultation again. These consultations tend to occur with units that have no ongoing mental health contact, such as on a ship. Common examples of this type of consultation are seen when there has been a problem such as a severe training accident, disaster, a number of suicides, or unit performance problems. A particularly exciting development in this type of consultation has been the concept of the U.S. Navy's special psychiatric rapid intervention team (SPRINT).[34] These teams are located at major U.S. Navy hospitals (Bethesda, Portsmouth, and Oakland) and are available to consult with commanders, usually on ships, when there has been a serious incident with the high likelihood of mental health consequences for the crew. SPRINT has been used following the collision between the USS *John F. Kennedy* and the USS *Belknap*,[35] the strike of the Exocet missile on the USS *Stark*, and the explosion aboard the USS *Iowa*.

An example of a problem-oriented consultation is provided by Crigler,[36] who described the results of part of a team consultation for a problem aboard an aircraft carrier:

> The aircraft carrier was having some friction between the air boss and the commanding officer of the ship. They wanted to know what was that about. The psychologist and psychiatrist took the tack of doing a full evaluation of both of them, and were getting lots of interesting data, but it was not relevant at the time, though some of it became more relevant as time went on. We decided we would split up and each do our own thing, getting together after dinner. What was interesting was that neither of us had ever been on a ship for an extended period of time, and had never seen the sort of personality dynamics that evolve on an aircraft carrier.
>
> There was a definite split between the "black shoe" navy which are the men who drive the boats and run them. They deliver the goods, whether it's people, airplanes or Marines, vs. the "brown shoe" navy which are the fly boys, the men in the squadrons. Very, very different kinds of people. When we went to the wardroom of the black shoe officers, they were cordial, polite, civilized, on their good behavior, as you might see in an officers' club. They had linen on the table, etc. The whole thing was genteel and the conversation was wide-ranging: music, literature, movies, politics. The next day, we had lunch and dinner with the brown shoe guys. They ate at plain long wooden tables with nothing on them but bottles of ketchup, mustard, and hot sauce, at least 50 people at a table. It was located right under the flight deck. The noise was bad and the jet fuel smell was pervasive. You would hear the planes slam into the deck as the hook caught the plane's cable. They all came in their flight suits, which were basically scruffy. They all looked like they hadn't shaved, washed, or combed their hair in two or three days. They were amazingly crass to me and to the male psychiatrist. Obviously, they were not trying to be anything they weren't; this was their normal style of camaraderie. I felt as if I were at a fraternity party in the middle of football season about an hour before the game starts when everybody is almost totally blitzed. These guys had not been drinking, but they were giddy. All they could talk about was "flying and broads." It was a fraternity, a rah-rah immature, bravado, narcissistic type of response. I admit that when you are trying to land a plane going 600 miles per hour on a postage stamp in a bouncing sea, you had better have a narcissistic trait or two or you are not going to do it very well and if you don't do it very well you are not going to live very long. It was easy to understand some of the differences, but it was also easy to see why these people were not getting along very well. They were operating out of two very different cultures. The commanders of both of the groups were as clearly dominant as you could find, so when we talked to the two commanders and the admiral, we said "Well, basically we have found a difference in personality styles and we are surprised that you are finding this a problem only on this particular ship." He said, "I picked one at random." Given that this situation is typically going to occur, we helped him find a way to institutionalize techniques to help those two very different kinds of people interact more effectively and smoothly. I don't know what happened to the study, but I know they did change the way they ran staff meetings and how the two admirals of the surface and squadron communities related to one another at headquarters.[36]

In some cases, the consultation may really be on system-oriented problems that are common to a number of units or types of people. Fragala[37] provided some examples:

> Part of the mystique of the fighter pilot rests in the congruence of her or his actions in terms of the legends of the old West. The heroic cowboy comes upon trouble alone and fixes it his way and on his terms. This kind of independence and autonomy used to be rolled into the idea that fighter pilots were to be trained to be "tigers." The problem is that "tigers" take big risks and don't generally operate well as part of a team. If you train people to be professionals first, think and talk to them as executives, issue them briefcases, etc., you end up with a different product. Even better, you teach that there is a time to be a tiger and a time to be an executive, and that *both roles* (along with others) are required; that is, that the roles really must be integrated to achieve the desired result.[37]

Primary Prevention or Public Health Consultation

In this situation, the consultant is asked to advise on policies or procedures that may affect large numbers of people. This type of consultation often depends on the consultant having specific scientific expertise in the area required. Recent examples have to do with advising command about continuous military operations and sleep discipline[38] and developing cohesive military units that are considered more combat effective than noncohesive units.[39]

Educational Consultation

A final type of consultation provided to commanders and units is one that has been frequently used to educate commanders about stress and mental health. During World War II, education was one of the goals of preventive psychiatry. Lectures to commanders were a part of preventive psychiatry, aimed at improved mental health and psychological education of officers. Today, there are several types of educational consultation. All of the services have requirements for classes on various mental health subjects to troops. For example, health promotion activities are required of all the services under Department of Defense (DoD) Directive 1010.10.[40] The elements of this program include smoking prevention and cessation, physical fitness, stress management, alcohol and drug abuse prevention, and early identification of hypertension. Three of these programs, suicide prevention, stress management, and combat stress, provide the opportunity for the mental health officer to come to the unit, teach a class, and attempt to form a consultative relationship with the unit officers and senior noncommissioned officers.

Gelles[41] described a consultation that developed from a request for stress management training:

> This consultation was to a medical command, one that deals with a combat unit. They were functioning inefficiently and then were stressing out the combat end of it [people they were serving]. They lost 13 of their people to Desert Shield [personnel who were deployed to Saudi Arabia from 1990 to 1991]. There was a problem in the unit which seemed to be some kind of acting out, a lot of stress. A lot of people had friends deployed and people were very anxious about this war. They wondered when they were going, too, and they had all kinds of excuses. I brought information on deployment and combat stress. I talked to people and found out there was gross inefficiency in communication in the command about the way people are feeling. They were not talking to their seniors because they thought their seniors were not effective. I tailored a lecture around communication and the feelings of stress about not being able to communicate about how they were feeling, the exacerbation of their own anxieties, the potential losses of friends deployed, and their own fears about being deployed. We talked about combat and delayed stress responses in anticipation of how they would manage friends or flyers that came back wounded. The other thing that was interesting was that there were some Vietnam veterans who had been corpsmen in Vietnam and had become officers and nurses. One doctor had bad experiences in Vietnam. The Persian Gulf war was exacerbating a lot of very uncomfortable feelings and they were not talking. They were looked at by the staff as role models for how you manage yourself during a war and they were actually role models for shutting down. I encouraged them to have their own group where they could talk with each other. In about a month, I made a follow up call. They said things were better. I sent them an after action report with recommendations, from clinical and organizational perspectives. They were encouraged to look and listen for the cues of what is symptomatic of dysfunction in the group and realize it may not be the individuals.[41]

Following the recent combat operations of the U.S. military, Operation Just Cause (Panama, 1989) and Operation Desert Shield/Storm (Persian Gulf War, 1990 to 1991), many mental health professionals have been called on to provide debriefings to returning units or classes on post-traumatic stress disorder (PTSD). In most of these situations, the mental health professional provides an attempt at prevention of later disorders through familiarizing troops and commanders with the usual sorts of symptoms that occur after a traumatic event. This approach is usually aimed at normalizing such symptoms as sleep disturbance, intrusive thoughts, dreams of the event, disturbances in interpersonal relationships, and understanding the need for a recovery time. Commanders often are very resistive to such interventions because they fear that such a class will traumatize their people by reopening subjects that they would like to see forever closed. Another common means that units use to deal with trauma is to make the training schedule very full. Consequently, anything that interferes with ongoing training activities is not allowed. Special programs, such as stress management classes or combat psychiatry classes, are often mandated by high-level authority, and units are required to make time for the consultant. In some cases, a meaningful dialogue can take place, but in others, the commanders are hostile and provide many obstacles to the consultant.

Fagan[42] reported that in the Persian Gulf War, perhaps as many as 1,000 units were given consultation for stress management, a need that the commanders of the units thought would be of help to the soldiers and was considered essential. In one sense, this might represent naïveté in that officers may see stress management functioning like a vaccination. On the other hand, it seems to be the first time that mental health resources have been requested on such a large-scale basis, indicating that officers and noncommissioned officers see mental health services as valuable to them.

PERFORMING THE CONSULTATION

Differences between Clinical and Consultation Questions

The consultation question is often framed in terms of one or more individuals but is also, to some degree, about the health of the command. An analogous process for psychiatrists may be school consultation and hospital consultation-liaison psychiatry. In both these cases, an assessment may be performed on an individual but also on the milieu in which the person interacts. In addition, in both cases, the clinician must serve the needs of the client and the system.

Clinical training frequently neglects the work environment, which probably reflects a devaluing of the ways in which work contributes to health. Work is often seen as a stressor, and not as something that maintains and sustains people. An example of this attitude was given by Ursano:[43]

> Clinicians ask, "Tell me what's going on in your family," but, unless there is something dramatic going on at work, they may not have a lot of interest in it. Command consultation, by definition, deals with the organization and looks at the work environment and its contribution to performance and health and is different from psychiatric care in terms of its focus on performance in addition to just health. For example, a healthy service member may present with depressive symptoms which are secondary to poor performance and disciplinary actions because he has personality conflicts with a supervisor.[43]

Cross-Service Consultations

For those persons making consultations across services, Ursano[43] described both advantages and disadvantages:

> There are frequently substantial advantages to wearing a blue suit [U.S. Air Force] when consulting with a green uniform [U.S. Army]. There can be disadvantages early on, it seems, in terms of getting into the system, because you have to give more explanation, but once you are in it is frequently an advantage because you are seen as someone who is not in the usual chain of authority or command. You are clearly identified as not a part of the usual chain in contrast to when a green suit consultant shows up, someone always wants to know "Where is it going to? Who is he or she reporting to? Which commander is going to hear about it?" When you are in a blue suit consulting to a green suit you are in fact already identified. You have trouble getting in, but once you are in, you may have a more clear definition in the eyes of the consultees which will assist their talking to the consultant. Being an outside consultant provides advantages and disadvantages; we can trivialize those issues if we think only of a consultant as working from inside. There is another aspect of being the outsider which is that the outsider provides a certain kind of validation to the experience of the consultees, which it is not obtained by someone on the inside.[43]

Uniform

The uniform of the consultant is of great importance. It is important to wear the same uniform as that worn in the unit. When the unit wears a work uniform, the consultant should wear the same. This is a nonthreatening way to begin a consultation and decreases the psychological distance between the unit members and the consultant, particularly important when psychiatric consultation is involved. When people hear that a mental health officer is coming to the unit, in most cases, they expect him to wear a white coat and are relieved when they find that such is not the case. However, there is a caution in wearing the same uniform as the troops being visited. Mateczun[44] noted that while a consultant may gain credibility by wearing the same uniform as the unit to which he is consulting, there is also a danger in thinking that you know what it is the unit does simply because you wear the same uniform.

Language

Using the language of the group to which one is speaking is a primary skill involved in being a consultant. Ursano[43] noted:

> Although we get kind of glib about that [the language], I think when we consult with commanders we sometimes act as if we already know it. I don't think that's true; I don't think the language of commander A is the same as that of commander B. The language of a commander of a hospital is not the same as the language of a troop unit, which is also not the same language as that of the commander of a support unit. The ability to identify what language is being spoken and to be able to speak that language becomes important. It is also important to remember that you can also fool yourself. You can learn the language and think that you automatically understand what it is that the unit does.[43]

Forming a Consultation Team

The U.S. Navy SPRINT is an example of a group brought together to perform a consultation but is not the only instance. More common is the ad hoc team that has been created for a specific consultation. When this is done, team composition must consider the expertise of each member, the group they represent, and the ability of each person to function in the type of team envisioned by the leader. In addition to the military personnel, team members may be needed who have special ability to understand the problems of members of other services, civilians, and family members. In a consultation that is expected to be lengthy and difficult, the ability of a group to work together and to support each other must be considered in addition to the other factors listed above. An organization is being created and then sent to do the consultation. For the SPRINT, no less than three people are sent out. In addition to the three traditional mental health professions, other line officers or noncommissioned officers and enlisted personnel, chaplains, nurses, and lawyers can be of assistance.

Formulating the Consultation Question

When a consultation has been requested, the consultant should help the requestor clearly formulate the goals of the consultation so that there are no unwarranted expectations. Leaders of military organizations often have very little idea of what they specifically would like you to do. Setting goals with the consultee is somewhat like making a therapeutic contract with a patient. You tell them what your limitations are, what you can and cannot do, and what it is that you have to offer them.

Gaining Entry to a Unit

The consultant who wishes to provide professional input for the purpose of improving the health and performance of the members of the unit must obtain a means of entry to the unit. The process of consultation may begin with a request for consultation from the unit commander or from an official outside the unit such as a higher level authority with an official interest in the unit. In addition to permission to visit the unit and talk to people, entry to the unit also means obtaining the willingness of individuals in the unit to disclose factual and emotional material on the subject of the consultation. This willingness seems to occur most easily when the following has occurred: the consultant has previously provided assistance to the unit, has spent time with members of the unit and is perceived as someone who is available and can be counted on to be around to discuss follow-on action, is not there to investigate or blame the unit for its problems, or is a well-recognized individual with outstanding credentials in the field in which he is asked to consult. Simply advertising oneself as a consultant in the military and having credentials to support that stance frequently leaves individuals disappointed when they are not called on.[45]

Explaining the Purpose of the Consultation

When the consultation involves an evaluation of one or more individuals, particularly in cases of fitness for duty, a question in the mind of the consultant sometimes is how much to tell the subject of the evaluation. Fragala[37] described the need for all parties in the evaluation to be clear about all the issues involved. Although these comments refer to evaluations of high-level personnel, they are generally applicable to all ranks in the fitness for duty type of consultation:

> I address that issue [the purpose and results of the consultation] right out of the box and tell them forthrightly that they will get to see and get a copy of everything I write, and that I will tell them who I talk to and about what. I also communicate the notion that, if indeed they are sent to me, I insist that they know who sent them so that I take of the purchase and the mantle of how ever many tea leaves [stars] it takes to get the person's attention. I insist, when I can, on a telephone or a face-to-face between the individual to be evaluated and the person who is referring them so it's real clear that somebody they respect is saying "Go do this and tell the doc the straight scoop." I will very often call the referring individual when first notified and say, "Look, please have the following conversation with the person that you are sending." I am not an MRI scanner.[37]

Approaching the Organization

A consultation usually begins with the head of the organization. Remembering the model of the consultation-liaison psychiatrist, just as in starting with a patient, his anxiety about being the subject of a consultation must be allayed. Mateczun[44] reported that he typically began with the question, "Tell me what it is you do and how do you do it. I'm here to learn about what it is you do."

The commander and others in the unit may tend to view themselves as passive recipients of the consultation process. It is preferable that they be active participants. Just as an understanding of the patient's concept of their illness is needed, that is, the chief complaint, so is getting the commander's view of what is happening. If the request for the consultation came from someone other than the commander, the initial concept of the problem will be that of the consultee, not the commander of the unit. There is usually a difference between the two. Each has his own perception.[44]

Understanding Unit Structures and Functions

For an unfamiliar unit, the first task of the consultant is to learn exactly what it is that the unit does. The formal structure of the unit is learned by looking at the unit organizational chart, but one can mistakenly believe that everything that goes on in an organization is listed on the organizational chart. In addition to the formal structure, the consultant must attempt to become familiar with the set of informal subgroups to understand how a unit really operates. For example, one must have some concept of the enlisted structure because enlisted personnel do most of the actual work in a unit. It is different in every service and is separate from the administrative structure. For example, in the army and the marine corps, the officers administer and the enlisted personnel fight; in the air force and navy, it is generally the opposite. One must also learn something about the enlisted working conditions, how communications flow up and down, and those who have power in the organization that comes from their own personality characteristics.[44]

Interventions

In doing a consultation, one must learn to distinguish between organizational consultation and intervention. Sometimes the process is an intervention or it can lead to a discrete intervention. For example, SPRINT has elements of command consultation built into it. They are not necessarily called that to the commander, but some of the concepts and techniques are the same. Mateczun[44] described the process of distinguishing between consultation and intervention this way:

> The intervention itself interacts with actually doing a consultation. When you are interviewing, you are performing a triage of your decisions and actions at the same point. You are constantly making decisions as you are finding out more information about where it is you are headed and what it is that you need to do. For instance, you may discover an individual who is obviously having problems of a suicidal, dangerous, or psychotic nature. You will make an intervention at that point and not wait for the process to end. You have to take a somewhat different framework with you. You have to know a little bit about systems theory and organizational psychology. The usual tendency is to frame things in terms of individual psychopathology, or organizational pathology, just as we sometimes want to deal with a client in a diagnostic sense. This is probably not the best approach. The tendency of many consultants is to use pathological language rather than a language that addresses function and ability which are more understandable to the consultee. You approach the consultee emphasizing that you are his or her consultant and, as such, are to be used as a resource to him. That is indeed what you are and failure to establish this understanding will likely result in a failure to establish rapport. The usual consequence is that your interventions will not be accepted. In other words, the likelihood of your interventions being accepted often depends as much on your style as it does on the perceived worth of your ideas.
>
> As an example, there is a squad where someone is being scapegoated. They have identified somebody as strange, different, or odd, and the squad is going through a process of group formation through exclusion of that individual or that has already happened and they have had a suicide. People may think that the person actually was odd or unusual and not understand the process of the group formation that went on or how leadership may not have been optimal during that process. To educate them you can say, "This is a process that can occur in groups, but you as the leadership can learn how to effectively intervene to educate people about this process and why it may endanger the function of the group." If they ask, "Why?", say, "Well, if this happens to an individual, the thought in everybody else's mind is that 'This may happen to me.' You have to keep this in mind in group formation." You may meet resistance from the other members of the squad, but the result should be a squad where soldiers feel safe. It should be emphasized that loyalty within the group to each is the basic strength of that group. Or, because of identification with the group, the leader may say "No, this guy really is weird." You have to work with them on that.
>
> You must continue that process as time goes on. Periodically check with them and remind them of your availability. You cannot just go off and never come back. One good method is to establish a regular meeting time. Your goal is to have the consultee

> value and appropriately seek your counsel, not create dependence on you.[44]

Terminating the Consultation

What happens at the end of the consultation depends on the type of consultation arrangement with the client. If it is a one-time consultation, the relationship usually ends at that point. If it is ongoing, you will close out a particular question, but you will continue the relationship that you have established with the consultee. Mateczun[44] described important aspects of the termination process of the "one-shot consultation" and its aftermath, particularly for the consultation team:

> In either case you may be required to do something such as provide a report, and you have to bring closure to the relationship or that phase of it. In this process you may have to close a lot of loops and talk to a lot of people. You have learned something from them, and they expect you to reciprocate. There are certain people to whom it is crucial to give some immediate feedback: the commanding officer or leader and the person who consulted with you originally. When you have finished, you want to debrief yourself and your team. This is crucial. Usually you have gotten very involved in the process. One way to look at it is as a "no fault" process for yourself and your team. Depending on the situation, you may have been exposed to a particular psychological trauma or been confronted with the stress of extremely unpopular recommendations to a hostile group. While you hope your recommendations will improve the function of the group and the individuals in it, there are always doubts. So you want to talk it over and debrief yourselves.[44]

Reporting the Consultation

The report prepared by the psychiatrist, in addition to being a legal document, is what the commander will pay the most attention to, and the success or failure of the consultation may ride on the ability of the officer to report his findings. If both sides are serious about solving problems, the report is a critical step in the consultation. Fragala[37] provided his views on preparing reports of consultations:

> Critical to the written report is the formulation of the case. The commander is trying to solve a problem first and foremost. Doctrinaire statements will often be followed by a return letter which says, "Please answer the question. . . ." The mental health professional must first be clear about what the real question is in a given case, and must also realize that it may not be the question that seems to have been asked. The consultation is a process. Once you decide that an Axis I mental disorder is or is not present, you need to realize that only if you are going to hospitalize the individual (and even then only if there is no chance that he or she will ever return to duty) is the commander not ultimately responsible for the health and welfare of the member. Commanders are selected, in part, because they take this kind of responsibility very seriously. They really do want to be given a professional's perspective so as to better understand who this person is, and how they work. Reporting Axis I as "Occupational Problem" doesn't quite do it.[37]

Mateczun[44] advised caution when preparing a report from an extended or a one-shot consultation:

> You need to exercise some caution before sending out a report from the unit. Usually someone else is there like the skipper, and he wants things to be finished and reports sent out and the case closed. Meanwhile, you have been working for 16–18 hours a day, constantly dealing with people, and you are tired. Your judgment is just not as good, and it is not wise to formulate your report until you leave the consultation site. Reflecting after you have left the place often gives you a great deal of information; you realize how enmeshed certain organizations are, what was going on and how you got involved in it. Consultation is not only a cerebral, objective process. We have to use ourselves as instruments, and measure how and why we respond to things.[44]

RISKS TO THE CONSULTANT AND ETHICAL ISSUES IN CONSULTATION

The Ex Cathedra Statement

Mateczun[44] cautioned the consultant in believing too much in his own infallibility:

> There is a tendency to see yourself as an expert, and as you become known in the larger, overall organization, you may tend to make pronouncements that are not warranted by the data. You have to constantly remind yourself not to make these ex cathedra statements. It will relieve your anxiety to believe that you possess this power and your consultees will likewise feel less anxious because of your certainty. It is, of course, delusional on your part and

theirs. Humility not only protects you but makes you less threatening to the consultees. Every problem is new and deserves the same approach.[44]

"Lone Ranger" Status and Low Rank

Military positions in which the incumbent has the best opportunity to consult are frequently entry-level positions for military mental health workers. Examples of these positions are the division psychiatrist, psychologist, or social worker in the army and the sole mental health provider at a clinic in the air force. These people are usually junior in grade to the commanders with whom they are asked to consult. Rosato[46] pointed out some of these demands on new mental health professionals:

> We have now about 121 USAF military treatment facilities and many are clinics with no beds at all. Of the ones that have beds, many of them are 25 or 50 bed facilities and smaller. These are smaller facilities than the other two services which have fewer facilities, but much larger facilities. What that can translate into is a lot of isolation among our people. Of those 120 facilities, about 35 have sole providers which means, at that particular installation, the mental health person operates all by him- or herself. They do all the psychiatric evaluations, they take care of the drug and alcohol evaluations, they take care of the child and spouse abuse problems, they take care of the exceptional family member program. They are Mr. or Ms. mental health for that base which means a lot of responsibility falls on their shoulders. It means often times that they may have to call and get consultation on things that are more complicated or beyond their level of expertise. At the same time, it allows them an especially close relationship, because they don't have as many medical colleagues. The tendency at smaller bases is to be more tied into the line community, to be more a part of the military community.[46]

In addressing the issue of how does a young officer consult with a relatively senior commander, Rosato[46] reported:

> Typically, I find new people or younger people a little ambivalent about consultation. They know that it needs to be done, but they are not sure how to do it. In these cases, you are talking about a lieutenant or a captain who might need to go into a squadron with a unit commander who is a lieutenant colonel or colonel. They are really not sure about how to approach that individual, whereas if that same lieutenant colonel or colonel were in their office and having a marital problem, they would have no problem. When you get into questions of managing people or organizations, then they are a little reluctant due to their inexperience within the organization.[46]

Breaking Boundaries

Mateczun[44] pointed out unexpected risks to the consultant in doing mental health work outside the patient setting where other than the usual roles apply:

> You have to go out and talk to people if you want to understand what's going on. Fortunately, the consultant can break boundaries with impunity. You walk all over a ship, or spend time with a unit that you would otherwise be unable to do. Usually in our day-to-day environment, we are in a very defined role and we interact with people in a very defined way. If you take the consultant's stance, "I'm here to learn what it is you do and how you do it," you go around and talk to anybody. There's an inherent danger in the consultative process. You may become involved, particularly when something bad has happened. You can lose objectivity, and it is very likely that at some point you could become enmeshed in the process and lose track of what you are doing there. It's important to constantly check yourself and debrief with your teammates. This is one of the many reasons to have teammates with you during this process. When you are out in a unit alone, you lose communication with everybody else that provides any kind of reality check.[44]

Double Agency

Adams and Jones[32] wrote on the dilemmas of evaluating pilots. Ursano[43] amplified their points:

> There is a dilemma for the person who serves as a consultant to a flight surgeon who is then a consultant to the commander of a flight line. When you evaluate a pilot for the presence or absence of psychiatric illness, you have the dilemmas of establishing rapport and getting information from the patient who sees you as the representative of the commander. You recommend medically to the commander and the pilot that the pilot should not fly. This is a dilemma because it seems that the recommendation would be different for the two. In fact, the best interest of the pilot and the unit are served when an honest evaluation is rendered. The pilot should not be placed in an airplane when not fit because of the danger to himself as well as the damage to the system. A parallel is security evaluations in which you are assessing the ability of some-

one to carry a weapon or their propensity for disclosure. The dilemma of the flight surgeon is similar to that, although maybe more so because the flight surgeon may also be the one treating the patient or having to recommend treatment. This is called double agency; one is representing two different organizations, goals, or tasks simultaneously.[47] One appears to be representing the organization against the individual. When the pilot says, "But you can't ground me. I've got to fly. It's what makes me happy. If I'm not flying, I'll feel even more depressed," it may be helpful to point out that "Flying was never meant to be a therapeutic activity." The consultant doesn't keep them in or out of their jobs. He simply renders a medical opinion. Another thing that is helpful in this setting is recognizing that one is dealing with ability to function and trying to maximize return to performance levels and functioning. You must remember and emphasize that removal from one's job based on psychiatric reasons is not an indictment or a declaration of lack of worth.[43]

Confidentiality

To some degree, confidentiality does not exist because the mental health professional works for the commander as well as the patient. The extent to which it exists is determined by the consultant who must frame the answer to the question, "What is it the person needs to know?" There is actually very little problem in preserving confidentially with commanders because they only want to know, "When can I expect him to be back at work, if at all?" and, "Is he going to continue to have problems?" You are dealing with issues of prognosis and performance. While you generally give a psychiatric diagnosis, you do not give the intimate details that are shared with you by the patient. For there to be a breakdown in confidentiality, the commander has to be asking inappropriate questions, and the consultant has to be answering inappropriately by providing information that is not needed.[48]

Another view of confidentiality addresses the needs of the consultant, the consultee, the patient, and the organization. Fragala[37] addressed this problem:

> Very often military mental health professionals who are at the beginning of their careers think of themselves as working for the patient's interests exclusively. This immediately leads them into difficulty since the service sees them as its agent as well. Splitting one's allegiance does no one a service. The professional must realize that she or he must arrive at a solution which serves both ends; the needs of the individual and the needs of the service. Any solution which respects the needs of only one agency is always the wrong solution.[37]

Community vs Patient

When consulting to an organization in your own military community, you have to be particularly sensitive to the danger of losing objectivity. One has to have an understanding of the community from which he operates. One way that this understanding occurs is through maintaining an intellectual distance from it. If the consultant is part of it, he not only has a sense of what the community needs and risks, but also a personal investment in that community. If there is too strong an identification with a community, one can lose track of the patient; if one lacks any identification with his community, he may not appreciate the seriousness with which the community views the issue. In the latter case, the consultant may be seen as a threat to the community and be devalued and dismissed.[49]

Closeness and Intimacy

As part of a military unit, one usually develops bonds or emotional ties to the unit and the people in that unit. On the positive side, because of this position, many informal mechanisms of consultation become available. However, it can be an extremely difficult task to remember which role one is operating in, comrade or consultant. An example is the flight surgeon, who is assigned to a squadron and flies with the people there. He is able to make use of informal consultation, such as suggesting that somebody not fly today rather than formally grounding them. That consultant must remember his responsibility to ground the pilot if the suggestion is not heeded.

When the consultant has developed a close relationship to a unit, as in the case of flight surgeons operating independently, he can be powerfully affected emotionally by losses. In addition to the family and other members of a squadron, the death of a pilot is also keenly felt by the flight surgeon.[50] This exemplifies the intimacy and closeness in these settings, particularly during combat when unit bonding typically becomes tighter. The consultant can also become a victim of the particular disasters or traumas of the unit to which he is trying to consult.[49]

Short vs Long Consultations and the Development of Relationships

The differences in a short- and long-term consultation may be related to the analogy of short- and long-term therapy.[51] Both short- and long-term consultative relationships have unique elements to them that are potentially very powerful and emotional, providing opportunities for self-disclosure and self-growth. In the short encounter, one may regret the brevity that precludes an enduring sense of relationship, but it frequently opens up avenues for self-disclosure by virtue of the expectation that the consultee will not have to interact with someone who knows too much about them. At times, there is an advantage to being a one-shot consultant where the subject of the consultation will never see the consultant again. It is a similar issue in assessing certain patients for psychotherapy where one needs to be somewhat confrontive and challenging. The confrontation may disrupt the ability to do ongoing work, but it brings the problem into awareness and makes future work on the problem possible. The recipient of the consultation may not be able to hear you later when you talk in a very different tone about information you want to provide to them. You have established a confrontational style of relating to them. This raises another parameter of being a consultant: that of duration and how that influences all one's behaviors, presentation of data and expectation of outcome provided in consultation.[49]

Shame, Guilt, and Victimization

When the consultant establishes an ongoing liaison with a group, he becomes familiar with all of its intricacies and informal systems used in its day-to-day operation. There is a disadvantage to this development because the consultant, based on what has been learned about the people, may carry senses of shame and guilt that the people in the unit may or may not carry:

> To help minimize this it is important to establish early on that you as the consultant are human with all the attendant frailties and shortcomings, but will try not to let these interfere in your work. However, if despite your best efforts they do, the consultees should feel free to let you know in order that you can take the appropriate corrective action. This should serve to let people know that you accept human weaknesses without being judgmental and models the attitude that the consultees should be open and help each other to work more effectively in an emotionally safe environment. Needless to say it is always helpful to remind ourselves that we are not employed to cast judgment but rather to assuage guilt in the interest of more harmonious human relations and more efficient organizational function. When you do become aware of personal issues that need to be addressed to individuals, remember that these issues are usually painful and should be treated with great sensitivity. One good way to highlight shortcomings to someone is to report one's own similar shortcoming in the past and your appreciation of the situation.
>
> In terms of disaster and trauma, when you are dealing with vulnerable individuals, this can affect the consultant's sense of himself or herself. If he or she is not able to provide something, and there is exploitation going on because of the victimization of people, the experience of the consultant is that of being someone who is also victimizing. That can be mitigated by the process of being able to provide something to them and thereby of experiencing oneself as helpful.[49]

Investigation vs Consultation

Consultation involves the collection of information and determining how to use it. While this aspect of consultation is rarely part of an actual investigation, it may appear as such to the consultee. Ursano[49] described some emotional and behavioral aspects of this sometimes subtle interplay between consulting and investigating:

> Another difficult aspect of being a consultant is that of balancing an investigative and a helpful mode because you are always collecting information. Whenever you meet somebody, there is always this sense of intrusion, that you are investigating. So one has to develop ways to deal with the anxiety from people that you are consulting to, particularly when the consultation occurs after a disaster or trauma, where investigations are being conducted to assess blame. The expectation is that you are also investigating something to find guilt, and you have to work to dispel that idea. The consultant usually has pieces of knowledge or information that can be given to provide consultees with something that they feel is helpful relatively early. It provides a certain sense of give and take that this is not going to be a one way street, that there is something coming back.[49]

RESISTANCES TO CONSULTATION AND SYSTEM LIMITATIONS

Changes in the military structure have to some degree conspired against both the mental health professional and the commander to create conditions where neither talks much to the other. Increasing centralization of support resources makes close associations difficult and thereby decreases the understanding built through frequent contact. The company mess hall became the battalion mess hall; the battalion surgeon and company medics relocated to a troop medical clinic rather than in the unit area; the battalion chaplain splits his time between the unit, the post chapel, and facilities such as a post family life center; and the division psychiatrist, psychologist, and social worker have been pooled at post level. All these assets are seen by the commander as having been taken away from him, leaving his unit to fend for itself while requirements have increased so that officers and noncommissioned officers may tend to see themselves as having little time to concern themselves with day-to-day troop matters.

With increasing automation in the military, the day is either here or very near when reports can be generated quickly on the referral rates by battalion, including comparisons with other units, all of which are unlikely to improve relations between the line and the mental health providers or consultants. Military units, like most organizations, do not like to make their inner workings and problems public. Commanders are acutely aware of negative indicators that may be taken by others as poor leadership on their part. Some indicators that make commanders nervous are poor performance on military tasks, unauthorized absences, courts-martials, venereal disease rates, police blotter reports, and mental health referrals. As a result, the consultant who notices that a unit has a high rate of mental health visits is not likely to be seen, at least initially, as bearing good news or offering a welcome service. Commanders are rated on their performance, and anything that reflects negatively on their unit is generally avoided and potentially reflects adversely on their leadership. As a result, it is important for the consultant not to appear as a critic or investigator, and thus a consultant stance is helpful.

Command consultation is not practiced as frequently as hospital-based mental health practice whether in psychiatry, psychology or social work. The limitation often seems to lie in the worker as well as in external constraints. The officer who wishes to spend time consulting with a unit is rarely forbidden from doing so, but usually he is not encouraged to do so either. The emphasis tends to be on the discouraging side rather than the encouraging.

Rodriguez[52] identified six resistances to involvement in community consultation programs: (1) ethical issues such as confidentiality; (2) time constraints; (3) discomfort with systems because of lack of familiarity with community-based programs; (4) fear or stigma by association with community programs, competition with nonmedical personnel, nontraditional identity, and political programs; (5) identification with the medical model of treatment with emphasis on individual treatment, hospital base, and medical therapies; and (6) role-identity conflicts related to public programs.

A very serious drawback to consultation by military mental health professionals is the lack of credit because of their efforts in terms of patient counts. With increasing emphasis on management in military medicine, the number of patients seen per provider is the basis for staffing and budgets. Preventive and consultative efforts produce few patient counts—little that the psychiatrist can take to his commander as evidence of his contribution.

In the air force, mental health professionals have a different distribution than they do in the army and navy. Often, only one psychologist or social worker is assigned to a clinic at a small air force base. Army and navy mental health providers are rarely totally professionally isolated. In these cases, the mental health service functions like a small town private practice. In some of these cases, the mental health professional must also provide specialized services to the community, such as drug and alcohol treatment and family advocacy. These services are required by the air force to be provided at every base and are staffed by or consulted to by psychologists and social workers and psychiatrists. Consultation is much more likely to occur in these locations than in the larger medical centers because there is a need for practitioners to help each other and there is more involvement with the line that does not usually occur at the larger medical centers.

Training programs have emphasized individual treatment and biologic approaches to psychiatric treatment.[52] A consequence of this emphasis has been less interest in community psychiatry and less attention to the importance of the family in sustaining the soldier than during the time when a preventive and community approach was emphasized. In an effort to indicate the current need for preventive programs, Rodriguez[52] noted that efforts to reduce family problems as a way to help reduce stress on the soldier are valid uses of a psychiatrist's time. Such family problems are often based on unit policies such as frequent deployments and field duty, irregular hours, and differences in policies toward married and single soldiers. Psychiatric consultation could benefit preventive as well as ameliorative efforts. Rodriguez[52] suggested five specific areas in which psychiatric leadership in the community could be affected: (1) weekly consultations at day care centers and schools including sessions with teachers, nurses, administrators, and students; (2) routine informal meetings with hospital physicians and nurses, monthly inservice education programs for staff, and special inservice courses for emergency room personnel on emergency and preventive psychiatric care; (3) alcohol and drug education at all commands; (4) lectures and discussions on television and radio and before community groups on mental health issues, such as alcoholism, isolation, and other military-related family problems, family stress, and child and spouse abuse; and (5) community seminars on subjects such as child-rearing, assertiveness training, women's issues, and relaxation techniques.

RESEARCH IN COMMAND CONSULTATION

Research in this area is hard to do, and most clinicians who perform consultation do not have the training or the time to do it anyway. Nevertheless, the Group for the Advancement of Psychiatry[19] identified some research needs that are still current. They recommended the following six areas as deserving of special consideration:

> (1) That statistical methods of the three branches of the armed services be made uniform; so that *experiences* and *methodology* can be readily compared.
>
> (2) That records be kept of policies, directives, or preventive and treatment measures that are initiated and might be expected to influence the indices of effectiveness.
>
> (3) That particular attention be devoted to factors that are emotionally supporting in the face of unusual stress; e.g., motivation, values, attitudes, needs, and communication, as well as environmental manipulation.
>
> (4) That the natural history of individuals undergoing basic training, overseas assignment, isolated assignment, and similar peacetime stresses be studied . . . to gain insight into the processes of adjustment and breakdown of individuals exposed to such situations.
>
> (5) That research teams be formed to function under operational conditions in the field and that, in the event of war, such teams be available to implement previously planned research studies.
>
> (6) That controlled studies be done using social science skills in the utilization of marginal manpower during peacetime . . . to avoid undue wastage of human resources during national emergencies.[19(pp296–297)]

SUMMARY

The task of consulting to command is not easy. The needs of the services have remained relatively similar over the years: Soldiers, sailors, marines, and airmen still have adjustment difficulties, and units still have difficult mission challenges, suffer disasters, and have leadership and performance problems. Ways of operating have changed both for military units as well as for the mental health community. For both, control has become more centralized, and more is demanded of officers. For example, automation has made it possible for people to count events in a way that was not possible earlier and has generated many more reporting requirements. Reporting takes time away from other activities. Within psychiatry and the other mental health disciplines, practice has changed. For psychiatry, the focus has gone toward biological and individual treatment rather than toward communities and group treatment. Of the other mental health professionals, social workers are the most likely to be interested in group and community processes.

Consultation started as a mass movement, at least in the U.S. Army. It has now become more of a specialty than it used to be, both in terms of the skills required and the number of people who attempt it. Today, the consultant must have a broad range of skills. He must know not only his own organization but also many others including other services. Such skill development takes time and, more important, the presence of a mentor who can teach younger people "the ropes" of consulting. Our impression is that most people who perform consultation successfully enjoy it and have a sense of having contributed something as well as having obtained something special that is not ordinarily encountered in clinical or administrative life.

Ultimately, consultation tasks are meant to improve the capability of the military unit to carry out its mission. This difference between civilian and military psychiatry has been noted in this chapter, but it may be of value to point out that the task of the consultant is not to please everyone.

The tasks for the mental health officer and consultant will not stay the same in future environments. Rather than applying principles without thought, the critical contingencies of conflicts must be observed and analyzed to apply mental health skills to their solution.

ACKNOWLEDGMENTS

The authors have benefitted from interviews with the following persons. They are, in alphabetical order, Patricia W. Crigler, Ph.D., Captain, Medical Service Corps, U.S. Navy, Chief, Department of Psychology, National Naval Medical Center; Joe G. Fagan, M.D., Colonel, U.S. Army, Chief, Department of Psychiatry, Walter Reed Army Medical Center, Washington, D.C. and former Psychiatry Consultant to The U.S. Army Surgeon General; Richard Fragala, M.D., Colonel, U.S. Air Force, Chief, Division of Mental Health, Malcolm Grow Air Force Medical Center, and Psychiatry Consultant to the U.S. Air Force Surgeon General; Michael Gelles, Ph.D., Lieutenant Commander, Medical Service Corps, U.S. Navy, Special Assistant for Behavioral Sciences, Naval Criminal Investigative Service; Richard G. Kurtz, Colonel, U.S. Army, Director of Human Resources, Office of the U.S. Army Deputy Chief of Staff for Personnel; John M. Mateczun, M.D., Captain, U.S Navy, Assistant Chief of Staff, Health Service Support, Headquarters, U.S. Marine Corps Forces Pacific; Ann Norwood, M.D., Lieutenant Colonel, U.S. Army, Department of Psychiatry, Uniformed Services University of the Health Sciences; Louis W. Rosato Jr., Colonel, U.S. Air Force, Chairman, Department of Social Work and Consultant in Social Work to the U.S. Air Force Surgeon General, Malcolm Grow U.S. Air Force Medical Center, Andrews Air Force Base; Robert J. Ursano, M.D., Colonel (Retired), U.S. Air Force, Professor and Chairman, Department of Psychiatry, Uniformed Services University of Health Sciences.

REFERENCES

1. Salmon TW. The care and treatment of mental diseases and war neurosis ("shell shock") in the British Army. In: *Neuropsychiatry*. Vol X. In: Salmon TW, Fenton N, eds. *The Medical Department of the United States Army in the World War*. Washington, DC: GPO; 1929: 497–523.
2. Menninger WC. Psychiatry and the Army. *Psychiatry: J Biol Pathol Interpersonal Relations*. 1944;7:175–181.
3. Glass AJ. Effectiveness of forward neuropsychiatric treatment. *Bull US Army Med Dep*. 1947;7:1034–1941.
4. Glass AJ, Artiss KL, Gibbs JJ, Sweeney VC. The current status of Army psychiatry. *Am J Psychiatry*. 1961;117:673–683.
5. US Department of the Army. War Department. *Nomenclature and Method of Recording Diagnosis*. Washington, DC: DA; 1945. Technical Bulletin MED 203.
6. Rioch DMcK. Problems of preventive psychiatry in war. In: *Psychopathology of Childhood*. Orlando, Fl: Grune and Stratton; 1955: 146–165.
7. Appel JW. Preventive psychiatry. In: *Zone of the Interior*. Vol 1. In: Glass AJ, Bernucci RJ, eds. *Neuropsychiatry in World War II*. Washington, DC: GPO; 1966: 373–416.

8. Menninger WC. *Psychiatry in a Troubled World.* New York: MacMillan Company; 1948.

9. Artiss KL. Human behavior under stress: From combat to social psychiatry. *Milit Med.* 1963;128:1011–1015.

10. Guttmacher MS. The mental hygiene consultation services. In: *Zone of the Interior.* Vol 1. In: Glass AJ, Bernucci RJ, eds. *Neuropsychiatry in World War II.* Washington, DC: GPO; 1966: 349–371.

11. Plesset MR. Psychoneurotics in combat. *Am J Psychiatry.* 1946;10:87–90.

12. Jones F. Personal Communication, 1991.

13. Hausman W, Rioch DMcK. Military psychiatry, a prototype of social and preventive psychiatry in the United States. *Arch Gen Psychiatry.* 1967;16:727–739.

14. Bushard BL. The US Army's mental hygiene consultation service. In: *Symposium on Preventive and Social Psychiatry.* Washington, DC: Walter Reed Army Institute of Research; 1958: 431–443.

15. Caplan G. *Principles of Preventive Psychiatry.* New York: Basic Books; 1964.

16. Cruvant BA. Replacement training center consultation service. *Am J Psychiatry.* 1943;100:41–46.

17. Appel JW, Beebe GW. Preventive psychiatry: An epidemiologic approach. *JAMA.* 1946;131:1469–1475.

18. Menninger WC. Psychiatric experience in the War, 1941–1946. *Am J Psychiatry.* 1947;104:577–586.

19. Group for the Advancement of Psychiatry. *Preventive Psychiatry in the Armed Forces: With Some Implications for Civilian Use.* New York: Group for the Advancement of Psychiatry; 1960. Report 47.

20. Lipowski ZJ. Consultation-liaison psychiatry: An overview. *Am J Psychiatry.* 1974;131:623–630.

21. Norwood A. Personal Communication, 1990.

22. Leamon MH, Sutton LK, Lee RE. Graduate medical educators and infantry commanders: Working together to train Army psychiatry residents. *Milit Med.* 1990;155:430–432.

23. Bey DR, Smith WE. Organizational consultation in a combat unit. *Am J Psychiatry.* 1971;128:33–38.

24. Sorenson E, Miles DA. Training mental hygiene consultation service (MHCS) personnel for combat readiness: The division social worker's responsibility. *Med Bull US Army Europe.* 1979;36(May/June):17–20.

25. Rahe RH, Looney JG, Ward HW, Tung TM, Liu WT. Psychiatric consultation in a Vietnamese refugee camp. *Am J Psychiatry.* 1978;135:185–190.

26. Daykin SP. The role of psychology and social work in the preventive medicine program of the armed forces. *Milit Med.* 1955;116:127–130.

27. Spencer CD, Gray BG. An approach to mental health consultation within the military. *Milit Med.* 1965;130:691–694.

28. Chapman RF. Group mental health consultation—Report of a military field program. *Milit Med.* 1966:131:30–35.

29. Satin DG. Allocation of mental health resources in a military setting: A community mental health approach. *Milit Med.* 1967;132:698–703.

30. Tyler MP, Gifford RK. Fatal training accidents: The military unit as a recovery context. *J Trauma Stress.* 1991;4:233–249.

31. McCarroll JE, Ursano RJ, Fullerton CS, Wright KM. Community consultation following a major air disaster. *J Community Psychol*. 1992;20:271–275.

32. Adams RR, Jones DR. The healthy motivation to fly: No psychiatric diagnosis. *Aviat Space Environ Med*. 1987;58:350–354.

33. Kurtz RG, Colonel, US Army, Director of Human Resources, Office of the US Army Deputy Chief of Staff for Personnel. 5 December 1990. Interview.

34. McCaughey BG. US Navy special psychiatric rapid intervention team (SPRINT). *Milit Med*. 1987;152:133–135.

35. Hoiberg A, McCaughey BG. The traumatic aftereffects of collision at sea. *Am J Psychiatry*. 1984;141:70–73.

36. Crigler PW, PhD, Captain, Medical Service Corps, US Navy, Chief, Department of Psychology, National Naval Medical Center. 22 March 1991. Interview.

37. Fragala R, MD, Colonel, US Air Force, Chief, Division of Mental Health, Malcolm Grow Air Force Medical Center, and Psychiatry Consultant to the US Air Force Surgeon General. 6 December 1990. Interview.

38. Manning FJ. Continuous operations in Europe: Feasibility and the effects of leadership and training. *Parameters*. 1979;9:8–17.

39. Ingraham LI, Manning FJ. Cohesion: Who needs it, what is it, and how do we get it to them? *Milit Rev*. 1981;61:2–12.

40. US Department of Defense. *Health Promotion*. Washington, DC: DoD; 1986. DoD Directive 1010.10.

41. Gelles M, PhD, LCDR, Medical Service Corps, US Navy, Department of Psychology, National Naval Medical Center. 22 March 1991. Interview.

42. Fagan JG, Chief, Department of Psychiatry, Walter Reed Army Medical Center, Washington, DC, and former Psychiatry Consultant to The US Army Surgeon General. 19 November 1990. Interview.

43. Ursano RJ, MD, Colonel (ret), US Air Force, Professor and Chairman, Department of Psychiatry, Uniformed Services University of Health Sciences. 28 November 1990. Interview.

44. Mateczun JM, MD, Captain, US Navy, Assistant Chief of Staff, Health Service Support, Headquarters, US Marine Corps Forces Pacific. 12 October 1990. Interview.

45. Fragala R. Personal Communication, 1990.

46. Rosato LW, Jr., Colonel, US Air Force, Chairman, Department of Social Work, and Consultant in Social Work to the US Air Force Surgeon General, Malcolm Grow US Air Force Medical Center, Andrews Air Force Base. 14 June 1991. Interview.

47. Ursano RJ, Jones DR. The individual's vs. the organization's doctor: Value conflict in psychiatric aeromedical evaluation. *Aviat Space Environ Med*. 1981;52:704–706.

48. Hausman K. Different practice pressures await military psychiatrists. *Psychiatric News*. 1990;25:6–7.

49. Ursano RJ. Personal Communication, 1990.

50. Jones DR. Emotional reactions to military aircraft accidents. *Aviat Space Environ Med*. 1982;53:595–598.

51. Sterlin H. Short-term versus long-term psychotherapy in the light of a general theory of human relationships. *Br J Med Psychol*. 1968;41:357–366.

52. Rodriguez AR. A community mental health approach to military psychiatry. *Milit Med*. 1980;145:681–685.

Chapter 10

PSYCHIATRIC SUPPORT FOR COMMANDERS

FARIS R. KIRKLAND, Ph.D.,* AND MOSS A. JACKSON, Ph.D.†

*Lieutenant Colonel (ret), Field Artillery, U.S. Army; Senior Research Associate, University City Science Center, 3624 Market Street, Philadelphia, Pennsylvania 19104–2614; Guest Scientist, Department of Military Psychiatry, Division of Neuropsychiatry, Walter Reed Army Institute of Research, Washington, D.C. 20307–5100
†Center for Psychological Services, 1125 Coulter Avenue, Ardmore, Pennsylvania 19003–2426

INTRODUCTION

Psychiatric support for commanders is an emerging approach to preventing psychological deterioration in key personnel and in units. The essence of the problem is that military service is noted for high stress, and leaders experience higher stress and lower levels of social support than do members of the rank and file in any vocation. The principal sources of stress for leaders are isolation, uncertainty, and responsibility. Current thinking on future warfare indicates that it will become more rather than less severe.[1,2]

Although there is no systematic documentation to define commanders' requirements for psychiatric support, almost any objective history of the U.S. armed forces in peace and war includes reports of deleterious effects on units of dysfunctional behavior by commanders. At the most superficial level, one need only recall the sorry parade of commanders of the Federal Army of the Potomac in 1861 to 1864 and the number of generals General Pershing relieved in 1917 to 1918 and General Marshall relieved in 1943 to 1945.[3–5] Blair has described in detail the inability of many commanders at battalion level and above to function effectively in the Korean conflict (1950 to 1953).[6(pp581–585,612–614)] Few senior commanders were relieved during the Vietnam conflict (1964 to 1972) because the bulk of the fighting comprised individual company and platoon actions. The breakdowns occurred among junior officers.[3–5]

The traditional solution to dysfunctional behavior by commanders has been to relieve those who display it. This approach accomplished three things: it got rid of leaders who failed, it deterred unwanted behavior, and it exculpated superiors by fixing blame on the identified problem. This philosophy of firing the failures is expensive in time and casualties, and it has tended to suppress initiative. In a world in which armed conflicts can explode overnight and in which early and competent application of force may be decisive, firing the failures must be the exception rather than the rule. An alternative, psychiatric support for commanders, acquired substantive potential in the 1990s because of developments in biopsychosocial theory and psychotherapeutic practice and because of a new awareness in the military community that psychological support can be useful and acceptable. A component of command consultation, it is a partnership between psychiatry and command to strengthen the masterful in contrast to the traditional psychiatric mode of healing the psychologically distressed. (See Chapter 9, "Psychiatric Consultation to Command," of this volume.) It offers an opportunity for psychiatrists in the field to assist commanders to strengthen the psychological readiness of themselves and their subordinate leaders to function under conditions of high stress.

HISTORICAL PERSPECTIVE

In the 18th and early 19th centuries, when American military traditions began, soldiers fought shoulder to shoulder. A company usually had a maximum strength of about 65 men. When it formed in two ranks for combat, the company had a frontage of about 30 meters.[7] The captain in command could shout instructions to his officers and noncommissioned officers (NCOs), and he could even run to any point in the line in less than half a minute. The colonel of a regiment of 10 companies could see his flank companies from his position on horseback and could gallop to the furthest one in a minute or two.

The principal tasks of the company commander and his lieutenants were to train their men in movements and discipline and see that they cared for their bodies and equipment so that they were fit to fight. The principal tasks of the regimental commander were to train his officers and see that his companies had food, clothing, lodging, equipment, and ammunition—the wherewithal to survive and fight.[7(pp128–131)]

Officers and NCOs faced the same risks as their soldiers in combat—they were in the line with them or in front in some cases. In addition to the danger of being felled by musket ball, saber, or bayonet, officers also ran the risk that their men might run away from the battle leaving them to death, capture, or disgrace. These uncertainties were somewhat palliated by the close proximity of all the members of a company; if a man quailed, an officer or NCO was not far away and could communicate with the faint-hearted lad by voice, boot, or flat of the saber. Moreover, the officers were available to each other for social support; they lived and ate together and interacted with each other throughout the day. Each was in sight of several other officers in combat and could hear each other shout commands. Evidence from memoirs reveals that the officers of a regiment in the 18th century were not necessarily always mutually supportive and trusting, but they were at least physically there for each other.[8(pp7–8,41,61–64,75)]

The Dispersed Battlefield and *Auftragstaktik*

With the advent of rifled cannon and small arms in the 1860s, shoulder-to-shoulder formations became suicidal, and a trend toward progressively greater dispersal on the battlefield began. In 1866, the frontage of a Prussian infantry company was 150 meters, a 5-fold increase, and one-half the width of an entire regiment 50 years earlier.[9(p84)] The company commander could no longer control his troops with his voice alone, and the regimental commander saw his force dispersed over one-half mile.

Even before combat began, the regimental commander would only be able to see a few of his companies and their commanders. Direct communication was impossible. Victory came to depend on junior leaders having the knowledge and confidence to act without reference to higher authority to capitalize on tactical opportunities they encountered. In response to this development, the Prussian army instituted *Auftragstaktik*,[10(pp22–27)] a complex set of behaviors on the part of commanders to develop in junior officers readiness and ability to act competently on their own initiative. *Auftragstaktik* was intended to make the army more effective in combat and had no psychological or ethical implications, but operationally it was the first systematic approach to providing psychological support for leaders.

Auftragstaktik was a function of command. It comprised behavior on the part of commanders to communicate to subordinate leaders that the senior had confidence in the junior's judgment, wanted him to exercise his initiative, and would support him in his actions. *Auftragstaktik* also included training to develop junior officers' judgment so that encouraging their acting on their own would lead to success more often than disaster. *Auftragstaktik* functioned as a process of psychologically supportive socialization that went on throughout an officer's career. Commanders did not scorn or belittle subordinates; neither did they overlook errors, inattention, sloth, or ignorance. When there were shortcomings in performance, the commander would use them as opportunities for transformational change. He would teach, orient, and strengthen his subordinates in the context of a partnership between the senior and the junior leader.[11(pp50–56)]

Psychological concepts were not part of *Auftragstaktik*; neither was coddling. Making war was a rough business. The Prussian leaders realized that the lower the echelon the rougher it got, and the more the leaders needed supportive chiefs. Although the junior officer was isolated on the battlefield, he had learned from his interactions with his commander that he was a valued member of a group whose leader respected and would support him. This social support, although less tangible than seeing and hearing his commander, often proved to be an operationally effective substitute on the dispersed battlefield.

Auftragstaktik served the Prussian and later the German army well. Although often outnumbered, it won decisively in 1866 against Austria, 1870 against France, 1914 against Russia, 1939 against Poland, 1940 against France, and 1941 against Yugoslavia and Russia. When Hitler took personal command of the armed forces in late 1941, *Auftragstaktik* faded away and, with it, the era of victories.

The U.S. Army in the 20th Century: A Culture of Anxiety

There have been individual commanders in the U.S. Army who practiced the essentials of *Auftragstaktik*, but even if they had been more common, the lack of any institutional understanding of the psychological stresses to which officers practicing this form of leadership were subjected would probably have doomed them to failure. Thus, *Auftragstaktik* has never become a way of life in the U.S. Army. The culture of the U.S. Army in the 20th century has been more nearly one of anxiety: Leaders feared their superiors would find fault with them, and they also feared their subordinates would let them down.[12(pp232ff),13(pp283ff)] Caught between the upper and the nether millstones, many leaders have sought to assure proper performance by intimidating their subordinates. To a major extent, the nature of U.S. military institutions between 1776 and 1945 made *Auftragstaktik* almost impossible and intimidation almost inevitable. Americans kept their peacetime military establishments extremely small. Expanding the army 20-fold to 40-fold in 1861,

1917, and 1942 allowed little time to develop subordinate leaders and imposed severe anxieties on regular officers shouldering new and heavy responsibilities.[14]

In 1940 to 1945, regular officers were forced to depend on inexperienced reservists, former NCOs, and officers commissioned directly from civilian life to fill most positions up through battalion commander and division staff. Many senior commanders used centralized control, minutely detailed orders, and close, coercive supervision to reduce the uncertainties they faced. Control rather than trust characterized professional relationships. Working together under stress united junior and senior officers and enlisted men in small units and staff sections, but there was no ethic of support for subordinate leaders.[15(pp71ff,384ff,413ff)]

The traditional practice of drastically reducing the officer corps after the war was not followed when World War II ended. The army was cut back to a little less than three times its prewar strength, but it retained almost five times as many officers as were on duty in 1939.[16(pp3,14)] Many of the officers on duty in 1947 could never have aspired to commissioned rank before the war. The army offered them undreamed of status and authority, but it could not make them secure in that status and authority. There had been social supports that sustained officers before the war. These supports included a small officer corps whose members knew each other personally, long assignments with the same colleagues, an atmosphere of study generated by a few bright and professionally oriented officers in the middle ranks, and social customs that encouraged interaction and mutual support.[8,17,18] These supports were attenuated during the wartime expansion. Officers commissioned during the war had never experienced those supports, and many did not feel fully assimilated in the less homogeneous and more fragmented postwar army. Some of them adopted authoritarian behavior patterns such as uncritical submission to superiors, hostility to innovation, and indifference toward subordinates.[19(pp258–265)] They did not trust their troops or teach small units how to act on their own. Together with those of their regular army colleagues who during the war had developed habits of not trusting their subordinates, these new officers structured human relations in the U.S. Army in an authoritarian mold.

According to the official historian, command during the initial phases of the Korean conflict was characterized by mistrust across ranks and episodes of leadership collapse.[20(pp84,698),21(p151)] As the war evolved, an extraordinary degree of micromanagement emerged.[12(pp262ff,460ff)] The post-Korean conflict era saw the full flowering of a culture of anxiety because the wartime mistrust was exacerbated by policies to reduce the size of the officer corps. New educational standards that were extremely difficult for officers to meet while performing their duties were imposed. A single efficiency report that was less than extravagantly complimentary could lead to termination of active commissioned service. Many officers who had won their commissions during World War II and the Korean conflict lost them. A culture of anxiety developed that taught officers to attract no attention, attempt no innovation, and take no action not specifically authorized by directives from higher headquarters.[12(pp291–292,314–315)] Some sought jobs with minimal exposure to responsibility, and this meant keeping away from troop command.

Vietnam and the Seeds of Reform

One consequence of the culture of anxiety was a reluctance on the part of midcareer officers to get involved with the comparative evaluations and technical disciplines associated with service in line units. When the conflict broke out in Vietnam, many field grade officers did not have the requisite professional knowledge to function effectively as battalion S–3, executive officer, or commander. They had isolated themselves so long from their basic branch skills that they no longer were able to teach or inspect the techniques of field service and combat. For example, in some infantry battalions and brigades, there was no officer who knew how to organize interlocking fields of fire, effective barbed wire obstacles, or indirect machine gun fire. Many field grade artillery officers did not know how to carry out meteorological and survey procedures. The company and battery commanders were, especially after 1966, mostly officers with less than 3 years of service; they needed older officers who could teach them the fine points of their profession.[22(pp208–209)] Instead, many got only imperious instructions about the results they were to produce and the fate that would befall them if they failed.[3(pp65ff),5(pp96ff)]

Of course, this approach to leadership was not unique to the U.S. Army. Many armies have been organized along rigidly authoritarian lines that allow little leeway for any but the most senior officers to exert any initiative. The underlying assumptions were that subordinate personnel were incapable of understanding the commander's intent and using their own intellects to carry it out, and subordinates had no reason to risk their lives other than fear of their commander. In past situations, these assumptions were often accurate. But, when they persisted into the 20th century, they were usually inaccurate.[23]

During the conflict in Vietnam, ignorance and the inevitable self-doubt and insecurity it entailed limited the ability of many career officers to provide psychological supports for junior leaders. Many junior officers lacked confidence in their superiors' judgment and in their readiness to back them up if they acted. The results in combat were often that junior leaders did not act. The leadership practices of an unusually large number of officers, particularly those in the field grades and higher, had deteriorated to the point that it caught the attention of senior commanders.[3–5] Lieutenant General William R. Peers, who had held divisional and corps-level commands in Vietnam, sent a memorandum to the Chief of Staff, General William C. Westmoreland, in which he pointed out that officers were shirking responsibility, lying, turning a blind eye to improper behavior by soldiers, commanding from a safe distance, ignoring their men's concerns, and failing to enforce measures to ensure the troops' safety.[24(pp195–198)] Although this type of behavior was not universal,[25(pp45–52)] it was sufficiently widespread for General Westmoreland to ask the U.S. Army War College to investigate the issues Peers had raised.

The War College's *Study on Military Professionalism*[26] of 1970 found that serving officers in all ranks perceived that if they were to achieve personal success, they had to please their superiors rather than meet the legitimate needs of their troops or attend to the good of the service. They saw themselves as compelled to attain trivial short-term objectives through dishonest practices that injured the long-term fabric of the organization. The pressure to behave in this way seemed,

> . . . to stem from a combination of self-oriented success-motivated actions, and a lack of professional skills on the part of middle and senior grade officers. . . . A scenario that was repeatedly described . . . [was] an ambitious, transitory commander—marginally skilled in the complexities of his duties—engulfed in producing statistical results, fearful of personal failure, too busy to talk or listen to his subordinates, and determined to submit acceptably optimistic reports which reflect faultless completion of a variety of tasks at the expense of the sweat and frustration of his subordinates.[26(ppiii-iv)]

The *Study on Military Professionalism*[26] described the gap between the official values of the U.S. Army and praxis—the way socialization processes taught leaders to behave. The gap was not new; describing it without euphemism was. The study recommended a number of actions focused on strengthening officers' technical and tactical knowledge, stabilizing command tours, and encouraging initiative and learning by experience. It described as counterproductive judgmental leadership and the use of statistical indicators as bases for evaluating units and commanders. Some of these recommendations were incorporated into policy. But research conducted between 1975 and 1990 indicated that behavior at variance with leadership policy continued.[27–30] Further, neither the study nor policy addressed the question of social supports for junior leaders.

The lieutenants and captains of Vietnam became lieutenant colonels and colonels in the 1980s and early 1990s. They were able to conceptualize the social and professional support they had wanted and had not gotten from their superiors in Vietnam, and many sought to give it to their own junior officers. Mentoring, empowerment, and providing space in which to fail while learning became active leadership principles in the mid-1980s.[31,32(pp33,36,39,47)] Within the limits of their own anxieties, and of the rapid turnover mandated by the U.S. Army culture for junior officers, the colonels of the 1980s and 1990s had an effect. They did not create an army-wide culture of *Auftragstaktik*, but some created climates of social support within their own units that led to unusually high levels of cohesion, competence, and morale.[33(pp3–16),34(pp68–74)]

The new culture made possible a fundamental change in army warfare doctrine, which first appeared in the 1982 version of Field Manual 100–5.[35] For the first time, a version of *Auftragstaktik* became official doctrine, as is apparent from such statements as "... initiative requires audacity which may involve risktaking and an atmosphere that supports it . . . [and] . . . it is essential to decentralize decision authority to the lowest practical level. . . . Decentralization demands subordinates who are willing to take risks and superiors who nurture that willingness and ability in their subordinates."[35(p15)] The U.S. Army's performance in the invasion of Panama and in the Persian Gulf War is a testimony to the success of the new doctrine, but much remains to be done to assure its full acceptance at all levels of command.

An important factor that made mentoring of junior by senior leaders more important—because it added to the stress of leadership at squad, platoon, and company levels—was a series of experiments with systems for stabilizing personnel. Under the names COHORT (Cohesion, Operational Readiness, and Training), New Manning System, and Unit Manning System, efforts were made to keep first-term soldiers together from their initial enlistment through entry training and for 3 years in a unit. The system offered the possibility of strong horizontal cohesion, and the reduced personnel turnover made possible progressive training in more sophisticated individual and unit skills. In field tests, the COHORT system proved to have the potential for making all units capable of strong cohesion, high morale, and outstanding performance. Whether it fulfilled its promise was a function of the leaders' abilities to rise to the challenge. They had to know three times as much about their profession to conduct 3-year training programs, and the emotional demands on leaders increased when they were with the same soldiers for prolonged periods.[29(pp49–50),33]

Psychological Supports for Soldiers but Not for Leaders

While these developments were taking place, officers in the 1980s and 1990s experienced increased intellectual and emotional demands, frequent and sudden calls to war or warlike deployments, and no sustained system for psychological sustenance from superiors. As operational and administrative demands grew, and the battlefield became more dispersed, social supports for officers in the U.S. Army were further attenuated.[36(pp16–17)] In European armies, the sense of belonging to a hereditary leadership class supported many officers. Others, not born to the officer class but assimilated, were able to draw some support from their achievement even though they were not part of the nobility. The officers' messes provided a daily source of social support in garrison and on campaign. In the U.S. Army, the officers' open messes gradually lost much of their potential for social support. During the 1950s and 1960s on many large posts, the officers' clubs became prestige symbols and entertainment facilities for the post commander. They were funded largely by obligatory contributions from the mass of junior officers, but they provided negligible social support for most of them.[12(p458)] In some cases, satellite beer halls functioned as after-hours gathering places for bachelor officers. When these had a battalion- or regiment-specific identity, they provided opportunities for officers to let their hair down, argue, complain, and share experiences informally. In the 1970s and 1980s, the movement for better health has led to alcohol consumption becoming a career liability rather than an asset, and the clubs and beer halls have waned further as sources of social support.

Throughout the history of psychiatry as an element of military medicine, the foci have been alleviating battle-induced psychiatric symptoms and screening out or eliminating individuals who gave indications that they were psychologically unsuited for military service.[37] Efforts to strengthen soldiers' resistance to combat stress have fallen under the rubrics of discipline and morale—functions of command rather than medicine. Psychological support has been primarily of a spiritual nature—the province of the chaplain. Military culture has defined leaders as not needing psychological support, and the higher the leader's position the more independent he is presumed to be. In military folklore, psychological neediness is a weakness that disqualifies an individual for leadership. For example, a field grade officer in a unit studied by the Department of Military Psychiatry of the Walter Reed Army Institute of Research had an impeccable record. He suffered a tragedy in his family, wept before his general, and was relieved of his command. Subsequently, he was passed over for promotion and separated without a pension.

In 1981, members of the military psychiatric research community undertook to collaborate with the Deputy Chief of Staff for Personnel in finding ways to enhance resistance to the stresses of combat. Experimentation, research, and/or evaluation have included pharmacological, organizational, and leadership approaches. The latter two domains have proved to be most promising, but their target was again junior enlisted personnel, not the leaders. Research on strengthening the psychological readiness, competence, and stamina of leaders was, until 1990, conducted only in the civilian sector.

PSYCHIATRIC PROBLEMS PECULIAR TO LEADERS

Because most of the available data on psychiatric problems of and support for leaders come from the civil sector, military psychiatry is initially dependent on civilian experience and research in designing programs to support commanders. It is helpful to have a starting point, but there are departures as well as correspondences between civilian and military executive roles. There are fewer levels of management in the civil sector that practice leadership per se. Officers in the combat branches of the army and marine corps have to become leaders within their first year. Officers in the navy, air force, and technical services acquire leadership responsibilities somewhat earlier than do their civilian peers. It is important to consider the differences and similarities of civilian and military executive roles and the processes by which individuals are prepared for such roles.

Stress Among Civilian Leaders

Research on stress management among leaders in the civil sector has focussed on chief executive officers and other senior managers. The reasons for this are obvious; stress breakdown in a top manager has more far-reaching effects than it does in a junior person, and with limited resources, it makes sense to take care of the people whose behavior has the most impact. The responsibility, isolation, and expectations associated with military leadership often are not present in civilian organizations except at the top levels. This fact in itself is a special source of stress for civilian executives because the training and experience that put them in line for promotion to a senior leadership position were technical skills, such as manufacturing, accounting, and sales, rather than leadership skills. They reach senior executive roles thinking they know the business and find they are in an entirely different set of psychological circumstances. In the words of one chief executive officer, "The development process short-changes the role of leadership. . . . Being a successful top manager means overcoming the limitations of becoming one."[38]

A review of civilian research on leadership and stress reveals four salient issues: isolation, competence, defenses, and support.

Isolation

Civilian chief executives find suddenly that they have no social supports within the organization. Relationships that were perfectly appropriate in a subordinate position can compromise an executive's authority. If a chief continues to confide his doubts and worries to a former colleague, it will probably lead to ill-feeling among other subordinates about the executive's playing favorites. If a relationship with a subordinate confidant includes romantic or sexual components, the effects could lead to a rapid deterioration of the executive's authority. His people want him to be a strong, autonomous leader, not one dependent on subordinates. This expectation, when combined with absence of social supports, is a burden peculiar to both military and civilian leaders.

Also waiting for the military and civilian executive is the trap of believing their own press releases. It is easy to fall prey to hubris. The executive-commander is the cynosure of all eyes, the fulfiller of all hopes, and the source of a great many fears. He must recognize that he is seen as larger than life. Every word he says will be the subject of interest and discussion among his subordinates. They will seek to anticipate his wishes and will, in many cases, go beyond the limits he intends. Understanding this amplification effect gives the executive-commander enormous power to influence events. However, becoming convinced of his own omnipotence and infallibility leads to further isolation. If a leader believes in himself totally and tolerates no one else's ideas, he will soon teach his subordinates to keep their mouths shut, and he will lose contact with what is going on in his organization.

A paradoxical corollary of the leader's position is that he is socially isolated among a large number of people seeking social contact. The problem is that the subordinates are seeking support rather than giving it, or if they are offering support, it is for the purpose of manipulating the leader—taking from him the autonomy essential to carrying out the particular functions of leadership. Subordinates clamor for decisions, approval, signs of favor, and hearings for ideas. The military and civilian executive must ration his time and energy so that none of the subordinates feel neglected, none acquire a predominant influence, and the executive's time and energy are not exhausted.[38]

All of these stresses arising from isolation are applicable to military and civilian leaders. The only difference is that they affect an infantry platoon leader when he is 22-years-old; they may not hit an executive in banking or the pharmaceutical industry until he is 50-years-old.

Competence

The civilian executive's and military commander's primary responsibility is to define the purpose and course of the organization. To carry out this responsibility, he must function concurrently in the present, the immediate future, and the distant future. He lives in a broad context of continuing uncertainty. Reassurance comes when his judgment proves to be correct, but the reassurance is only momentary; the future continues to be full of uncertainties. The ability to function effectively in such an environment is called vision. Vision is an intangible quality difficult to define precisely, but it includes knowledge, judgment, courage, and close contact with reality.

Knowledge comes from experience and study. It includes detailed information about the financial, material, and human resources required and available, and how requirements and availability are changing. With respect to people, the executive needs to know what skills and temperaments are most productive in the context of the organization, how to attract them, and how to capture their interest and commitment. Many of these kinds of knowledge a budding executive or commander acquires in fulfilling a variety of assignments at progressively greater levels of complexity. Many large companies and the armed services deliberately rotate junior and middle leaders through different functions.

Judgment is the faculty that assigns weights and priorities to incomplete and often conflicting fragments of evidence. Making decisions with incomplete data is the woof and warp of the civilian executive's and military executive's life. One definition of good judgment is guessing what works. There are both stress and zest in living with perpetual uncertainty. An infrequently recognized component of judgment is the ability to detect when one is becoming addicted to the zest and taking the organization into risky ventures for the thrill of having one's judgment validated more dramatically.

Courage is an essential aspect of vision, and one that is often degraded by experience. A leader must pursue new and uncharted ventures and must terminate popular, familiar, and comfortable activities that are reassuring and familiar to the members of the organization. Any change will provoke resistance, and the leader becomes a focus for hostility arising out of members' fears that they will not be able to cope with the changes, will lose status or influence, and may even lose their jobs. They will act out their feelings of helplessness and fear by opposing, vilifying, and undermining the chief. It takes courage to persevere, especially since the best way to neutralize the subordinates' hostility is with forbearance and understanding. Middle managers and officers who take unpopular positions or challenge their superiors' policies usually have short careers. Aspirants for promotion must, therefore, develop their courage privately or exercise it discretely.

Vision is not the province of visionaries; it is a function of leaders who are in close contact with the capabilities of their subordinates and the realities of the situation in which they work. An executive's vision is meaningless unless subordinates can understand it, believe they can carry it out, and see how it can pay off for them as individuals and as members of the organization. When the members of an organization embrace his vision, it alleviates the leader's isolation by bringing all members of the organization together in a common enterprise.[39(pp269–274)]

The leader's words and behavior create a climate in the organization that can impede or facilitate the implementation of his policies. A leadership climate can emphasize, for example, a spirit of being on the crest of a wave of new developments or of self-conscious belt-tightening or of commitment to precision. But creating and maintaining a particular kind of climate requires the leader to be consistent. There is a risk of sending inadvertent messages that are contrary to his intentions. The executive must learn to monitor constantly the possible second- and third-order consequences of words, acts, and policies. Keeping watch over one's casual remarks and gestures is fatiguing and stressful, and when the leader makes a slip, it can be personally demoralizing as well as operationally disadvantageous.[40]

Defenses

The executive, because he is the one responsible for setting the course of the organization, rarely has clear and specific guidelines about what to do. The role is inherently ambiguous. The executive can only get validation of his judgment by events that may not unfold for years. The executive lives in a world of permanent uncertainty. Events today can demonstrate the correctness of the executive's judgment, but it is judgment that was exercised months or years ago. A vast array of decisions is always awaiting validation. To alleviate the inevitable anxiety inherent in executive roles, executives may unconsciously make use of maladaptive defenses.

The chief is perpetually caught between the Scylla of symbolism and the Charybdis of detail. If he goes too far in the direction of generality, he will give subordinates the impression of being in another world that has nothing to do with problems that subordinates face. On the other hand, if the boss gets enmeshed in micromanaging, he will lose sight of the overall purpose of the organization. The problem lies in the leader going to one extreme or the other for unperceived psychological reasons. Abstraction can be a welcome respite from the need to make specific decisions. When a chief gets hooked on the freedom of dealing in airy generalities, it may become hard to get back to business, and his usefulness may be ending. Just as seductive to the executive or commander who feels the burden of making plans the fruits of which may not be apparent for years is getting down to the workers or troops and making little improvements in technique. Such interventions are gratifying because they show results immediately, but they are the province of front-line supervisors. Some executives find so much satisfaction in "helping" their subordinates do their jobs that they neglect their own job of looking into the future and making long-range decisions.

Uncertainty combined with isolation and responsibility can impose stresses that will make the most stable and mature personality grope unconsciously for succor. The most obvious need is for companions who will reassure the executive about his wisdom and worth and help deny the evidence of advancing age. These companions may be compliant subordinates—the "yes-man" phenomenon or sexual partners who restore the executive's faith in his lovability—or intellectual confidants. It is appropriate for leaders to treat their subordinates with respect and friendliness. It is, therefore, extremely easy for a chief to become involved in a dependency or sexual relationship with a subordinate, thinking all the while that he is engaging in appropriate role behavior. The key variable of which the executive is usually unaware is his own need for emotional support, reassurance, and sustenance.

Closely linked with sexual adventurism is recreational risk-taking. Hunting, racing cars and boats, climbing mountains, and other high-risk sports expand the arena of a leader's uncertainty. (They also expose the organization to an increased likelihood of suddenly needing to find a new chief.) Their practitioners describe these activities as "relaxing," but a more accurate description is that they are distracting. They take the executive's mind off the uncertainties in the organization, but they do not bring him any closer to confronting, understanding, or neutralizing the anxieties that may distort his judgment.

Another defense is the omnipotence referred to earlier. The executive got to his position through being a highly successful manager. Why should he not have complete confidence in himself? Total belief in one's own judgment is inherently reassuring; it gives the chief and his subordinates the illusion that everything is under control. But omnipotence is an exercise in self-deception to hide from oneself feelings of inadequacy, insecurity, and vulnerability. The more precarious the chief's ability to tolerate uncertainty, the more he is likely to cling tenaciously to a conviction of omnipotence. Operationally, it closes the executive's data receptors, and he loses control.

Supports

An executive or commander can find social supports and psychological security among members of his family, friends, peers, and psychiatrists. The first three of these categories of relationships have important limitations. While relationships with spouse, children, and parents may include mistrust, jealousy, or antagonism, often there will be one or two in a familial constellation who can be supportive. Friends often combine a limited interest with an unspoken agenda. Peers are almost always competitors, at least in achievement if not for markets. This situation leaves the psychiatrist, who ironically is often least able to help a leader before a breakdown because acceptance of one's psychic vulnerability is incompatible with the self-confidence that chief executives and commanders are expected to display.

Recent work by Jackson[41] with corporate executives has indicated that a combination of psychotherapist and peers in a group setting oriented toward strengthening the strong rather than curing the sick can be both acceptable to executives and effective in protecting them against stress breakdown.

Case Study

In 1982, a dynamic young general at the Pentagon became concerned that some of his most able commanders were becoming disabled or dying from myocardial infarctions. He organized a three-pronged approach: physical assessment (the "over 40" physical examination including a stress electrocardiogram); physical conditioning; and stress management exercises (relaxation, group discussion, and so forth) led by organizational effectiveness personnel. The program identified a number of colonels at risk and probably saved their lives. The outcome of the stress-management intervention is harder to assess.

Comment: This approach, couched in terms of fitness, if institutionalized, might be a method by which commanders could get psychological support without stigma.

Stress Among Military Leaders

There are three major differences between the stresses military leaders experience and those their civilian counterparts encounter. First, the risks in the military are higher. Failure, loss of status, and dismissal face both soldiers and civilians. But the officer's competitors are, during wartime, seeking to kill him and those for whom he is responsible. Second, the character of the relationship between leader and subordinate is many times more comprehensive in the military than it is in the civil sector. A civilian executive is responsible for providing direction to his subordinates in accordance with an overarching design and for developing his subordinates in a vocational sense. The military officer has these responsibilities and also is responsible for feeding, housing, and clothing subordinates; for assisting them with personal and familial problems; and for protecting them against the efforts of the enemy to kill them. The third difference in civilian and military leadership stresses is the age at which they begin. Many military officers find themselves in their first vocational experience as platoon leaders or division officers responsible for training, motivating, punishing, and comforting 20 to 40 enlisted personnel. It is instructive to review for military officers two of the issues—isolation and competence—identified as salient in the research[38] on stress among civilian executives. The defenses and supports available to both civilian and military leaders are generally similar.

Isolation

"The lonely splendor of command" is an accurate cliché for both military and civilian leaders. But for many military leaders, the isolation begins with the first duty assignment. There is an immediate legal and social gulf between the officer and his enlisted personnel. In wartime, the officer is alone in the responsibility of doing everything he can to keep his subordinates comfortable, healthy, and alive while directing them to undertake missions that put their lives at risk. In peacetime, the officer is alone in the responsibility for his subordinates' personal, professional, and familial welfare while directing them to undertake tasks that may appear purposeless and that keep them from their families and personal development.

In common with the civilian chief executive, the military leader must keep his fears and doubts from subordinates and must avoid getting involved in dependency relationships with them. Also in common with the civilian executives, the officer needs to be wary of believing in his omniscience. Being the sole authority figure in a group of 30 or 40 at the age of 22 is heady business, and the readiness of some subordinates to curry favor can easily unbalance a young officer's judgment. Isolated as he is, it is often hard to find corrective perspectives. The officer's immediate commander may be physically remote and is certain to be inundated with work. Research has shown that he is unlikely to have much time or energy to provide balance, reassurance, or psychological sustenance.[36(pp15–17),42(p118)] Other junior officers are each surrounded by their own subordinates and have little time to support each other.

One factor can mitigate the junior officer's isolation and is not generally available to the civilian executive. It is love. Students of superior-subordinate relations in the civil sector usually insist that intimate, or family-like, relationships are inappropriate in vocational settings.[38] But small military units are, psychologically, families. The members are physically close together, experience fear and hardship together, and are dependent on each other for survival in the face of the enemy and for avoidance of harassment in garrison. The leader, although socially and legally segregated, often becomes a psychologically integral member of the group. The leader comes to love his subordinates and to be beloved by them, all the while holding extraordinary powers over them. The love has nothing to do with sexuality or the sexual composition of the unit. It has to do with trust, respect, and interdependence developed during shared experiences. The degree to which military leaders can derive support from intimacy with their subordinates is a function of several complex factors. The prerequisite is time together pursuing common goals under stressful conditions. If, in such a setting, a junior officer demonstrates that he will share all the risks and discomforts, take action to protect his subordinates and alleviate their discomforts, attend to their distress before his own, and contribute to accomplishing goals valued by the group, intimacy can develop. If the leader is sufficiently secure to accept the risks of intimacy, it will develop. Although there have been a great many words written about how authority and discipline are degraded by familiarity between leaders and subordinates, the most thoughtful writers[43–45] have recognized that intimacy brings strength. A U.S. Army Regulation[46] adopted in 1915 states:

> Officers will keep in as close touch as possible with the men under their command and will strive to build up such relations of confidence and sympathy as will insure free approach of their men for counsel and assistance. This relationship may be gained without relaxation of the bonds of discipline and with great credit to the service as a whole[46(p11)]

Research during the 1980s indicated that in the most cohesive and effective military units, there is intimacy between leaders and followers, without the least diminution of obedience or respect for authority.[33] In fact, it is the trust and respect that the members of the unit have come to feel for each other as a consequence of the suffering they have endured and the things they have done in each other's presence—and often for each other's benefit—that are the bases for both discipline and love. In cohesive units, the leader's authority rests on the confidence his subordinates have in his ability to lead them in ways that will maximize damage to the enemy and minimize injury to them and on their trust that the leader will never abandon them. Subordinates in cohesive units may call their officer by nicknames, they may feel comfortable arguing with him, and they may disregard rituals of subordination, but they execute his orders immediately, creatively, and with full commitment. Junior military officers who experience such mutual trust and confidence are not isolated; many report leading a platoon or being a division officer on a ship as being the richest experience of their lives. Some have lifelong friendships with the members of their platoons.

Commanders at higher levels have progressively fewer opportunities to share daily and directly in the lives of their private soldiers. Company-level commanders and department heads, with 50 to 200 subordinates, can know all of them and can do informal things with many of them. They can interact as quasi-equals in such activities as the unit softball team, talking during a long night vigil, or sweating out the birth of the subordinate's child. Combined with competent performance of his duty and attention to the needs of his subordinates, these informal activities enable a unit commander to contribute to a climate of trust and respect in the unit, and the commander will feel the goodwill, the support, and even the love of his subordinates. Commanders of battalions, squadrons, and ships have 300 to 1,000 subordinates; they can rarely know all of them and can only interact informally with a few. The unrelieved nature of their isolation resembles more closely that of the civilian chief executive. Commanders at the colonel/navy captain level and general/flag officers also experience unrelieved isolation. They interact socially and professionally with a great many other officers, but they are alone; they cannot have close experiences with any of their subordinates without presenting a confusing image to them.

A paradoxical aspect of military commanders' isolation is the need for a clearly understood system for succession. Because of the violent nature of military activities, each commander must keep his immediate subordinates sufficiently aware of his intentions so that they can act independently in accordance with his plan even when out of communication for prolonged periods or when the commander is killed. This requirement entails intimacy between a commander and his subordinates on a professional level; the paradox is that the ultimate purpose of the intimacy is to facilitate pursuit of the mission when the senior partner in the relationship is dead. The loss of a beloved leader, however, can have devastating effects.

Competence

On the strictly vocational level, the officer's technical knowledge is the foundation of his authority. This is true for the civilian executive also but in a more restricted sense. If a civilian chief executive lays out a marketing and production plan that fails, the stockholders lose dividends; if a commander lays out a battle plan that fails, his soldiers lose their lives. Even in peacetime, the stakes riding on a commander's knowledge are higher psychologically than they are in a civilian organization. Members of a military unit identify with it; they derive their sense of worth from it. Soldiers confer authority on a commander who "knows his stuff," who can lead them in the way of success, and who knows how to take care of them. They find ways of evading or undercutting the orders of an ignorant leader. Civilian subordinates also are involved psychologically and practically with their organizations, but their involvement is not as intense. Civilians can quit a company without leaving their field. For civilians, the job is largely a way of earning money, and in our culture, an individual's sense of worth is often associated with the amount he earns rather than what he does. Frequently, the way to increase income is to move to another firm. For a soldier, the military provides a living, but the soldier's sense of worth is based more on the importance of his role and the reputation and mission of the unit. Identity as a soldier/sailor/airman/marine confers a sense of personal significance.[47(pp218–219)]

Lack of knowledge is a severe source of stress for newly commissioned officers. They know less about the army than their subordinates, yet they are in charge. Most officers never feel fully prepared for their jobs, and spend most of their careers studying. The armed services recognize that officers need to know a great deal about many fields and fields in which there are rapid changes; every 5 years or so, they give officers an academic year off to study at a military school.[48]

The range of knowledge an officer requires can best be illustrated with vignettes.

Vignette 1—The Reversed Screw. A lieutenant in an air defense battery found that the tractors with which the unit was equipped would only go 10 miles per hour when they were supposed to be capable of 30. None of her maintenance people could fix the tractors. She had them explain how they adjusted the engines and then went over the procedures in the technical manual. They were doing everything as the manual prescribed. One of the adjustments involved turning a screw clockwise for maximum performance, but the screw was under a floorboard and faced downward. The lieutenant visualized the problem from the perspective of the screw rather than the mechanic. She showed the mechanics what to do and the tractors performed correctly.

Vignette 2—Taxes Everywhere. A new company commander in a foreign country got a notice from the host government that his unit had failed to pay social security taxes for indigenous kitchen helpers for more than a year, and he would be imprisoned if the arrears were not paid within 10 days. He had to find the appropriate office and official, find out what the tax law required, learn how to comply, and figure out what the back taxes were—all in a foreign language.

Vignette 3—Chaperonage. An officer in a unit that included both men and women was periodically on duty in Saudi Arabia. He learned that the Saudi religious police would arrest any woman who appeared in public without her husband. Because the women in the unit wanted to tour the city, the officer proposed that each woman pair up with a man who would say he was her husband. The religious police accosted several couples, received reassuring answers, and left the women alone.

Vignette 4—The Covenant of the Arc. A staff officer was detailed to investigate the shelling of a friendly village by American artillery. He identified the battery that had fired, interviewed its personnel, and found that no one knew how to calculate corrections for the effects of weather on artillery shells. He subsequently found that no one in higher headquarters knew how either. In the melee of charges and countercharges about who would be court martialed for the incident, he was the only one who had facts or an understanding of the facts. Several people in the chain of command who were exposed to responsibility sought to get him to alter his findings, and failing that, to discredit him.

These vignettes illustrate the range of knowledge officers must acquire. Two of the vignettes also illustrate how lack of knowledge can be a source of intense stress. It is a double-acting source. Efforts to learn more put pressure on an already packed schedule, and lack of knowledge is not an excuse for inaction. The officer must act and endure the stress from making a decision on the basis of inadequate information.

The military leader's judgment is put to the test more often than is the civilian executive's because the officer operates in an arena in which there are more unknowns. Judgment is a learned faculty; experience and knowledge sharpen it. But frequent exposure to having to act in a climate of multiple uncertainty with severe penalties for failure does not necessarily "hone" judgment. A leader can protect himself from the psychological stress of making such judgments by becoming fatalistic—a process that does not enhance the rational content in judgment. Some leaders burn out and opt not to make judgments. Some convince themselves that they will win some and lose some. When they are wrong they repress the memory and drive on. Making demands on judgment is always psychologically expensive. When, in combat, the enemy defeats an officer's judgment and kills his people, the emotional cost escalates rapidly. Because they must use judgment early, often, and for mortal stakes, comparatively few officers become addicted to risk as some executives do, but many become reluctant to make decisions.

In his very first assignment, the military leader needs the kind of moral courage the civilian executive needs when pushing through changes to popular and familiar procedures. The officer needs a second kind of courage when leading his subordinates into danger that he shares. The military leader needs a third and most demanding type of courage to order his subordinates into danger that he will not share. The commanders of units from platoons on up normally direct the maneuvers of their subordinate elements from at least somewhat protected command posts. The officer seeks to coordinate the movement of subordinate units with fire support in ways that neutralize the ability of the enemy to harm them and maximize the damage done to the enemy. This is the essence of the military commander's version of vision, and it takes a special kind of courage to carry it out when his subordinates are facing enemy fire.

People who have never experienced military command may perceive that officers do not exercise vision because they are merely executors of plans developed at remote headquarters. It is true that most military operations are carefully planned to bring as many uncertainties as possible under control, and battles are controlled by phase lines, boundaries, schedules, and the like. The military passion to plan is driven by the fact that there are more numerous and more dangerous uncertainties in war than there are in corporate operations. Vision is essential to the military commander in three respects. First, the apparently simple act of putting an armed force in position to confront an enemy entails forward thinking about tons of food, ammunition, and fuel; hospitals, tents, and spare part stocks; air and sealift capacity; terrain, enemy forces, and weather; and the numbers, equipment, and training of friendly units. The plan requires vision. Second, orders assign missions; it is up to the subordinate commander to figure out how to accomplish them. Battles may take minutes or hours, but for the participants, they last an eternity. The visualization at the small unit level of who does what, when, and how; what enemy reactions might develop and how they might be countered; and how to keep balanced in case of unexpected developments must be carried out minute by minute in advance. Third and probably the most critical facet of military vision, and the one that most closely resembles the chief executive officer's vision, is developing forces in peacetime. Commanders at all levels set goals for the long term development of their units knowing that at any time they may be called into combat. The kind of battle they will be called for is never known, personnel are coming and going, new equipment is due in and personnel will need to practice with it but no one knows when it will arrive, and funds for training and travel are unpredictable. A lot of vision is required.

Stress on Military Leaders in Modern Warfare

Military service has evolved into a generalized readiness to engage at short notice in a wide range of predictable and unpredictable missions involving danger, discomfort, and separation from families. There is no permanent enemy that soldiers and leaders can learn to visualize as evil; there will be a series of temporary adversaries, generically described as "the bad guys." Military personnel will have to fight members of an armed force defined as enemy and, then after defeating them, often succor them.

The nature of military action may be nonviolent, as in stabilization, peace-keeping, or nation-building operations. It may involve low-level violence, as in counter-insurgency or counter-terrorist operations. Or the intervention may be against a modern armed force capable of high-intensity combat operations possibly including chemical, biological, or nuclear weapons. The nature of an operation may change, as it did in the invasion of Panama in 1989 and the Persian Gulf War in 1991. The first began as medium-intensity combat using minimal force to limit enemy as well as civilian and friendly casualties, but it quickly became a civil government and institution-building operation.[49–51] The U.S. Army's involvement in the Persian Gulf War began as a show of force to deter Iraqi moves into Saudi Arabia. A buildup and embargo culminated in an ultimatum for Iraqi withdrawal from Kuwait. When this was not forthcoming, the American and allied involvement escalated into a high-intensity conventional air attack, then ground-sea-air attack, then into a relief operation for Iraqi minority groups.[52–53] The leaders had to have sufficient knowledge, common sense, and flexibility to sustain their soldiers' morale and persistence in the face of changing missions that were difficult to perform, obscure in purpose, and always dangerous. Their success was a consequence of changes in U.S. military doctrine,[35] and in the organization, manning systems, and leadership training to support them. The interlocking patterns of stress that commanders in such operations have to endure will be evident from the discussion that follows.

The nature of low-intensity and counter-insurgency operations entails the deployment of very small numbers of military personnel in the midst of populations that are either skeptical or hostile and whose language most soldiers do not understand. The soldiers' anxiety is very high because there may be no apparent danger and when it comes, it will be a surprise. They are completely dependent on each other's alertness and on their leader's judgment to survive and accomplish their missions. Squads or platoons will be out of sight of each other and out of range of supporting weapons. In a sea of people, any of whom could become lethally hostile at any moment, the leader is under perpetual stress. Commanders know that any of their units could be snuffed out in a moment before they could intervene.

At the other end of the scale of violence is high-intensity war. Technology makes possible almost continual pulses of combat involving weapons of extreme lethality. Surveillance systems make it difficult to conceal units and weapons, and the only hope for survival lies in a high degree of dispersal. Electronic warfare will normally interdict electrical communications. The leaders of small units will be isolated and out of contact with supporting headquarters for prolonged periods. Commanders will have very little information about their subordinate elements and will live in advanced states of anxiety. The psychological effects on units, even well-equipped, battle-seasoned, elite units, were demonstrated in the collapse of many Iraqi units under allied air, sea, and ground attack in 1991.[52]

The stress on leaders in forces that must be prepared for an overnight deployment to engage in such a wide range of military actions is high in peacetime as well as wartime. Measures to improve the fighting capacity and psychological readiness of units may enhance the gratifications inherent in military command, but they do not mitigate the strain. Research[29,54] on cohesive, high-performance military units in which the first-term soldiers were stabilized for 3 years revealed that the demands on leaders were increased. These demands were of three basic types—intellectual, behavioral, and emotional. The demands were interactive; to describe them, it is necessary to outline the relational system within such units. The descriptions are derived from research done by teams from the Walter Reed Army Institute of Research during the 1985 to 1991 time period, but the same patterns are reported by other observers in other countries and services.[29,33,54,55]

In several cohesive, high-performance units, soldiers bonded strongly with each other during their basic and advanced individual training. They came to trust and depend on each other, to be concerned about each other's welfare, and to share values throughout the unit. Because of their mutual concern and common values, if a superior did something the privates thought was unfair to one soldier, that superior became the target for the enmity of the whole unit. Similarly, if a leader went out of his way to help a soldier, all would know about it and approve. Leaders lived in a goldfish bowl in which all of their actions were judged by all of their subordinates—even if only one member witnessed an action.[29,56]

One of the values the soldiers developed in their initial training was interest in military matters and in being effective soldiers. They judged each other on their military aptitude, they helped each other to become proficient, and they reserved their scorn for the soldier whose ineptitude was a consequence of lack of effort or attention. They looked to their leaders to be experts, to teach them, and to respect their interest by talking army to them. Leaders found themselves burning the midnight oil to keep ahead of their soldiers and to develop training experiences they would find challenging and professionally meaningful.[29,33]

The soldiers devoured their leaders' time and energy. They had ideas; they wanted to be in on planning so that they could learn about what goes into an operation. They perceived themselves to be full members of the unit and, as learning professionals, to deserve their leaders' attention. They expected their leaders to be able to teach them how to cope with the problems of being husbands, fathers, and householders. The leaders had to be endlessly accessible, and they still had to find the time to become the physical, moral, and intellectual models in which their troops could have confidence.[29]

The interdependence between leaders and followers, the satisfaction they experienced together when they accomplished a task through joint effort, and the misery they shared getting those jobs done forged links of mutual respect and trust. Respect and trust were supplemented by affection when leaders and followers went out of their way to say or do something to ease or recognize another. Intimacy, a readiness to make oneself vulnerable to someone for whom one has strong trust and affection, emerges spontaneously in many units that are successful in combat. In units that can go into combat overnight, it is desirable to develop intimacy across ranks in peacetime. But it is difficult for most leaders and commanders to tolerate the vulnerability and the feeling of being exposed that intimacy entails. Treatises on civilian leadership proscribe intimacy between the chief and his subordinates. The primary reasons are that the chief is expected to project an image of strength and autonomy, and intimacy appears to be favoritism if bestowed on only a few. In a military platoon, company, small vessel, or aviation unit, intimacy is possible for all members, irrespective of rank. The members are together 24 hours a day for days on end, not just for 40 of the 168 hours in a week. Their lives depend on each other, and the closer they are to each other the more effective they will be in battle.

Intimacy for many leaders is one more source of stress; they have to fend it off, or if they succumb to it, they feel guilty. A paradox of intimacy in military organizations is that it is almost impossible for it to compromise the leader's authority. Here is the dynamic. If subordinates have sufficient trust and respect for a leader to be intimate, his authority is beyond challenge. If he feels sufficiently secure in the authority his troops have conferred on him to be intimate with them, the circle of mutual trust, respect, and affection is complete. The much-maligned "familiarity breeds contempt" is a totally different system of relationships. It begins with a superior who does not feel competent and does not believe he has his subordinates' respect and trust. He wishes to purchase their support with friendly behavior. The subordinates, perceiving both the leader's incompetence and neediness, make use of his overtures to manipulate him. The difference in relational processes between a unit in which informality and affection between leaders and subordinates are based on trust and respect and one in which they are based on scorn is apparent in a few moments of observation.

The cost of fending off intimacy that has been earned and is appropriate is additional stress for the leader and a lower level of cohesion for the unit. The cost of accepting intimacy is negligible. The soldiers have too much affection for their leader to embarrass him in front of a less secure superior who might consider the intimacy within the unit to be inappropriate. Intimacy with subordinates of the kind that is available to a military leader is one of the two most powerful stress buffers available to him. The other is intimacy with his commander. Each leader must have the conviction that his boss is thinking about him, wants him to succeed, will do everything in his power to help him succeed, and will not abandon him on the battlefield. In most combat scenarios, the junior and senior commanders will rarely see each other and sometimes will not even be able to communicate for long periods. Because they are totally dependent on each other, the trust between them that the other is competent and is doing his best needs to be as complete as possible. The higher commander, who rarely sees the battlefield but who is responsible both for his subordinates' accomplishing their mission and for their welfare, can come to hate his subordinates because of his isolation and impotence. Similarly, the junior commander can come to hate his superior for failing to do enough to take care of him and his troops. Commanders at all levels need help in empathizing with those above and below them, in recognizing and accepting their own feelings, and in managing the uncertainty and isolation they will experience.

THE PSYCHIATRIST AND THE COMMANDER

By the time the battle is joined, the opportunity for preventive psychiatry has passed. The partnership between psychiatry and command, like the trust between senior and subordinate leaders, must be forged in peacetime. The commander is responsible for creating the trust and respect necessary to support cohesion and resistance to stress. This has never been considered a medical problem. The psychiatrist cannot be criticized if he deals only with those who break down. Indeed, in combat, the slender mental health resources of a division can be immediately overwhelmed with psychiatric casualties. Before the battle, however, it is possible for the psychiatrist to take a proactive role. He can strengthen the ability of commanders to build relationships with subordinate leaders that will enable them to persevere, command effectively, and create climates that reduce the incidence of stress casualties.

The situational vulnerability of military leaders is not balanced by any system for selecting the psychologically most hardy individuals for leadership positions. In the first place, six decades of research have not turned up reliable screening systems.[57] In the second place, the army is imbued with the democratic ideal that leaders are made, not born.[58(pp251ff),59(pp58ff)] The only screening that differentiates leaders and followers are civilian education and brief military training programs.[60(pp132–133)] Most officers have college degrees, NCOs are expected to be high school graduates, and college credits help enlisted soldiers rise through the ranks. Soldiers selected to be NCOs and college students in military academies or other officer programs receive special training, some of which is designed to test and/or develop ability to persevere through exhaustion, pain, and frustration.[61(pp166ff),62(pp25ff)] In wartime, even these requirements are often waived; the leaders face isolation and responsibility with little preparation and haphazard support.

There are four primary issues the psychiatrist must consider in providing support to military commanders: resistance, military efficiency, modalities of intervention, and the appropriateness of civilian models to the military setting.

Resistance

There is strong resistance among civilian executives to any activity that smacks of psychology or "touchy-feely" approaches. Researchers[38] have found that executives feel uncomfortable unless they are measuring their strength against each other and do not want to reveal private feelings of fear, doubt, or vulnerability. When such topics come up, they typically protect themselves with sarcasm. They feel at ease talking about money, achievements, and victories over competitors, regulatory agencies, and lawyers. Military personnel are, if anything, more resistant to things psychological. Studies in 1987–1990 by the Walter Reed Army Institute of Research[54] showed that even after traumatic combat or surviving a catastrophic accident, neither soldiers nor their leaders wanted mental health professionals in their units. Soldiers in units that suffered casualties during the invasion of Panama in 1989 said afterwards, "The psychiatrist offered to come to the unit, but command dragged its feet." "People fear mental health workers. They might make them look at themselves." "We don't say nothing about our nightmares. It might get into our records."[54]

There are related processes behind soldiers' fear of "shrinks"—mental health theory and mental health professionals. The most fundamental process is a reluctance to upset a psychic system that is working albeit imperfectly. Those soldiers who have been willing to talk about themselves indicate that they have some sense that they have conflicts and problems hovering just beyond awareness and indicate that they would rather not know more about them. To probe them and to penetrate the defenses around them would be to invite pain. Often, membership in a military organization is a part of a defensive system to avoid awareness of feelings of vulnerability, to help control hostile urges, or to achieve a sense of adulthood or potency.

A derivative process is fear that having psychological problems would damage a military career. The fear is accurate. Any evidence of "mental instability" is a mandatory ground for revocation of security clearance. Beyond the fact that no military person can hold a position of responsibility without access to classified information, the stigma of unreliability that accompanies loss of a clearance is enough to stifle any military career. Predictability, stability, and hardiness under stress are essential characteristics of a soldier and particularly of a leader. No one wants to go into combat with an individual labeled as psychologically unstable.

Psychological problems are in a realm of vulnerabilities that cannot be strengthened by working out in the gym or corrected by surgery. They are particularly threatening because they are unknowable, they can manifest themselves without warning, and their effects are unpredictable. To express symptoms of mental illness or to acknowledge a need for psychiatric help is, in most units, a manifestation of weakness that would destroy a male soldier in his own eyes. It would be unthinkable even to admit to himself, and it would certainly be punished forthwith by his superiors and peers. For example, in 1991, a captain with an outstanding record was experiencing symptoms of a psychiatric disorder. He sought inpatient treatment at a military hospital. On discharge he was relieved of his position, given a relief-for-cause efficiency report, and directed to appear before a board of officers to show cause why he should not be eliminated from the service. None of his peers or superiors, all of whom had esteemed him before his hospitalization, would make statements in his behalf.

Because psychological problems are so ephemeral, devastating to a professional military man's sense of himself, and destructive of military careers, few military personnel willingly acknowledge them. Many soldiers have concealed their psychological distress for years; others have acted it out on their subordinates or families or pursued solace through alcohol or drugs. For generations, in armed services throughout the world, alcohol has been an acceptable, if not obligatory, way of avoiding psychological pain.

The challenge is to demonstrate that psychological services can strengthen the masterful, not just cure the needy. It is a legitimate question for the military psychiatrist, given the position of military folklore and culture with respect to his profession, whether he should bother to undertake anything more than recovery of the wreckage of the battlefield and the elimination of those who demonstrate their "unfitness" by seeking help before the battle. However, another given is the psychiatrist's potential for strengthening leaders' ability to create climates in which their subordinates can resist the stresses of combat more successfully. This potential is a strong argument for psychiatrists to make every effort to show the commanders in their units how they can use mental health staff and psychological principles to enhance the psychological readiness of their commands. Each psychiatrist must make his own decision on how much effort he is willing to expend based on the climate in the command in which he is serving.

Military Efficiency

The effect of an insecure commander on subordinate leaders is usually detrimental. As the commander acts out his insecurities through authoritarian, paranoid, or withdrawal behavior, communications dry up, morale among junior leaders plummets, and the efficiency of the organization flags. Junior leaders get out of the service at the first opportunity, abandoning a calling that they had once found highly attractive. Research[63(p77)] has revealed that commanders who are not comfortable with making decisions and accepting responsibility have inefficient units or ships, poor retention among their officers, and high incidence of psychological behavior dysfunction—spouse/child abuse, substance abuse, and inability to commit to the military profession in many subordinates. Under stressful conditions, the greater the complexity of the tasks, the more severe the degradation of performance.[64,65]

Modalities of Intervention

The basic mode of intervention used with civilian executives has been peer workshops. In the few workshops on which data are available, the participants, all of them men, were selected on the basis of being chief executive officers roughly comparable in achievements and reasonably open as human beings. The essential character of the workshops has been developmental, an orientation toward mastery, growth, and empowerment. There is never any mention of therapy or cure. The assumption is that the men are superbly functioning people who want to enhance the richness of their lives and the scope of their competence.

In most of the workshops, the men begin by relating to one another with sarcasm and put-downs. They subtly flex their psychological muscles at each other. The group facilitator works toward introducing the notion that there are new things to be learned—growing, relating, and empowering. He moves the structure of the group from leader-directed to a horizontal, collegial arrangement in which the facilitator is a participant. He can thereby serve as a role model for new ways of relating. He raises questions to encourage the members to understand and appreciate where others are coming from in a pluralistic as contrasted to a right-wrong way. Initially, the members are uncomfortable with open-ended and personal issues. They want structure, an agenda, and closure. The leader challenges them—do they want to play it safe or go for bigger stakes? Do they want to go where they have never been before or not? Gradually, they begin to see that each has vulnerabilities, and the bolder ones lay them out. As they come to feel safer with each other, they open up to new ideas. They begin to look at themes associated with power and intimacy—how they are antithetical and how they can be mutually supportive.

In a second phase, the therapist introduces possible paradigm shifts. The participants come to see the workshop as an opportunity to define themselves as men, and to define their missions in life. Questions arise such as "Could something come out of this other than that I am just stronger? Could I be actually different?" "Can we create something new, question our roles as men?" "Can we reexamine how we have been trained by our culture, parents, school, career?" "Can we develop and pass along the capacity to have more satisfaction?" More complex and conflicting themes emerged—failure, relationships with women, raising children. Gradually, they come to dare to venture into troubling territory and trust the integrity of the group to see them through.

One group, after 7 months, went on a wilderness experience. The group leader hired a ropes expert as an instructor. None of the men had any experience with rock climbing or rappelling. They were terrified. The ropes instructor made his pitch, and no one volunteered. At length, one man said he would do it. He was drenched with sweat and could not repeat the instructions he had been given. The group analyzed what was going on. The man said he was willing to risk his life to look good in front of the other men. He guessed he could do it, but he did not know; he had not been listening to the instructor. He had slipped into a regressive mode; he would do anything to have the illusion of control. The members talked about how this kind of regression could be self-destructive. They were able to understand how the process works because they had seen it and felt it. They explored how it could affect their behavior as chief executive officers or as fathers or husbands. As chief executive officers, they were supposed to know what they were doing, but if they got into a regressive mode, they would be blind to information and ideas. The experience of taking new kinds of risks brought them to see the faces of fear and shame and brought new readiness to accept new ideas.

On one occasion, the group facilitator proposed that the members spend a week observing themselves. They were not to do anything different; they were to respond and behave as they always had but to observe the difference between how they normally reacted and the impulses they had now. They came back furious. They hated the facilitator. It was stupid to deny themselves a breakthrough they had discovered. They discussed the sources of the anger. They came to realize they were imprisoned in the "real man" paradigm, were used to selling out for approval, and would do anything for psychological survival. When this group went on a wilderness experience, one of the men sat against a tree at the bottom while the rest climbed a cliff. He refused to do it. At the debriefing, they all talked about their feelings and he was excited about what he had done. "I had two feelings. One was shame and embarrassment that I had wimped out. The other was pride that I could say 'no,' that I didn't have to look good." The group acknowledged his courage to stand against the real man paradigm. His behavior changed; he became less angry and belligerent and was a more effective leader. Acknowledging and owning his fear and making his own choice had empowered him in a fundamental way.

In a late stage, the groups raised the question of whether they were designing their lives or their lives were designing them. They had worked on leadership, effectiveness, and satisfaction. They were ready to try the leap from being reactive to proactive. A first step was to explore what each was doing to help the other men in the group. They developed a shared vision and then worked to realize it. What they were doing was using the workshop as a case study in generativity. They then applied their discoveries to empowering their subordinates and the members of their families. They also used the concept of a community vision that they had developed in the group to buffer the isolation they experienced in their corporate roles.

They then went on to explore resiliency, the ability to bounce back from a defeat. They practiced in the group turning frustrations and disappointments into opportunities to learn and transferred the technique to their businesses. They learned how to absorb defeats without suffering damage to their senses of self. The basic objective was to maintain a context in which to look at a crisis or a failure as an opportunity for breakthrough into growth.

Psychological resiliency, the ability to persevere and maintain a balanced perspective under stress, has been the subject of research focused on children and civilian executives. The salient findings from studies[66–68] of children are that the resilient ones have interactional histories that have led them to believe they can trust adults to provide guidance, nurturance, and information; have experienced gratification, support, and comfort after deprivation, frustration, and pain; and have identified with competent, supportive adult figures.

Studies[69,70] of adults indicate that the so-called "invulnerables," having experienced repeated successes in the intellectual, physical, and interpersonal aspects of their lives, expect to succeed. They identify with older people who have worked hard and mastered pain, defeat, and loss to achieve important goals. Their commitment to their work is a function of the pleasure they derive from its content and challenge; they are not driven. Maddi and Kobasa[69] have defined "the hardy executive" as one who has a "vigorous sense of commitment, control, and challenge"[69(p32)] and who "reacts to stressful events with transformational rather than regressive coping."[69(p32)] Transformational coping comprises becoming actively engaged with the stressor, understanding and acting on it, and ultimately changing it to reduce its stress potential. The hardy executive recognizes stressors that he cannot alter in an objective sense, and that alteration consists in changing his own attitudinal valences. Transformational coping does not, however, include denying the reality of the stressor, or withdrawal through acting out.[69,70] The evidence indicates that resilience develops throughout adulthood and that hardiness can be learned. Social supports, mastery experiences, and trustworthy adult figures in the vocational and counseling environments can build resilience.[69]

SUMMARY

Military commanders, even more than civilian executives, need to be resilient, invulnerable, transformational copers. They have already experienced substantial success through the process of selection for command. Although not all are invulnerables, many may be on the threshold. The role of the psychiatrist is to work with senior commanders—those commanding ships, battalions, squadrons, and higher level formations—to enhance their sense of invulnerability. They, in their turn, can then create command climates in which resilience and hardiness can develop in their subordinate leaders. The bottom line will be tighter cohesion, stronger commitment, more open communication, and higher levels of resistance to combat stress breakdown within their commands.

The challenges of applying the techniques developed by civilian psychiatrists and psychologists in a military setting are daunting. The resistance of both individuals and the military culture, the frequent absences of commanders from their home station, the 2-year turnover of commanders, and the commanders' and the psychiatrists' workloads all provide excuses for dropping any project of psychiatric support for commanders. One could argue that the importance of being proactive is self-evident for the chief of a corporation but might doubt that it was necessary for a colonel—a leader near the middle of an immense hierarchy. Considering the stress on commanders and leaders at all echelons and the role each plays in creating a climate for his subordinates that either strengthens or compromises resistance to combat stress breakdown, growth workshops for commanders would probably prove useful. Only a few would be interested, but the pattern of predispositions inherent in participating suggests they would profit immensely. And, for every brigade commander who learns that he does not have to look good all the time, 3,000 subordinates will have a better chance of surviving combat physically and psychologically. Psychiatric support for commanders is an idea whose time will come when creative pioneers put it into effect.

REFERENCES

1. Jones FD. Neuropsychiatric casualties of chemical, biological and radiological warfare. In: Jones FD, Sparacino LR, Wilcox VL, Rothberg JM, eds. *War Psychiatry*. Part 1, Vol 6. In: *Textbook of Military Medicine*. Washington, DC: Office of The Surgeon General, US Department of the Army and Borden Institute; 1994: Chap 4. In press.

2. Jones FD. Psychiatric principles of future warfare. In: Jones FD, Sparacino LR, Wilcox VL, Rothberg JM, eds. *War Psychiatry*. Part 1, Vol 6. In: *Textbook of Military Medicine*. Washington, DC: Office of The Surgeon General, US Department of the Army and Borden Institute; 1994: Chap 5. In press.

3. Cincinnatus [pseu]. *Self-Destruction*. New York: Norton; 1981.

4. Gabriel RA, Savage PL. *Crisis in Command*. New York: Hill and Wang; 1978.

5. Hauser WL. *America's Army in Crisis*. Baltimore: Johns Hopkins University Press; 1973.

6. Blair C. *The Forgotten War*. New York: Doubleday; 1987.

7. US Continental Congress. *Regulations for the Order and Discipline of the Troops of the United States*. Part 1. Philadelphia: Styner and Cist; 1779.

8. Millett AR. *The General: Robert L. Bullard and Officership in the United States Army 1881–1925*. Westport, Conn: Greenwood Press; 1975.

9. Prussia. Army. *Drill Regulations for the Infantry, German Army, 1906*. Translated by Behr FJ. Washington, DC: War Department, Office of the Chief of Staff; 1907.

10. Nelsen JT, II. "Auftragstaktik": A case for decentralized battle. *Parameters*. 1987;17(3):22–27.

11. Echevarria AJ, II. "Auftragstaktik": In its proper perspective. *Milit Rev*. 1986;66(10):50–56.

12. Hackworth DH. *About Face*. New York: Simon and Schuster; 1989.

13. Sheehan N. *A Bright Shining Lie*. New York: Random House; 1988.

14. Weigley RF. *History of the United States Army*. Bloomington, Ind: Indiana University Press; 1984: 596–600.

15. Stouffer SA, Suchman EA, DeVinney LC, Star SA, Williams RM, Jr. *The American Soldier. Vol 1: Adjustment During Army Life*. Princeton, NJ: Princeton University Press; 1949.

16. US Department of the Army. *Strength Reports of the Army*. Washington, DC: Office of the Army Comptroller; 1948.

17. Coffman EM. *The Old Army: A Portrait of the American Army in Peacetime 1784–1898*. New York: Oxford University Press; 1986.

18. Elting JR. *American Army Life*. New York: Scribners; 1982.

19. Dixon NF. *On the Psychology of Military Incompetence*. London: Jonathan Cape; 1976.

20. Appleman RE. *South to the Neutong, North to the Yalu, June-November 1950*. Washington, DC: Office of the Chief of Military History; 1961.

21. Fehrenbach TR. *This Kind of War*. New York: Macmillan; 1963.

22. Lunding FJ, Clements GL, Perkins DS. Everybody who makes it has a mentor. In: *Harvard Business Review—On Human Relations*. New York: Harper and Row; 1979: 207–226.

23. Kirkland FR. Combat leadership styles: Empowerment versus authoritarianism. *Parameters*. 1990;20(4):61–72.

24. Peers WR. Leadership requirements in a counter-insurgency environment. Enclosure to memorandum for Chief of Staff, U.S. Army, Subject: The Son My Incident, dated 18 March 1970. In: Cincinnatus [pseu]. *Self-Destruction*. New York: Norton; 1981: 195–198.

25. Carafano JJ. Officership 1966–1971. *Milit Rev*. 1989;69(1):45–52.

26. US Department of the Army. *Study on Military Professionalism*. Carlisle Barracks, Pa: U.S. Army War College; 1970.

27. Ingraham LH. *The Boys in the Barracks*. Philadelphia: Institute for the Study of Human Issues; 1983.

28. Marlowe DH. *New Manning System Field Evaluation*. Washington, DC: Walter Reed Army Institute of Research; 1985. Technical Report 1 (ADA 162087).

29. Kirkland FR, Furukawa TP, Teitelbaum JM, Ingraham LH, Caine BT. *Unit Manning System Field Evaluation*, Washington, DC: Walter Reed Army Institute of Research; 1987. Technical Report 5 (ADA 207193).

30. Kirkland FR. The gap between leadership policy and practice. *Parameters*. 1990;20(3):50–62.

31. US Department of the Army. *Leadership Makes the Difference*. Washington, DC: DA; 1985. DA PAM 600–50.

32. US Department of the Army. *Soldier Team Development*. Washington, DC: DA; 1987. Field Manual 22–102.

33. Kirkland FR. *Leading in COHORT Companies*. Washington, DC: Walter Reed Army Institute of Research; 1987. WRAIR Report NP–88–13 (ADA 192886).

34. Kirkland FR, Katz P. Combat readiness and the Army family. *Milit Rev*. 1989;69(4):68–70, 73–74.

35. US Department of the Army. *Operations*. Washington, DC: DA; 1986. Field Manual 100–5.

36. Schneider RJ, Kirkland FR. Training lieutenants. *Milit Rev*. 1992;72(5):10–21.

37. Jones FD. Traditional warfare combat stress casualties. In: Jones FD, Sparacino LR, Wilcox VL, Rothberg JM, eds. *War Psychiatry*. Part 1, Vol 6. In: *Textbook of Military Medicine*. Washington, DC: Office of The Surgeon General, US Department of the Army and Borden Institute; 1994: Chap 2. In press.

38. Mechanick PG. Psychological considerations for executive leadership. Department of Psychiatry, University of Pennsylvania. Undated. Author's unpublished briefing notes.

39. Covey SR. *The Seven Habits of Highly Effective People*. New York: Simon and Schuster; 1989.

40. Gal R, Jones FD. Psychological aspects of combat stress: A model derived from Israeli and other combat experiences. In: Jones FD, Sparacino LR, Wilcox VL, Rothberg JM, eds. *War Psychiatry*. Part 1, Vol 6. In: *Textbook of Military Medicine*. Washington, DC: Office of The Surgeon General, US Department of the Army and Borden Institute; 1994: Chap 6. In press.

41. Jackson MA. *Corporate Initiatives*. Ardmore, Pa: Center for Psychological Services; 1994.

42. Oliver D, Jr. Growing. *US Naval Instit Proceed*. 1990;116(12):117–118.

43. Ashley-Montagu MF. *Touching*. New York: Columbia University Press; 1971.

44. Lyon HC, Jr. *Tenderness Is Strength*. New York: Harper and Row; 1977.

45. Morris D. *Intimate Behavior*. New York: Random House; 1971.

46. US War Department. *Regulations for the Army of the United States*. Washington, DC: GPO; 1913 with change to US Army Regulation No. 35, 5 November 1915 applied to p11, para 3.

47. Kirkland FR. Men, women, and the Army reserve. In: Goldman NL, ed. *Women in the United States Armed Forces: Progress and Barriers in the 1980s*. Chicago: Inter-University Seminar on Armed Forces and Society; 1984: 218–219.

48. Crocker LP. *The Army Officer's Guide*. 43rd ed. Harrisburg, Pa: Stackpole; 1985.

49. Donnelly T, Roth M, Baker C. *Operation Just Cause: The Storming of Panama*. New York: Macmillan; 1989.

50. McConnell M. *Just Cause*. New York: St. Martin's Press; 1991.

51. Watson BW, Tsouras PG. *Operation Just Cause*. Boulder, Colo: Westview Press; 1991.

52. *Conduct of the Persian Gulf War: An Interim Report to Congress*. Washington, DC: GPO; 1991.

53. Friedman N. *Desert Victory: The War for Kuwait*. Annapolis, Md: Naval Institute Press; 1991.

54. Kirkland FR, Ender MG, Gifford RK, Wright KM, Marlowe DH. Human dimensions of rapid force projection: Operation Just Cause, December 1989. *Milit Rev*. 1994;74(11):in press.

55. Gal R. *The Israeli Soldier*. Westport, Conn: Greenwood Press; 1989.

56. Kirkland FR. Assessing COHORT. *Army*. 1990;40(5):44–50.

57. Jones FD. Psychiatric lessons of war. In: Jones FD, Sparacino LR, Wilcox VL, Rothberg JM, eds. *War Psychiatry*. Part 1. In: *Textbook of Military Medicine*. Washington, DC: Office of The Surgeon General, US Department of the Army and Borden Institute; 1994: Chap 1. In press.

58. US Department of the Army. *Military Leadership*. Washington, DC: DA; 1983. Field Manual 22–100.

59. US Department of Defense. *The Armed Forces Officer*. Washington, DC: DoD; 1975. DA PAM 600–2.

60. Bassford C. *The Spit-Shine Syndrome*. New York: Greenwood Press; 1988.

61. Atkinson R. *The Long Gray Line*. Boston: Houghton Mifflin; 1989.

62. Barkalow C. *In the Men's House*. New York: Poseidon Press; 1990.

63. Oliver D, Jr. Keeping the campers happy. *US Naval Instit Proceed*. 1991;117(2):76–78.

64. Manning FJ, Ingraham LH. Continuous operations: Who melts, when, and why? *Field Artillery J*. 1981;49:13–18.

65. Manning FJ. *Human Factors in Sustaining High Rates of Artillery Fire*. Washington, DC: Walter Reed Army Institute of Research; 1985. WRAIR Report NP. 84–7.

66. Anthony EJ. Risk, vulnerability, and resilience: An overview. In: Anthony EJ, Cohler BJ, eds. *The Invulnerable Child*. New York: Guilford Press; 1987: 3–48.

67. Moriarity AE. John, a boy who acquired resilience. In: Anthony EJ, Cohler BJ, eds. *The Invulnerable Child*. New York: Guilford Press; 1987: 106–144.

68. Musick JS, Stott FM, Spencer KK, Goldman J, Cohler BJ. 1987. Maternal factors related to vulnerability and resiliency in young children at risk. In: Anthony EJ, Cohler BJ, eds. *The Invulnerable Child*. New York: Guilford Press; 1987: 229–252.

69. Maddi SR, Kobasa SC. *The Hardy Executive: Health Under Stress*. Homewood, Ill: Dow Jones-Irwin; 1984.

70. Peck EC, Jr. The traits of true invulnerability and posttraumatic stress in psychoanalyzed men of action. In: Anthony EJ, Cohler BJ, eds. *The Invulnerable Child*. New York: Guilford Press; 1987: 315–60.

Chapter 11

EDUCATING MENTAL HEALTH WORKERS

RONALD J. KOSHES, M.D.,* JOHN M. PLEWES, M.D.,† BRIAN G. McCAUGHEY, D.O.,‡ AND JAMES STOKES, M.D.§

*Medical Director, Adult Services Administration, Commission on Mental Health Services, Department of Human Services, District of Columbia, Washington 20032; Guest Scientist, Department of Military Psychiatry, Walter Reed Army Institute of Research, Washington, D.C., Clinical Assistant Professor of Psychiatry, Uniformed Services University of the Health Sciences, Bethesda, Maryland; President, Society of American Military Psychiatrists

†Lieutenant Colonel, Medical Corps, U.S. Army; Chief, Department of Psychiatry, Fort Bragg, North Carolina, and Clinical Assistant Professor of Psychiatry, Uniformed Services University of the Health Sciences, Bethesda, Maryland 20889–4799

‡Captain (ret), Medical Corps, U.S. Navy; Naval Health Sciences Education and Training Command, and Assistant Professor of Military Medicine and Psychiatry, Uniformed Services University of the Health Sciences, Bethesda, Maryland 20889–4799

§Colonel, Medical Corps, U.S. Army; Chief, Psychiatry and Neurology Branch, Behavioral Sciences Division, Academy of Health Sciences, Fort Sam Houston, Texas 78234–6133

INTRODUCTION

Mental health workers play a unique role in military organizations. They work with families, military units, individual soldiers, sailors, and airmen to promote cohesive working and family relationships, improve morale, and maximize unit effectiveness. They also provide direct services to individuals with psychiatric or emotional problems. Finally, mental health workers consult with leaders about effective strategies to support military units during war and peace. In these varied roles, military mental health workers focus especially on occupational health.

Military and civilian mental health professionals differ in many respects. For one, the arena of practice is different. Military mental health professionals must not only aggressively intervene with units and individuals during war but also provide a greater focus on families, assist in stress reduction within units, raise morale issues, and explore other preventive mental health concerns during peacetime. Civilian practice provides few models for military mental health workers. The calmness of garrison life may be interrupted at any time by a national emergency, requiring mobilization of individual units or entire armies that must face dangerous missions and uncertain futures. Mental health workers are often part of the mobilization and share the same risks and uncertainties of their client population. In addition, practitioners of various disciplines are required to work together within the military rank system. Mental health professionals, although experts in their field, often work under the jurisdiction of higher ranking officers in command of the fighting forces.

Stress is inevitable in combat and often decides success or failure. This recognition makes the military mental health provider unique from his civilian counterpart. Training, therefore, must reflect this difference in preparation for battle.[1] To improve training of psychiatrists to work with infantry commanders, Lee devised a course for psychiatry residents to participate in the activities of light combat infantry battalions at Fort Ord, California.[2] The first residents in the course (Leamon and Sutton) found that familiarity with the mission of the units helped them in providing effective psychiatric interventions.[2] The equally impressive finding was that all three battalion commanders involved in the project expressed "enthusiastic support" for the program and requested that their units remain involved in the subsequent years. That program has not continued, but a conceptually similar program has been sustained at Schofield Barracks, Hawaii.

Although these special courses are novel and important, they are often carried forward by the enthusiasm and drive of their originators. The military unit consultation training must compete for time with other parts of the psychiatric curriculum that are required for accreditation of the residency program. The training may lapse unless other faculty members support it actively.

New army doctrine has been written that requires the intimate involvement of mental health personnel in the work of units. The Army Medical Department operational concept for combat stress control (CSC) and Field Manual 8–51[3] specify that each maneuver brigade in a division needs a dedicated brigade CSC team consisting of one mental health officer and one behavioral science noncommissioned officer (NCO) from the division mental health section. Before combat, the brigade CSC team must be proficient in field and survival skills and knowledgeable about combat stress reactions and general mental health issues. The CSC personnel must know the equipment and mission of the supported units. They must interact with and teach all of the brigade's leaders, chaplains, and medical personnel to enhance combat performance and control stressors. The officer-NCO team from the division mental health section must be trusted as a cohesive part of the brigade and participate early in all operational planning.

If the mental health section officers and NCOs are to accomplish these requirements, they cannot remain in a clinic. They must go out and meet the unit leaders and soldiers in their work areas, motor pools, and barracks. They must sometimes take physical training with those units early in the morning. They must meet with the unit's spouses in the family support group meetings. They must live with the units overnight in field exercises. They must ride in the unit's vehicles and go with the soldiers as observers in their lines training and live fire drills. They must practice conducting unit survey interviews (structured small group discussions) to assess unit morale, horizontal and vertical bonding, trust and information flow, and the strengths and shortfalls of leadership. Based on these interviews, the CSC teams provide consultation to the unit leaders on how they can capitalize on their units' strengths and fix the shortfalls—being careful to safeguard the confidentiality of the sources.

Ultimately, the brigade CSC teams must deploy with their brigades' rotations to the National Training Center (NTC), Fort Irwin, California; the Joint Readiness Training Center (JRTC), Fort Polk, Louisiana; or the Combat Maneuver Training Center (CMTC), Hohenfels, Germany. These 2- to 3-week exercises have the realism, fast pace, and high stress provided by a highly trained and experienced opposing force (OPFOR) and the Multiple Integrated Laser Engagement System (MILES), which tells when each vehicle or soldier has been hit by enemy (or friendly) "fire." These exercises provide sufficient real-world fatigue and stress (including, sometimes, fatal training accidents) for the CSC teams to practice their real-world combat consultation and treatment missions under tactical conditions. Full involvement of the division mental health sections in these exercises must become standing operating procedure.

With this preparatory training accomplished, the mission of the mental health workers can be focused with specific emphasis on combat readiness. The following standards must be part of the working agenda for combat: provide far-forward triage and intervention to immediately return to duty over 50% of battle fatigue cases and prevent misconduct as a result of combat stress; supervise recovery of the battle fatigue cases with rest, nutrition, and expectancy of return to duty in their own units; supervise restoration or referral of battle fatigue casualties at the forward support medical company to assure 70 to 85% return to duty within 3 days; assure that recovered battle fatigue casualties are returned quickly to their units and keep relapse below 15%; assist units who have lost soldiers to battle fatigue in reconstitution to rapidly restore combat power; supervise or conduct unit after-action stress debriefings to prevent disabling post-traumatic stress disorder in effective soldiers; and serve as point of contact for other medical personnel assigned to the CSC teams from the echelon above division who will reinforce the brigades.

The army's new active and reserve component medical CSC detachments and companies, at the echelon above division, should also coordinate to send teams to reinforce the exercises at the NTC, JRTC, and CMTC (as well as to lesser field training exercises at the division and brigade posts). These units are discussed in the second part of this chapter. The air force's four-person combat stress units from the 50-bed air transportable hospitals could also receive excellent training at the JRTC; they could work at the Fort Polk airfield, which serves as the entry point into the exercise. Navy mental health teams might also have the opportunity to work with marine or army units at the JRTC. All services' combat stress teams should be deployed in the major joint field exercises, such as Team Spirit in Korea and Ocean Venture in the Atlantic Command.

In peacetime and military operations other than war, as well as in war, the cohesion, trust, and involvement of mental health personnel with line units (both active and reserve) are important for controlling stress and maintaining readiness in the evolving post-Cold War force. This can only be accomplished by close working relations with those units and their unit families. The driving model must be one of proactive, primary and secondary prevention, conducted on the line unit's own ground, rather than the reactive patient-care model in a clinic or hospital.

One problem with achieving the required capability is that the military and civilian professional training programs do not provide sufficient hands-on experience with the military community and the prevention model. Therefore, most graduates do not overcome their initial hesitancy about trying it. No one likes to feel and appear ignorant or incompetent—especially not physicians or other mental health professionals. The graduates naturally feel more comfortable with, and gravitate to, the familiar direct patient care model in which they have trained. This occurs even when the graduates are assigned to division mental health or CSC unit slots where the community-oriented mission should be the highest priority. Their own natural tendency is reinforced by the pressure of full clinic appointment schedules and the natural desire of short-staffed garrison medical facilities to coopt the unit mental health personnel onto their clinic and oncall rosters. We must give the future practitioners sufficient baseline knowledge and confidence about CSC and preventive unit consultation during training so that they take the first steps toward learning to do by doing.

This chapter examines the unique role of military mental health providers and delineates the process of teaching them the principles of combat psychiatry. The essentials of combat psychiatry, the type of practitioners involved in treating combat victims, and suggested methodologies for teaching combat psychiatric principles are also presented.

ESSENTIALS OF COMBAT PSYCHIATRY

The practice of military mental health is grounded in the principles of community mental health that emphasize primary prevention, group dynamics, healthcare delivery system issues, and individual treatment.[4,5] Most military mental health professionals are trained in nonmilitary settings where they primarily learn to diagnose and treat individuals. Most military mental health practitioners must augment their training to be effective in a military setting. In the early European mobilizations of World War II, it was evident that while the number of military psychiatrists (most of whom were on-the-job trainees with 90 days of education) was adequate, most did not have the background to prevent what we now call combat exhaustion.[6] This is because the psychiatrists, most of whom had no prior psychiatric training and had been drafted from civilian practices, were not trained to deal with this problem. Because of this, dysfunctional soldiers were inappropriately evacuated from combat zones to the United States, which decreased unit morale, cohesion, and fighting strength and caused long-term morbidity among these psychiatric patients.[6,7] Under the leadership of Roy Halloran, William Porter, and William Menninger, programs were established to train on-the-job psychiatrists to triage and treat military psychiatric casualties.[8]

The following sections describe the unique principles of combat psychiatry. Not merely a collection of techniques, the field of combat psychiatry involves the training of the mental health worker as a military professional whose knowledge-base and attitudes reside within the military organizational structure.

Situational Aspects

Anyone who has taken a course in either creative writing or public speaking knows the importance of understanding one's audience. If asked to give a banquet speech, the logical questions are, "Who will be in attendance and what is their level of interest in this subject matter?" Likewise, mental health professionals must know their military organization to be effective. "How large is the unit; what is its mission, location, composition, and recent deployments?" These are just some beginning questions to ask. More sophisticated ones include: What are the demographics of the group? Are most married? Single? Is this the first assignment for most of the members? Where do they come from? What has been the particular history of the unit throughout its command and leadership? Insight into these particular features of the military organization can make the mental health worker more effective. The process of finding out this information can also promote effective liaison between caregiver and unit personnel.

During the time-consuming process of information gathering, the worker has an opportunity to get to know the people who make up the unit and to learn what their jobs are and the problems they face. A military police unit, for instance, may have frequent, short-term deployments that come unexpectedly and have high visibility within the community. This may predispose them to higher rates of alcoholism or other dysfunctional ways of dealing with stress. This instability will be stressful for their family members. A personnel agency may have a high degree of stress during mobilizations but be bored the rest of the time. This can promote job dissatisfaction and frequent work conflicts.

A failure of the mental health worker to understand the work environment of the personnel he is responsible for can result in distrust and anxiety on the part of the unit. Recommendations concerning management style or retention of personnel may be ignored. As a result, mental health workers may deal more with the frustrations and emergencies of a unit, leaving little time to deal with morale or unit effectiveness.

Mental health workers in the military must also deal with unique administrative issues. They must be familiar with key regulations[9–11] to be able to effectively provide militarily unique services, such as forensic evaluations, clearances for specialty schools, or how to initiate the removal of commanders from their positions because of alcohol or drug abuse or psychiatric illness.

Understanding the importance of what constitutes good military leadership is crucial to the work of the mental health worker. While many for-profit, civilian organizations emphasize individual and central responsibilities to increase productivity, a military organization needs cooperation among its members for it to function properly. Effective military leaders understand this principle. During peacetime as well as during conflict, effective communication among members of the unit is paramount. The training and relationship building that occurs during peacetime within the unit prepares that organization for rapid assumption of its mission during armed conflict or mobilization. Mental health workers can help leaders to maximize cooperation among their personnel and consequently improve productivity.

An understanding of leadership also allows the head of a mental health team to deliver services more efficiently to the unit. For all military organizations, strict adherence to the chain of command, as well as obedience to leadership, is essential for the morale and effectiveness of that organization. Mental health workers cannot act as individual parties in the treatment of patients, but they must recognize the responsibilities and authority of the unit's commander and be able to work effectively with him. In this way, the mental health worker functions as a consultant.

Individual/Role Aspects

Mental health workers often function as liaisons to units and advisors to commanders, in addition to being individual caregivers. The mental health worker must be knowledgeable of the principles of primary prevention and community psychiatry, including the importance of stress reduction techniques, as well as the importance of family and other support structures available at the base or post. Often, a mental health worker can learn a great deal about the functioning of the unit by reading police reports, knowing the number of referrals for alcohol and drug treatment, and learning about disciplinary actions. At training sites, the pass rate of a particular unit may reflect not only the difficulty of the subject matter but the general morale of the group.

During combat, the liaison role is especially important and onsite presence of the mental health worker is essential. Contrary to most civilian mental health practices, military workers have an onsite mission, and they must be proactive; they should not wait for patients to come to them. These principles have been most clearly articulated in contemporary community psychiatry doctrine[12] that applies to working with chronic mental illness in the community, as well as the management of disaster victims that requires an onsite intervention approach. A mental health worker must give up his office for the onsite field environment.

Mental health workers can be troubled by their own anxieties and frustrations during combat. The leader of the mental health team is responsible for the morale of his workers and must emphasize the need for debriefing, rotations, rest time, and proper medical and nutritional support during these periods. Mental health workers are at risk for burnout; they must monitor themselves for signs and symptoms of decreased effectiveness and personal stress.

Perhaps the most difficult of the mental health worker's roles is being a command adviser. Commanders may excessively depend on the advice that is given by mental health workers, placing unrealistic demands and expectations on them, and thereby abdicating their own responsibility as leaders. Another possibility is that mental health workers may be branded as causing the problem rather than contributing to the solution. In the case of military trainees, a rising number of suicide attempts was blamed on the presence of a mental health worker operating on the training post. Only after discussion with commanders were a variety of environmental stresses identified as the actual causes of the increased suicide attempts, namely a war mobilization, incapacity of several drill sergeants due to alcohol and drug problems, unrealistic expectations of soldiers during the war effort, and an increased training mission and increased standards for training.[13]

In much the same way that a unit's commander and executive staff may depend on a mental health worker, so too can command actions and decisions be delayed until the counsel of the worker is obtained. While in many instances information provided by the workers may directly impact command decisions, some military leaders may excuse their own inability to make decisions based on "expert advice" from mental health workers. Specific aspects of this point are well documented by Bion in his work with leaderless groups during the 1950s.[14–21] He found that in a leaderless situation, group members can become dependent on each other, suspicious and distrustful, or apathetic. Bion's thesis was that in the work group, certain basic assumptions such as dependency, paranoia, and expectancy decrease the efficiency and effectiveness of the group.

Mental health workers may be the first to identify dysfunctional groups. There are several examples. In dependency groups, commanders will make decisions that can be made by the first sergeants or other operational personnel. A "fight or flight" group may have members that are so competitive that they are paranoid. A "pairing group," or one that is incompetent without a leader, will push off decisions until a commander returns from vacation or temporary duty, thereby paralyzing any work progress within that group. An essential element in all these situations is that the group leader's anxiety will determine how effective the unit can be. The mental health worker may be chiefly responsible for relieving the leader's anxiety through whatever means are available.

Educational Principles

The principles of immediacy, proximity, and expectancy in managing combat stress casualties deserve another airing. Removing an individual from stress is the goal of modern psychiatric hospitalization. In contrast, during combat, rest and return of the individual to his military unit have been shown to decrease long-term psychiatric morbidity, improve morale, and promote unit cohesiveness and effectiveness.[22–25]

There are important differences in the kinds of casualties that occur during various types of combat. High-intensity conflict, in which there is either a rapidly mobile land force or a static battlefield, tends to produce combat exhaustion characterized by anxiety and confusion disorders. Low-intensity garrison warfare can produce "nostalgic" types of combat reactions that include alcohol and drug abuse, depression, and suicide. The mental health worker needs to be aware of the variety of stress responses that result from the different types of combat.[26–28]

Command consultation is another essential principle of combat psychiatry. The process of getting to know a unit and providing effective consultation involves a slow, steady progression of meetings, often held weekly with key leaders in a military unit, to discuss the needs of those leaders. Just as medical consultants would behave improperly if they took over complete care of a consultee's patient, it would also be inappropriate if the mental health worker attempted to gain control of the unit. Mental health workers, although they possess unique professional abilities, must be replaceable at any time during the life of a unit. A unit cannot grow too dependent on the worker, nor can the worker see the unit as his command. Specific techniques to be used in command consultation include involving the chain of command in any presentation made to the organization, deferring to the authority of the command structure in any decision regarding personnel retention or separation, allowing commanders to initiate requests for consultation, being available as consultant on a regular or predictable basis, responding aggressively and appropriately to a commander's request for help, and providing feedback to commanders on referrals or treatment of an individual unit member as needed.

SPECIFIC AUDIENCES

The education of mental health personnel occurs in a variety of settings and utilizes many techniques. This section will describe the specific audiences for which training in combat psychiatry is necessary.

The most often neglected individual who needs to be properly educated to maintain the mental health of a unit is the individual soldier, sailor, or airman. Several pamphlets have been produced that emphasize the need for the "buddy system" in promoting unit morale and cohesiveness. Simply put, each soldier should look for dysfunction in his comrades. Isolation, decreasing attention paid to uniform cleanliness and personal hygiene, and insubordination may indicate that a problem exists. Unit members may often be the first ones a troubled soldier turns to, and education of all unit members about the importance of referring him to appropriate personnel within the command is essential.

Medics, those enlisted personnel who function mostly as licensed practical nurses, medical technicians, and orderlies, are also part of the military mental health team. While these medics are not always practicing in the field of mental health, it is important that they understand the basics of psychiatric triage. Important concepts for them to learn are the difference between neurotic and psychotic behavior, the characteristics of psychiatric illness that can masquerade as physical illness, management of anxiety, management of suicide, management of combat stress reactions, and substance abuse disorders. For the most part, the medics who specialize in mental health will learn how to work with patients in their first assignment while under the supervision of a psychiatrist or social worker.

Psychologists and social work officers work closely with psychiatrists in the care of emotionally disturbed patients. Although these individuals may be credentialed to provide unsupervised care, the care of patients on medications and those who require hospitalization must be supervised by a physician. The psychologist and social worker should have a working knowledge of the latest Diagnostic and Statistical Manual of Mental Disorders (DSM), be able to conduct a comprehensive interview of a patient, make a provisional diagnosis, and develop a diagnostic or treatment plan. By the nature of their education and training, the psychologists and social workers will have an advanced academic degree in the field of mental health.

Medical students are often challenged by learning psychiatry. For a military medical student population, introducing the concepts of battlefield management of combat stress reactions is crucial. Participating in field exercises that realistically include battle fatigue cases and cases that mimic battle fatigue will prepare the practicing physician to make cogent and useful referrals to his psychiatric colleague. A model program for the education of medical students is described in the next section.

Nonpsychiatric physicians are the usual source of referrals for psychiatrists, and they may be the first physician practitioners to come in contact with combat stress casualties. Educating these professionals must be an ongoing enterprise.

Psychiatric residents can learn about combat psychiatry by first learning how a military unit functions. Electives should focus on field placement of residents for a realistic experience in the practice of military mental health. In the next section, a model for the education of psychiatric residents is proposed. Residency is also an opportune time to teach the techniques of psychiatric debriefing, a process by which survivors of trauma or combat begin a reintegration into their communities and units.[29]

Nursing staff have the most contact with patients when hospitalized, and during combat this contact is probably increased. Military nurses in all areas of specialty should be taught how to recognize and treat combat stress reactions. Part of any military nursing continuing education conference should include update, review, and latest techniques for managing these disorders.

METHODS OF TEACHING

The following section describes three programs designed to educate military personnel in the field of combat psychiatry. The first is primarily aimed at medical students, the second is for psychiatric residents, and the third is a field exercise that tests the overall medical and mental health capabilities of a medical unit. While these programs are far from ideal, we feel these are the best educational models tested to date.

Medical Students

A course for medical students concerning the practice of medicine during combat was designed by McCaughey at the Uniformed Services University of the Health Sciences. A basic concept about the course is that there is a stepwise approach to the training.[30,31] Exhibit 11–1 is a comprehensive description of this course that gives students the ability to learn basic concepts, practice them, and make evaluation and management decisions under simulated wartime conditions.

Some institutions may not be able to adapt all aspects of this course because of their limited capabilities. For instance, it may not be possible to get all of the equipment that is necessary to conduct certain parts of this course in the field. But this should not prevent the faculty from doing the best that can be done. Even with a very limited amount of equipment, a worthwhile field exercise can still be conducted.

The planning faculty includes a course director and several other faculty members who can act as advisers to help develop and revise the course as needed. They should be motivated to teach and be knowledgeable about battle fatigue or be willing to learn. Initially, they need to meet to establish the goals and objectives of the battle fatigue course and decide how it is going to be taught in their institutional setting. Later, they should meet periodically to look for ways to implement improvements.

The teaching faculty conducts the teaching. Training them properly is critical to the success of the course. This group will present the lecture and conduct the case discussions groups and testing in the classroom and the field. Like the planners, they should have an interest and ability to teach and should be knowledgeable about battle fatigue. This group may include members of the planning faculty. This course was originally designed to teach medical students, but if modified, it could be used to teach other groups.[30,31]

If others are to be included, the next step is to identify the students and construct a course that will fit their background, needs, and interests. The course can be basic and still benefit a group with

EXHIBIT 11–1

PSYCHIATRY TRAINING COURSE

Phase One: Providing Information

Information should be provided in three forms: handout, lecture, and videotape presentation.

1. *Handout.* The handout should include information about battle fatigue and how the course will be conducted. Information about battle fatigue should include published articles from various perspectives, one of which is historical. It is important to convey to the students that battle fatigue is not just a recent problem but that it has been around as long as wars themselves. There should be case examples from the American Civil War, Russo-Japanese War, World Wars I and II, the Korean and Vietnam conflicts, and the Arab-Israeli wars. The various names that have been given to designate battle fatigue (nostalgia, shell shock, and so forth) and how it was managed for each of these wars should be included. Other topics should include how to deal with battle fatigue management and prevention today and the application of battle fatigue management principles in other settings, such as civilian disasters.

   The handout should be distributed well in advance of the course so that the students have enough time to read the background material. Any additional instructions, such as the name and telephone number of a person to contact if there are questions, should also be included with the handout.
2. *Lecture.* The lecture should include the following topics: types of battlefield stressors and the reactions of service personnel to these stressors; description of battle fatigue and its extremely variable presentations; physical and psychological symptoms associated with battle fatigue; a sample case; theories about the cause of battle fatigue; battle fatigue epidemiology; importance of battle fatigue to the serviceman, combat unit, and medical facilities; a list of the groups of medical personnel that need to be informed about battle fatigue; management of battle fatigue; prevention; and uses of the battle fatigue management principles in the peacetime setting.
3. *Videotape presentation.* The videotape presentation is given immediately following the lecture. It should show various types of actual battle fatigue casualties. After each case is shown, the presenter should stop the tape and discuss the case with the students. A suitable videotape, edited from a World War II documentary black and white film, is entitled *World War II U.S. Army Battle Fatigue Cases—Combat Exhaustion* (A1701–90–0059). It is available from the Army Medical Department Center and School for restricted use in training military and medical and mental health workers.

Phase Two: Practicing

The students use the information they have learned about battle fatigue in the following settings: pretest, case discussion groups, and the classroom testing.

1. *Pretest.* The pretest is taken after the lecture and graded by the students. It is then discussed in a classroom setting.
2. *Case discussion groups.* Five to seven students meet with a mental health professional for about 2 hours. Individual cases, found in the handout, are discussed. The focus is on the identification of battle fatigue, differentiation of battle fatigue from other problems, management, and returning to duty. Students, in pairs, also practice interviewing skills by having one student conduct the interview while the other one plays the role of a battle fatigue casualty. The rest of the group has the opportunity to observe the interview and participate in the critique.
3. *Classroom testing.* Just before going on to the field exercise, the students are tested in a classroom setting. This is a pass-fail test whose purpose is to see if the students have gained the basic skills and knowledge they need to effectively evaluate and manage battle fatigue cases. The students are tested in pairs. They alternate roles as an interviewing physician or a battle fatigue casualty while a faculty member evaluates the interaction. The faculty member also asks general questions about battle fatigue. If the students demonstrate that they have minimal competence, they can go to the next phase.

Phase Three: Testing

There are two parts for the testing: written test in the classroom and practical testing of simulated battle fatigue casualties in the field.

EXHIBIT 11–1 (*continued*)

PSYCHIATRY TRAINING COURSE

1. *Written test.* The test includes material from the lecture, reading material, videotapes, and the case discussion groups.

2. *Testing in field under simulated wartime conditions.* A field exercise is the last part of the training program. The students are evaluated on their ability to evaluate and manage simulated battle fatigue cases. If possible, this should be part of a larger field medical exercise that includes a variety of other surgical and medical problems to add to the realism.

   Simulated battle fatigue casualties are trained before the field operation starts. They are introduced into the medical care system and, through triage, are sent to a combat stress center that is manned by students who are supervised by faculty. The interview of the battle fatigue casualty is observed by a faculty member. After this, the faculty member meets with the student to discuss the case and ask general questions about battle fatigue. The student is evaluated on the following points: orienting the casualty to the interview, identifying the reason for referral, conducting past history and mental status examinations (adapted for the battle fatigue situation), formulating the problem (diagnosis and differential diagnosis), developing the intervention, ability to elicit information, and general knowledge about battle fatigue and leadership. Students should be evaluated individually and feedback given at the end of their rotation at the combat stress center.

mixed backgrounds, such as one that includes physicians, nurses, physician assistants, corpsmen, medical service personnel, and so forth. Alternatively, the course can be designed for specialized groups, such as just psychiatrists, just psychiatric residents, or any one of the other groups mentioned above.

All courses, no matter who the audience is, should use a phased approach, in which each phase prepares the students for the next phase. The first phase provides information through reading material (handout), lectures, and videotapes. In the next phase, the students practice the use of battle fatigue identification and management techniques using the information they have learned. The last phase is testing, which occurs in the classroom and in the field.

The students should be given the opportunity to provide feedback about the course. This feedback is best done at the end of the course. Forms with open-ended questions and or scales that indicate how well teaching objectives were met can be used. The feedback should be submitted anonymously. Changes to the course should be based on the faculty's observations and the student feedback.

Psychiatric Residents

The following is a model for a residency elective in community psychiatry. The goals of the elective are to attain the skills necessary to function as a military psychiatrist, especially during combat, and

TABLE 11–1

ELECTIVE IN COMMUNITY AND MILITARY PSYCHIATRY

Component	Comments
Course Directors	Insert names of individuals who will be responsible for the training: one a member of the medical center faculty, the other the onsite director.
Place	Provide the exact location of facility.
Duration	This will usually be 2 weeks to 2 months depending on extent of material covered.
Participants	Will be selected from appropriate level psychiatry residents.
Housing	Arranged by the onsite director.
Cost	Per diem costs and transportation expenses will be covered.
Rationale	While military psychiatrists function in a variety of settings (divisions, research, and hospitals), most graduating residents are assigned to community hospital/clinic settings. This training prepares them for their initial practice experience.

to develop strong collegial relationships with commanders and other unit personnel. Tables 11–1 and 11–2 are examples of a proposal that could be developed for this elective, along with a discussion of the aspects of the field setting.

Field Training Exercises

The U.S. Army usually conducts one large-scale medical field exercise each summer except when world events such as the Persian Gulf War or budget limitations have taken precedence. Since 1984, these field training exercises (FTXs) have rotated among several medical brigades (headquarters units). Each of these FTXs has involved between 3,000 and 9,000 medical troops. The medical brigade headquarters commands two or three medical group headquarters. Each medical group controls two to four hospitals (usually evacuation hospitals, combat support hospitals, and mobile army surgical hospitals). The hospitals do not come at full strength and usually are staffed for 50 to 100 medical and surgical beds.[32–38]

Each medical group headquarters also usually controls one or more medical clearing companies (with 50 to 100 of its 250 patient cots). The medical battalion, or an evacuation battalion headquarters, also controls several helicopter and ground ambulance companies and detachments.[32–38]

Additional medical and surgical specialty detachments augment the hospitals. Preventive medicine, dental, and veterinary detachments are assigned to the medical brigade or the medical groups to provide area support. Simulated and actual medical supply and logistics for the many medical units are provided as they would be in a combat zone by medical supply units.

In all of these FTXs between 1984 and 1992, there has been at least one U.S. Army Reserve "OM team"

TABLE 11–2

ASPECTS OF THE FIELD SETTING

Component	Comments
Background	Describe the training site and its unique features.
Elective Experience	Residents working under the chief of psychiatry will experience all levels of patient care to include consultation-liaison, outpatient and inpatient evaluations and treatment, supervision of social workers, psychiatric technicians, and the psychologists. Emphasis will be placed on providing the resident with an opportunity to observe and participate in the operation of a full-scale, multiservice psychiatric practice, as well as interact with crucial hospital personnel supporting that practice. The resident will attend the usual departmental meetings, as well as hospital governance boards, and meet with officers in logistics, administration, resource management division, and clinical support.
	A major feature of this field elective will be command consultations and unit visits. This will be accomplished under the auspices of the community mental health service. If timely, the resident can participate in the post's chief of staff briefings.
Patient Population	The profile of the patient population should be described here.
Supervision and Evaluation	All patient care supervision will be provided by the chief of the department of psychiatry. A meeting of all practitioners in the department will be scheduled at the end of the resident's stay to gather performance data. The final rating of the resident will be done by the chief, department of psychiatry, and returned to the training director at the medical center in a timely fashion. Additionally, the resident will have the opportunity to rate the program as a part of his or her semi-annual evaluations conducted by the medical center staff.
Requirements	The training director at Medical Center X will review this proposal and contact the chief, department of psychiatry, regarding appropriateness for training and seek clarification if needed.
	The training director and chief, department of psychiatry, at Medical Center X must formally approve the elective and schedule the first resident participant(s).
Time Table	Give time that the program will be operational.
References	Provide pertinent references for the proposal.

(the designation for a psychiatric medical detachment) to fulfill the CSC mission. The OM teams served in the Persian Gulf War but have since converted to the new CSC companies or detachments. An OM team at full strength had 48 persons. It included five psychiatrists, six social workers, two psychiatric nurses, a clinical psychologist, enlisted psychiatric and behavioral sciences specialists, and administrative support personnel. In practice, most OM teams came to these FTXs with between 20 and 35 personnel with only one psychiatrist and no psychologist. They were augmented by volunteers from the other OM teams and by active duty, U.S. Army Reserve, and U.S. Air Force occupational therapists and by occupational therapist enlisted specialists. The occupational therapists were especially eager to demonstrate their field role in promoting return to duty of battle fatigue casualties. The OM teams also had some (but usually not enough) vehicles, tents, and equipment.[32–38]

One of the best features of these field exercises is the opportunity they provide for individuals or small teams from other organizations to reinforce or fill out the CSC unit that has been programmed into the FTX. The operational concept for CSC calls for the capability to concentrate CSC personnel and expertise rapidly at sites of acute need by having them temporarily reinforce the small CSC teams already near the site. The CSC personnel themselves need to be highly adaptable and able to integrate new team members quickly. Cross-attaching personnel among active duty or reserve CSC units in FTXs practices this critical skill. It has the added benefit of sharing ("cross-fertilizing") practical experience and initiating networking. The FTXs also provide an economical way for mental health interns, residents, and practicing clinicians who are slotted as PROFIS (Professional Filler System) fillers in CSC units to receive high-quality, emotionally positive, field experience.

In most of the FTXs, the OM teams operated according to evolving U.S. Army CSC doctrine. The OM team headquarters were assigned directly to the medical brigade headquarters. The detachment divided into smaller, dispersed teams. Depending on the numbers of each professional discipline and the vehicles available, the CSC unit tried to provide CSC support to one or all of the subordinate medical groups in the medical brigade.

Because these FTXs were played at the level of the medical brigade in support of a corps, the OM(CSC) detachment had as one mission the staffing of a reconditioning center. *Reconditioning* by definition[3,39,40] is the 4 to 14 day treatment of battle fatigue casualties who do not return to duty in the first 3 days of restoration treatment. Reconditioning cannot be simulated in real time in a 4 to 5 day FTX. However, the staff can do the admissions workup and then go through the daily schedule of structured activities in "quick time" or "time compression" in which 10 minutes equals 4 or 6 hours.[3,39,40]

In the FTXs, as in evolving doctrine, the OM(CSC) reconditioning facilities collocated with an evacuation or combat support hospital. They were dependent on the hospital for food, water, fuel, medical records, and often tents and cots. This was as it would be in real combat. The CSC teams must establish duty-sharing arrangements with the host hospital without letting their personnel and equipment be absorbed into that hospital. Absorption would rightly happen to a hospital-augmentation detachment like a neurosurgery team, which becomes an integral part of the hospital, but must not happen to a mobile CSC team. The CSC team uses the hospital as a base of operation but must deploy its teams elsewhere, often on short notice. Even those treatment functions such as restoration and reconditioning must, by doctrine,[3] maintain a separate "nonhospital" identity and atmosphere.

Experience has shown that the reconditioning center is best set up in the hospital staff quarters area, near the kitchen and mess hall, laundry, and motor pool. It should not be among the triage or ward tents, and it must maintain a nonpatient, soldiering milieu. The patient role players simulating battle fatigue can be assigned to assist the host hospital with real work details, as well as being fed, showered, rested, and involved in recreational, physical fitness, and group debriefing activities.

In these FTXs, other subteams of the OM detachment were normally deployed to one or more of the medical clearing companies under the medical battalion in the medical groups. These teams usually attached to the medical company for support and remained with it 24 hours a day to triage, evaluate, and provide restoration treatment for locally generated battle fatigue cases (both simulated and "real"). *Restoration,* by definition,[3,39,40] is the 1- to 3-day initial treatment of battle fatigue soldiers and is best done at the medical treatment or clearing company closest to the soldier's own unit, not at a "hospital." Restoration requires a reasonably sized tent, preferably with cots, dedicated to the recovering battle fatigue casualties.

The CSC teams at the clearing companies also provided actual preventive consultation, education, and case evaluations to the medical company and all other nearby units. In some FTXs, when there were too few CSC personnel to provide a continuous presence at the medical companies, the CSC team instead provided a regular schedule of circuit-riding. The team spent the night at the OM team headquarters or reconditioning center (base camp) and drove to visit one clearing company in the morning, then on to another each afternoon. The teams were prepared to spend the night at a clearing company as the workload or the tactical situation required. In this situation, the patient-holding sections and medical treatment teams of the clearing company were trained to manage and restore all but the problem cases. The problem cases were evaluated by the CSC team each day, and, if necessary, they were taken back to the reconditioning (and restoration) center by the team as it completed its daily rounds.

The medical FTXs also routinely included nonmedical combat support and combat service support units, especially signal battalions and detachments to set up and operate the communications equipment. Some FTXs also had military police companies to provide rear area security and manage enemy prisoners of war. Engineer units may be available to assist with hospital site preparation and personnel replacement elements to coordinate the return to duty of simulated casualties.

At some of these FTXs the U.S. Air Force provides C141 and/or C130 aircraft to conduct simulated air evacuation from the combat zone (taking off with the simulated patients, flying around, and landing nearby so that the patients can be "recycled"). The air force also provides a mobile air staging facility with medical and nursing staff to hold and prepare the patients for the flight. In the future, it may be possible to involve a navy hospital ship in these exercises.[41] Having a hospital ship offshore was considered for Wounded Warrior '92, part of which took place at Camp Pendleton and involved a marine medical battalion working under an army medical group headquarters. However, it was not feasible then because of expense.

A few of the FTXs in California and Mississippi have combined the medical brigade's exercises with the annual training of the states' national guard division or separate brigade. In some instances, the maneuver brigade or division medical companies and organic battalion assets were included in the medical evacuation play.[33,34,36] On those occasions, the OM team has fulfilled its forward CSC mission by sending mobile teams forward to reinforce the division and brigade medical companies.

The virtue of such large-scale medical exercises for training in CSC is that the exercises suggest the magnitude and complexity of the real combat mission. The FTXs illustrate the real-world problems of exercising command and control through multiple layers of headquarters, communicating with dispersed teams over other units' overworked and breakdown-prone field switchboards and radio nets,[41] traveling and navigating to find unfamiliar units, and negotiating allocation or loan of scarce resources such as tents, food, water, and vehicle maintenance. All of these problems must be overcome in the combat theater.

The larger FTXs provide actual supported units and audiences for staff briefings, command consultation advice, and preventive educational presentations. They may provide extensive patient play that can include simulated stress and neuropsychiatric cases. Invariably, they also provide actual overstressed soldiers who need individual case evaluation and, when appropriate, onsite treatment. Exercises of this size also always provide one or more true neuropsychiatric cases, usually with a preexisting disorder, who decompensate and must be evacuated to the supporting hospital system.

The shortfall of these FTXs is that, large as they are, they are still only a small-scale model of a real U.S. Army area of operations. The medical units are not surrounded by the many more nonmedical combat service support units with which they would be aggregated into base defense areas and base defense clusters. The distances between clusters during actual combat would be much greater than can be achieved at some of the posts hosting the FTXs. The rear battle threat may be simulated by OPFOR attacks, but there is little real danger or difficulty when going from unit to unit, which may create a false sense of security. Still, such FTXs are much better preparation for learning to live and function in the field as part of a huge system than are purely individual or small unit training exercises.

The major medical FTX typically has between 300 and 600 personnel assigned to play the simulated casualties. The FTXs generally try to achieve a mixture of simulated surgical wounds and injuries plus nonbattle diseases (including neuropsychiatric disorders), which conforms roughly to the expected incidence in mid- to high-intensity conflict. They may include battle fatigue casualties. Chemical casualties are usually included and nuclear casualties may be included.

Role players who simulate soldiers who have diseases or minor injuries can be briefed quickly at the FTX patient operations center (POC). Role players with simulated surgical wounds must receive extensive make-up ("moulage") from a trained moulage team at the POC. Make-up artists do a remarkable job of mimicking serious and even grossly deforming wounds.

The realism of the moulage is one of the factors (along with sleep loss, field sights, sounds and smells, and sometimes the sound of actual artillery firing in the distance) that has provoked distressing and even temporarily disabling post-traumatic stress syndrome symptoms in some medical personnel who have had previous combat experience in Vietnam or other conflicts. Such persons may request help themselves or be referred to the CSC teams to help them deal with their memories. Many more may simply "tough it out" and then perhaps decide to leave the army, national guard, or reserves rather than face another painful training exercise. This is one of the reasons why the CSC teams have active and visible outreach programs.

Most of the simulated patients are picked up at the patient moulage center and taken directly to one of the medical treatment facilities by the helicopter or ground ambulances that are dispatched to transport them. A few patients may be taken by truck to remote field sites, where the ambulances must find them. The patient players in these FTXs may be made up and sent out once, twice, or even three times in a 12-hour shift. The number of times depends on how extensive their make-up is and the prognosis of the injury. Those who can be treated and released quickly, or who are "dead on arrival" or "die" soon after they reach the clearing company, can be returned to the POC by a shuttle service and be recycled quickly. For the role players, the experience can be tiring and uncomfortable. They are covered with make-up and prosthetic rubber or plastic, strapped to a litter, and then transported in the summer heat in a vibrating helicopter or bouncing ground ambulance to one or more medical facilities where they may wait for minutes to hours to be examined. It is a demanding job.

The patient players are often members of another medical unit within the medical brigade's area (such as a general hospital) that has been tasked to provide "patients" as its part in the FTX. They usually serve as patients for the entire 4 to 5 days of continuous scenario operations. They are "guaranteed" time to eat and sleep, but that guarantee may be disrupted by transportation difficulties or the inhospitable field or barracks environment. In other FTXs, the patient players may be borrowed from the participating hospitals and other medical units on a day-by-day basis. When national guard divisions or brigades have been involved in the FTX, some line unit soldiers may be declared casualties and be evacuated through their organic medical platoons and companies to the corps facilities one time only. These soldiers will not have extensive moulage make-up unless a moulage team is deployed forward. In some FTXs, there may also be volunteer role players from other organizations, such as the state's national guard cadet program. These details of where and how the role players are obtained have proved very relevant to the real-world stress control missions of the CSC teams.

A recurrent finding[32–38] is that both the role players and the medical units become involved in the scenario portion of the FTX with enthusiasm. However, for the medical units the novelty of realistically moulaged patients wears off after a while because the triage and surgical teams only pretend to start the intravenous infusions and insert the nasogastric and chest tubes and only get to explain what surgical procedure they would be doing. The triagers, operating room teams, and ward staffs themselves become progressively more sleep deprived, hot, dirty, and uncomfortable.They become increasingly short-tempered with and even negligent toward the role-playing patients. That increases the stress and undermines the motivation of the already uncomfortable patients.

Those role players who have been assigned to serve the full duration of the FTX (and even some of the volunteers) begin to grow weary of the exercise. Some may actually require the attention of mental health workers for the transient exercise fatigue they suffer. They begin to find ways to delay or evade being made up and sent out again. By the last night, a few may even become "combat refusers," flatly declaring to the POC (or telephoning home tearfully to family) that they will resign from the army if forced to go out again as surgical patients. The result has been that the CSC teams have performed excellent service treating the battle fatigued surgical moulage players.

Anecdotes from actual exercises help to underscore important points about these experiences. During MEDEX [medical exercise] '86 (Camp Shelby, Mississippi, 1986), the OM team elements at the clearing companies established ongoing "ventilation/gripe" sessions for the surgical and medical role players. These sessions were reported by the role players as being very helpful to them. A memorable moment in the FTX occurred during a brief afternoon thundershower when lightning struck a pine tree that fell and barely missed the tent in which such a session was going on.

During the Dusty Bull FTX (Fort Hood, Texas, 1988),[35] the OM team is credited by the 807th Medical Brigade's chief of the patient operations (moulage) center with "saving" the FTX.[42] The moulage role players became very disgruntled by the evening of the fourth day, and the corps surgeon and POC leader consulted the OM team. They immediately implemented the recommendations to call a temporary halt to give all role players food and sleep. Meanwhile, the OM team sent a contingent on night convoy to the POC and, early in the morning, initiated a concentrated schedule of debriefing sessions mixed with entertainment that had the role players ready to continue the FTX soon after sunrise.

Wounded Warrior '92 (Camp Roberts, California, 1992) provided an even more dramatic real-world demonstration of the value of a multidisciplinary, multipurpose stress control team. The 12-person CSC team was composed of a psychiatrist, psychiatric nurses, social workers, and enlisted behavioral and psychiatry specialists from three reserve OM teams. No simulated combat stress casualties were scheduled among the surgical and medical patient play because there was a shortage of patient role players. The "patients" were male and female members of a state cadet organization, aged 11 to 19 years. The cadets had been enlisted initially to play only a 1-day, joint military/civilian disaster medical assistance team earthquake scenario. They had agreed to continue through a 4-day continuous (12-hour shifts) battle casualty scenario. By the first day of the army exercise, it was clear that the cadets' cadre were not able to keep the adolescent cadets sufficiently occupied (on an old army post) while they were offshift. A social worker and two technicians from the CSC team, who had civilian expertise with adolescents, were pulled in from the field to advise and train the cadet cadre, to establish a program of recreational activities, and to maintain order in the barracks' dormitories.

One of the young female cadets became extremely agitated while she was being driven out to the field in an ambulance as a surgical wound case. She had asked to be allowed to use one of the portable latrines and had then perceived the behavior of the male medics as a sexual assault. The cadet reported this perception by telephone to her mother, and the post provost marshall was notified. Fortunately for all, the female social worker was able to work therapeutically with the cadet that evening. Several years earlier, that cadet had been molested in a public restroom, which made her especially sensitive to the threat of sexual assault. The next day, when the formal hearing was held, the girl's testimony of what the ambulance medics had done and the testimony of the medics themselves were sufficient to convince everyone that only poor judgment, not wrongful intent, had been involved. The timely assistance of a trained mental health worker helped the cadet work through a psychological trauma—and also arguably saved the careers of more than just the ambulance medics if the accusations had reached the news media.

Thus, the psychiatric (stress control) detachments can be fully and profitably occupied in these FTXs by concentrating on their real-world preventive and treatment missions. Unlike the surgical teams (and like the dental, preventive medicine, and veterinary food inspection teams), they have plenty of real-world missions, provided they are proactive, mobile, and helpful. They must not remain in their tents waiting for "patients" to be sent to them. Indeed the people who would send such cases to them (or come on their own behalf) are more likely to misunderstand and mistrust the mental health teams if those teams are relying only on their professional reputations.

In fact, too much simulated stress casualty play may actually be counterproductive. It may keep the mental health teams so busy (doing what they already know fairly well how to do) that they put off undertaking the new challenges of going out, meeting, and forming trusting professional relationships with all of the units that they should be supporting. They need to become fully familiar with the missions and stressors of the supported units.

The major medicine FTXs (especially the earlier ones—Dusty Bull '84 and '88, Wounded Warrior '85, and MEDEX '86) did have extensive simulated stress casualty play. A mobile training team (MTT) from the Behavioral Sciences Division, Academy of Health Sciences, U.S. Army (San Antonio, Texas), was requested through command channels[41] by the medical brigades to assist in training the OM teams and guiding their employment. The MTT also assured that a suitable number and variety of simulated battle fatigue and neuropsychiatric casualties were played.

The moulage source book[43] provides very few neuropsychiatric and combat stress roles (with sample field medical cards). The battle fatigue cases are mostly the dramatic (but actually rare) and problematic cases. The recommended treatment (contrary to current doctrine) is to prescribe diazepam (Valium) or chlorpromazine (Thorazine). The neuropsychiatric cases are also rather limited. For example, the alcoholic with impending delirium tremens has physical findings (such as a large and tender liver with ascites). That would be common, perhaps, in a big city hospital emergency room but would not be typical of the heavy drinking but otherwise successful army NCO or officer who might go into delirium tremens if he suddenly cuts back from his regular heavy daily drinking. The soldier-alcoholic's general health and physical fitness might appear good with only the more subtle signs of heavy alcohol use.[41] The army's programs of physical fitness testing, weight control, the mandatory physical periodic examination, annual performance appraisals with interim counseling sessions, plus the Alcohol and Drug Abuse Prevention and Control Program are usually sufficient to detect the gross signs of chronic physical deterioration because of alcohol abuse.[41]

To provide a wider variety and more representative sample of battle fatigue and neuropsychiatric cases, the MTT has fielded and tested a set of role player instruction sheets. Examples are given in Figures 11–1, 11–2, and 11–3.

Each instruction sheet included the field medical card (DA Form 1380) entries and physical findings. It included general instructions to the role players plus a checklist of recent stress events they should incorporate into their story about themselves. It gives specific instructions on what to do, how to look, and what to say, plus further instruction on how to change or not change the scenario based on how they are treated.

The battle fatigue cases have been written in sets of 20 cases. Each case is unique, but in each set, there are three simple exhaustion/sleep deprivation cases, five with primarily anxiety symptoms, five with primarily depressive and/or survivor guilt symptoms, three variations on dissociative (memory loss) symptoms, and four variations on conversion symptoms. This breakout still somewhat favors the dramatic and problematic end of the battle fatigue spectrum at the expense of the more common exhausted, anxious, and depressed forms. However, that shift is appropriate for corps-level or division rear-level exercises, where most of the simpler cases can be assumed to have been treated and released further forward.

The instructions deliberately omit the stereotypical "pseudopsychotic," "acting out," and potential violent types of battle fatigue cases. This omission was done for two reasons. First, they are actually rare, and it is important to counteract that stereotype lest it become a self-fulfilling prophecy as soldiers become overly suggestible with battle fatigue. Second, there will always be a few role players who will overact or use this opportunity of playing a stress casualty as a license to play "psycho," in spite of warnings not to.

In addition to the 60 variations on battle fatigue, instructions were written for neuropsychiatric cases, including a manic episode, paranoid schizophrenic-like psychoses, acute organic brain syndromes (atropine or anticholinergic type), alcohol withdrawal, and other substance abuse problems. Some of these cases require additional administrative or legal action. Some of these cases do provide for the players to become threatening and disruptive. This will give the medical or psychiatric triagers and treaters the opportunity to practice safe management and restraining techniques without erroneously targeting battle fatigue as the likely cause. The players of these roles must be strongly instructed not to continue their resistance to the point where they or others get hurt.

Interestingly, there was a case during MEDEX '86[34] when one of the nonviolent battle fatigue cases—a soldier with psychogenic deafness who was pretending to be unable to hear instructions or questions—was wrestled to the ground and his eye glasses broken by overzealous triage and security personnel who mistakenly identified him as either a "psycho" or an enemy infiltrator. All of the observer and controller personnel in the FTXs must be trained to intervene to prevent such unnecessary safety violations by the role-playing patient or the treaters.

Several "special combat stress cases" that involve misconduct and other legal issues have also been prepared as role player instruction sheets. Examples are the soldier who confesses that the guilt he is feeling comes from having participated in the commission of an atrocity or the "combat refuser" who describes a pacifistic religious conversion experience while under extreme stress. These cases provide training not only in clinical management but also in the administrative actions that should be initiated and followed through the system.

The role player instruction sheets are sufficiently detailed that a reasonably literate and motivated

Casualty Tag No:

Name:

SSN:

Rank:

Job title:

Unit:

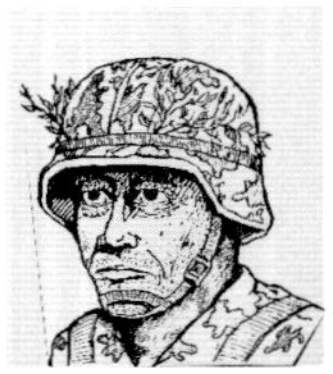

MOS/ADC:

( )	Walking	( )	Litter
( )	Injury	( )	Disease
( )	"Fatigue"	( )	"Psych"
( )	In restraints	( )	Under escort
( )	Simulated	( )	Constructive

DIAGNOSIS: BATTLE FATIGUE
( ) mild, ( ) moderate, ( ) severe
( ) Hold for Trtmnt ( ) Hold, Evac

Rule out:

EVALUATOR may detach this part and give information to whoever does examination.

SIGNS/SYMPTOMS AND PHYSICAL FINDINGS

Paralysis, both legs at knee and below.

Oriented and cooperative. Not ambulatory but can low crawl; capable of limited self-care. May have bruises & scratches, but no major injury. No sign of head, back, or leg injury. Chest, abdomen OK. Pupils equal, large; react to light and accommodation. No blood or fluid is dripping from ears or nose.

Total loss of voluntary movement of knees, ankles, toes, bilaterally. Tendon reflexes and Babinski normal. Loss of joint position sense: knees, ankles, toes. All other sensory modalities normal. Does not appear to be deliberately faking. No sensory or motor changes in the upper extremities.

HR 90-105, regular   RR 20
BP 115/81   Temp 98.8 oral
BF 20

BATTLE FATIGUE CASUALTY ROLE PLAYERS, READ ALL THESE INSTRUCTIONS FIRST

You are to play a normal, good soldier who has just had too many bad things happen at once. You will show one of the many forms of "battle fatigue."

Read what to DO, LOOK, AND SAY. Also read how to RESPOND TO HOW YOU ARE TREATED. When the instructions say you can tell people what has happened to you, you need to describe what you would have seen and done if this exercise had been a real war.

First, check this sheet to learn your soldier's rank, MOS (job duties), and unit. Adapt the story of the soldier on this sheet to fit that information. You can add background details to the basic story, including events from the following RECENT STRESS CHECKLIST. Especially use events marked with an X.

- Under artillery or bombing attack
- In chemical, smoke, or flame attack
- Caught in minefield or ambush
- Unit was harmed by friendly fire
- Friends, leader, or women and children killed or horribly wounded
- Had a close call with death
- Very heavy work or responsibilities
- Could not get needed information or support
- Have gotten very little sleep
- New to the unit, do not know anybody
- You may also be worried about home:
  - Recently got bad news
  - Received a "Dear John" letter
  - Just married or became a parent
  - Have a sick parent or child
  - Job, money, or legal problems
  - Not sure your family is safe

Do play the basic role on this sheet. Use your imagination to add details, but do not overdo it. Keep it realistic for a normal person like yourself.

If you are given a Field Medical Card (DA form 1380), which says you have received some treatment, change how you act now to fit what it says last.

SHOW THIS SHEET ONLY TO EVALUATORS.

DO, LOOK, AND SAY THE FOLLOWING
(BF20, weakness, both legs)

You cannot walk because you cannot get your legs to move, although you can drag yourself along in a low crawl.

Say that you suddenly could not move your feet and lower legs at all.

You can still feel touch, pain, temperature, and vibration in your legs, but cannot tell which way your toes, ankles, or knees are bent.

You do not know why this happened and are worried (but not frightened or agitated) that you will stay paralyzed.

If asked what was happening when this started: describe the stressful events without showing much emotion. (See RECENT STRESS CHECKLIST for ideas of bad things that happened in battle and at home.)

RESPOND TO HOW YOU ARE TREATED

IF hassled, set aside to wait, or evacuated and treated as if "sick": do not get better.

IF only given medicine: get somewhat better over hours. You can walk with assistance, but your knees stay wobbly and your ankles are limp. Continue to worry about why.

IF treated as a soldier, examined, and told nothing serious is physically wrong, and that this is not uncommon with battle fatigue, and will get better soon: improve very slowly.

IF hypnotized: walk perfectly and remember the bad events with feeling.

OR IF given food and water, chance to clean up, sleep, work to do, and help to talk about what happened: improve slowly. Talk about it with feeling. Cooperate slowly in work details.

THEN IF reminded that unit needs you: say you are ready to return, but worry what unit thinks of you.

Fig. 11–1. Battle fatigue casualty instructions used during FTXs. Instructions delineate role-playing behaviors of the casualty and provide a simulated casualty tag. The primary presentation for the example in this scenario is weakness in both legs. Source: Training materials developed by the Psychiatry and Neurology Branch, Behavioral Science Division, Army Medical Center and School, Fort Sam Houston, Texas.

Casualty Tag No:

Name:

SSN:

Rank:

Job title:

Unit:

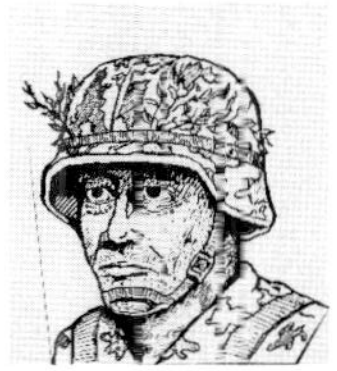

MOS/ADC

(X)	Walking	( )	Litter
( )	Injury	( )	Disease
( )	"Fatigue"	( )	"Psych"
( )	In restraints	( )	Under escort
( )	Simulated	( )	Constructive

DIAGNOSIS: BATTLE FATIGUE
( ) mild, ( ) moderate, ( ) severe
( ) Hold for Trtmnt ( ) Hold, Evac

Rule out:

EVALUATOR may detach this part and give information to whoever does examination.

SIGNS/SYMPTOMS AND PHYSICAL FINDINGS

Anxiety with fine tremor of fingers, startle reactions, and autonomic signs (palpitations, diarrhea, sweating); onset while under stress. "Phobic" about artillery. Oriented and cooperative. Ambulatory, capable of self-care. May have bruises and superficial scratches, but no major injury.

Pupils equal, large, react to light and accommodation. Ears, nose OK. Chest, heart, lungs, abdomen OK. No signs of chronic alcohol abuse.

HR 125-135, regular — RR 30/min, shallow
BP 117/82 — Temp 99.1

BF5

BATTLE FATIGUE CASUALTY ROLE PLAYERS, READ ALL THESE INSTRUCTIONS FIRST

You are to play a normal, good soldier who has just had too many bad things happen at once. You will show one of the many forms of "battle fatigue."

Read what to DO, LOOK, AND SAY. Also read how to RESPOND TO HOW YOU ARE TREATED. When the instructions say you can tell people what has happened to you, you need to describe what you would have seen and done if this exercise had been a real war.

First, check this sheet to learn your soldier's rank, MOS (job duties), and unit. Adapt the story of the soldier on this sheet to fit that information. You can add background details to the basic story, including events from the following RECENT STRESS CHECKLIST. Especially use events marked with an X.

X Under artillery or bombing attack
— In chemical, smoke, or flame attack
— Caught in minefield or ambush
— Unit was harmed by friendly fire
X Friends, leader, or women and children killed or horribly wounded
X Had a close call with death
— Very heavy work or responsibilities
— Could not get needed information or support
— Have gotten very little sleep
— New to the unit, do not know anybody
— You may also be worried about home:
  — Recently got bad news
  — Received a "Dear John" letter
  — Just married or became a parent
  — Have a sick parent or child
  — Job, money, or legal problems
  — Not sure your family is safe

Do play the basic role on this sheet. Use your imagination to add details, but do not overdo it. Keep it realistic for a normal person like yourself.

If you are given a Field Medical Card (DA form 1380), which says you have received some treatment, change how you act now to fit what it says last.

SHOW THIS SHEET ONLY TO EVALUATORS.

DO, LOOK, AND SAY THE FOLLOWING
(BF5, anxiety, tremor)

Look and act anxious (scared). You can walk and talk and are cooperative.

Make your hands tremble.

Say that you cannot get ahold of yourself. "It's the shelling. I can't stand the shelling."

Say that you are afraid you cannot do your job and will let the unit down but feel terrified every time you hear artillery fire or incoming rounds.

Say (and act out, when you can) that you have these symptoms:
— Heart pounding, may skip a beat
— Sweating
— Frequent urination, diarrhea
— Startle (flinch) at any sudden sound or movement

IF asked, you are not a heavy drinker.

RESPOND TO HOW YOU ARE TREATED

IF hassled, set aside to wait, or evacuated and treated as if "sick": do not improve. Continue anxious, shaky, and jumpy. Be unable to sleep, or wake up with a terrifying dream.

IF only given medicine: go to sleep (without dreaming) and be somewhat less shaky on awakening but still very unsure you can do your job.

IF treated as a soldier and told you just have battle fatigue, and will recover soon, and your unit needs you: worry about it, but go back to duty.

OR IF given food and water, chance to clean up, sleep, work to do, and help to talk about what happened: improve, talk about it, and cooperate in work details, but worry that your unit will think you are a coward for breaking down this way

IF given reassurance: return to duty.

Fig. 11–2. Battle fatigue casualty instructions used during FTXs. Instructions delineate role-playing behaviors of the casualty and provide a simulated casualty tag. The primary presentation for the example in this scenario is anxiety and tremor. Source: Training materials developed by the Psychiatry and Neurology Branch, Behavioral Science Division, Army Medical Center and School, Fort Sam Houston, Texas.

Casualty Tag No:

Name:

SSN:

Rank:

Job title:

Unit:

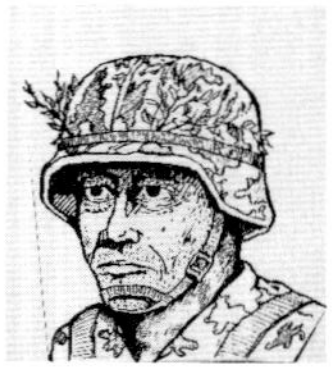

MOS/ADC:

( ) Walking	( ) Litter
( ) Injury	( ) Disease
( ) "Fatigue"	( ) "Psych"
( ) In restraints	( ) Under escort
( ) Simulated	( ) Constructive

DIAGNOSIS: BATTLE FATIGUE
( ) mild, ( ) moderate, ( ) severe
( ) Hold for Trtmnt ( ) Hold, Evac

Rule out:

EVALUATOR may detach this part and give information to whoever does examination.

SIGNS/SYMPTOMS AND PHYSICAL FINDINGS

Fatigue, 1,000 yard stare. Describes typical visual misperception and/or hallucination of the sleep-deprived. Oriented and cooperative, although tired and has difficulty concentrating and remembering. Ambulatory; capable of self-care. Mild-moderate psychomotor retardation.

May have bruises and superficial scratches, but no major injury.

Pupils equal, large, react to light and accommodation. Ears and nose OK. Chest, heart, lungs, abdomen OK.

HR 85-95, regular — RR 18/min
BP 119/86 — Temp 98.1, oral

BF23

BATTLE FATIGUE CASUALTY ROLE PLAYERS, READ ALL THESE INSTRUCTIONS FIRST

You are to play a normal, good soldier who has just had too many bad things happen at once. You will show one of the many forms of "battle fatigue."

Read what to DO, LOOK, AND SAY. Also read how to RESPOND TO HOW YOU ARE TREATED. When the instructions say you can tell people what has happened to you, you need to describe what you would have seen and done if this exercise had been a real war.

First, check this sheet to learn your soldier's rank, MOS (job duties), and unit. Adapt the story of the soldier on this sheet to fit that information. You can add background details to the basic story, including events from the following RECENT STRESS CHECKLIST. Especially use events marked with an X.

— Under artillery or bombing attack
— In chemical, smoke, or flame attack
— Caught in minefield or ambush
— Unit was harmed by friendly fire
— Friends, leader, or women and children killed or horribly wounded
— Had a close call with death
X Very heavy work or responsibilities
— Could not get needed information or support
X Have gotten very little sleep
— New to the unit, do not know anybody
— You may also be worried about home:
  — Recently got bad news
  — Received a "Dear John" letter
  — Just married or became a parent
  — Have a sick parent or child
  — Job, money, or legal problems
  — Not sure your family is safe

Do play the basic role on this sheet. Use your imagination to add details, but do not overdo it. Keep it realistic for a normal person like yourself.

If you are given a Field Medical Card (DA form 1380), which says you have received some treatment, change how you act now to fit what it says last.

SHOW THIS SHEET ONLY TO EVALUATORS.

DO, LOOK, AND SAY THE FOLLOWING
(BF23, simple exhaustion)

You are very tired, but keyed up. You can walk and talk and are cooperative.

IF asked: give your name and unit, and describe the recent combat, but have trouble paying attention, with a poor memory for details.

Keep your facial expression blank, with a wide-eyed ("1,000 yard") stare. Move and speak slowly, with long pauses.

Say that you have only slept a few hours in the past week and have been under constant heavy pressure and danger. You do not have any energy.

Say that last night you thought you saw enemy infiltrators and opened fire. Your unit said it was only shadows, but they sure looked exactly like real enemy soldiers to you. That really shook you up.

RESPOND TO HOW YOU ARE TREATED

IF hassled, set aside to wait, or evacuated and treated as if "sick": fall asleep. Be more alert on awakening. Tell them that you are not sure you can handle duty anymore.

IF only given medicine: go to sleep (without dreaming) and be more alert on awakening. Say you feel better but are afraid you are going crazy and should not return to duty.

ONLY IF treated as a soldier, and told that sleep-deprived brains often "see things", and you just have battle fatigue, and can still fight, and your unit needs you: say you want to go back.

OR IF given sleep, food and water, chance to clean up, work to do, and help to talk about what happened: improve, talk freely, and cooperate in work details, but worry that your unit will not want you back.

IF reassured: return to duty.

Fig. 11–3. Battle fatigue casualty instructions used during FTXs. Instructions delineate role-playing behaviors of the casualty and provide a simulated casualty tag. The primary presentation for the example in this scenario is simple exhaustion. Source: Training materials developed by the Psychiatry and Neurology Branch, Behavioral Science Division, Army Medical Center and School, Fort Sam Houston, Texas.

soldier could take one out of his pocket, read it carefully, and know how to play a fairly detailed case using his imagination to fill in the necessary details. However, experience shows that it is best to invest more effort in the selection and training of battle fatigue and neuropsychiatric role players. If there are psychiatric nurses as members of the moulage team, they may be recruited and trained to choose only those role players who are themselves mentally stable and able to act the part. Otherwise, members of the MTT must be detailed to do this.

SUMMARY AND CONCLUSION

Military mental health providers function differently from their civilian counterparts. During peacetime missions, they may deal with service members who are lonely and frustrated and have any number of family, occupational, or financial problems. During combat, the provider is likely to provide care to patients who are acutely anxious and exhausted. Therefore, not only does the scene of practice change for the military mental health provider, but the type of pathology is likely to be different depending on the setting.

Taken together, this situation means that the practice of military mental health is grounded in the principles of community mental health. The providers perform an occupational health role, focusing on preventing combat stress casualties and determining the fitness of the individual to function at his given job.

Training military mental health providers starts at the entry level. For specialists, technicians, social workers, and psychologists, training is available in the recognition and treatment of combat stress casualties. Most other providers, such as physicians, and specifically psychiatrists, often have not been trained in medical school to treat battle fatigue casualties. An innovative course for medical students has been described in this chapter. In addition, a model proposal to teach psychiatry residents how to interact with commanders and hospital personnel in the field is included. Last, the major medical FTXs have been described in detail. These FTXs are important in the preparation and training of all healthcare personnel in the proper management of battlefield stress casualties. For most mental health personnel, on-the-job training is the best possible way to learn about the practice of military mental health.

Recommendations for training must take into account military structure. Put simply, the management of combat stress cannot be taught in the medical center. Psychiatric residents and allied mental health professionals must have exposure to officers and enlisted service members in a variety of military settings.

With this in mind, the following four specific recommendations can be made: (1) Develop a short course and training packages in combat stress management that are mandatory for personnel assigned to troop mental health support slots. Include as many allied healthcare personnel as needed. To be sure, nurses, chaplains, and hospital commanders should be specifically asked to participate in this training. (2) Require inclusion of brigade combat stress teams in FTXs, especially at combat training centers. (3) Increase combat stress training in core career courses armywide to the level of application in practical exercises. (4) Train and program unit medical and mental health personnel to give sustainment training to unit leaders in the garrison and field.

REFERENCES

1. Wise MG. The past, present, and future of psychiatric training the U.S. Armed Services. *Milit Med.* 1987;152:550–553.

2. Leamon MH, Sutton LK, Lee RE. Graduate medical educators and infantry commanders: Working together to train Army psychiatry residents. *Milit Med.* 1990;155:430–432.

3. US Department of the Army. *Combat Stress Control in a Theater of Operations.* Washington DC: DA; In press, 1994. Field Manual 8–51.

4. Hausman W, Rioch DMck. Military psychiatry: A prototype of social and preventive psychiatry in the United States. *Arch Gen Psychiatry*. 1967;16:727–739.

5. Bushard B. The U.S. Army's mental hygiene consultation service. In: *Symposium on Preventive and Social Psychiatry*. Washington, DC: Walter Reed Army Institute of Research, Walter Reed Army Medical Center, and the National Research Council, 15–17 April 1957.

6. Glass AJ. 1966; Lessons learned. In: *Zone of the Interior*. Vol 1. In: Glass AJ, Bernucci RJ, eds. *Neuropsychiatry in World War II*. Washington, DC: Office of The Surgeon General, US Department of the Army; 1966: 735–759.

7. Glass AJ. Army psychiatry before World War II. In: *Zone of the Interior*. Vol 1. In: Glass AJ, Bernucci RJ, eds. *Neuropsychiatry in World War II*. Washington, DC: Office of The Surgeon General, US Department of the Army; 1966: 3–23.

8. Menninger W. *Psychiatry in a Troubled World*. New York: McMillan; 1948.

9. US Department of the Army. *Neuropsychiatry and Mental Health*. Washington, DC: DA; 10 August 1984. Army Regulation 40–216.

10. US Department of the Air Force, Army, and Navy. *Psychiatry in Military Law*. Washington, DC: DAF, DA, DN; 25 September 1981. Training Manual 8–240.

11. US Department of the Army. *Alcohol and Drug Abuse Prevention and Control Program*. Washington, DC: DA; 21 October 1988. Army Regulation 600–85.

12. Goldman HH, Morrissey JP. The alchemy of mental health policy: Homelessness and the fourth cycle of reform. *Am J Public Health*. 1985;75:727–731.

13. Koshes RJ., Rothberg JM. Parasuicidal behavior on an active duty Army training post. *Milit Med*. 1992;157:350–353.

14. Bion WR. Experiences in groups, I. *Human Relations*. 1948;1(3):314–320.

15. Bion WR. Experiences in groups, II. *Human Relations*. 1948;1(4):487–496.

16. Bion WR. Experiences in groups, III. *Human Relations*. 1949;2(1):1322.

17. Bion WR. Experiences in groups, IV. *Human Relations*. 1949;2(4):295–303.

18. Bion WR. Experiences in groups, V. *Human Relations*. 1950;3(1):3–14.

19. Bion WR. Experiences in groups, VI. *Human Relations*. 1950;3(4):395–402.

20. Bion WR. Group dynamics: A Re-view. *Int J Psychoanal*. 1952;33(2):235–247.

21. Bion WR. *Experiences in Groups and Other Papers*. New York: Basic Books; 1961.

22. Artiss KL. Military combat and social psychiatry. Presented to the Psychiatry Staff, Tripler Army Medical Center, Honolulu, Hawaii; 12 December 1984.

23. Artiss KL. Human behavior under stress. *Milit Med*. 1963;128(10):1011–1015.

24. Hibler RJ. Battlefield stress: Management techniques. *Milit Med*. 1984;149:5–8.

25. Solomon Z. Benbenishty R. The role of proximity, immediacy and expectancy in frontline treatment of combat stress reactions among Israelis in the Lebanon War. *Am J Psychiatry*. 1986;143(5):613–617.

26. Jones FD, Crocq L, Adelaja O, et al. Psychiatric casualties in modern warfare: I. Evolution of treatment. In: Pichot P, Berner P, Wolf R, Thau K, eds. *Psychiatry: The State of the Art*. Vol 6. New York: Plenum Publishing Corporation; 1985: 459–464.

27. Jones FD, Johnson AW. Medical and psychiatric treatment policy and practice in Vietnam. *J Soc Issues*. 1975;31(4):49–65.

28. Jones FD. Lessons of war for psychiatry. In: Pichot P, Berner P, Wolf R, Thau K, eds. *Psychiatry: The State of the Art*. Vol 6. New York: Plenum Publishing Corporation; 1985: 515–519.

29. Hales RE, Jones FD. Teaching the principles of combat psychiatry to Army psychiatry residents. *Milit Med*. 1983;148:24–27.

30. McCaughey BG. Role players: A brief intensive training program to portray acute psychological distress. *J Traumatic Stress*. 1991;4(4):595–599.

31. McCaughey BG. Observations about battle fatigue: Its occurrence and absence. *Milit Med*. 1991;156:694–695.

32. Stokes J. Personal Observations, June 1984. Fort Hood, Tex: Dusty Bull '84.

33. Stokes J. Personal Observations, June 1985. Camp Roberts, Calif: Wounded Warrior '85.

34. Stokes J. Personal Observations, June 1986. Camp Shelby, Miss: MEDEX '86.

35. Stokes J. Personal Observations, June 1988. Fort Hood, Tex: Dusty Bull '88.

36. Stokes J. Personal Observations, June 1988. Camp Roberts, Calif: Wounded Warrior '88.

37. Stokes J. Personal Observations, 1989. Camp Shelby, Miss: MEDEX '89.

38. Stokes J. Personal Observations, 1992. Camp Roberts and Camp Pendleton, Calif: Wounded Warrior '92.

39. US Department of the Army. *Health Service Support in a Theater of Operations*. Washington DC: DA; 1991. Field Manual 8–10.

40. US Department of the Army. *Leader's Manual for Combat Stress Control*. Washington DC: DA; In press, 1994. Field Manual 22–51.

41. Stokes J. Personal Observations.

42. Boatright C. Personal Communication, June 1988.

43. US Department of the Army. *Patient Play in Exercises*. Washington, DC: DA; 1991? GTA 8–12–3(17).

Chapter 12

A MODEL COMBAT PSYCHIATRY TRAINING PROGRAM FOR DIVISION PERSONNEL

R. GREGORY LANDE, D.O.*

*Lieutenant Colonel, Medical Corps, U.S. Army; Chief, Outpatient Psychiatry Service, Walter Reed Army Medical Center, Washington, D.C. 20307–5001

INTRODUCTION

When the training program described in this chapter was conducted, the U.S. Army Third Infantry Division (3ID) was a primary bulwark against aggression in Europe. Since the breakup of the Warsaw Pact and the Soviet Union, 3ID (and other divisions like it in Korea and the continental United States) must continue to train for missions that range from peacekeeping and peace enforcement in ethnic conflicts, which involve appalling atrocities, to nuclear, biological, and chemical regional wars. Combat psychiatric and stress casualties will be a significant area of concern in any future conflict. A simple statement, yet how to address this concern remains elusive. The members of the 3ID mental health team consisting of the division psychiatrist, the division social worker, and the division psychologist conducted a program evaluation in an attempt to answer this concern. The research consisted of a critical evaluation of present capabilities, field problems to assess the degree of difficulty in treating and identifying casualties, and a thorough review of the literature on combat psychiatry. In addition, line commanders' opinions were solicited, as were opinions and practices in other divisions in the U.S. Army relating to combat psychiatry.

This material was compiled and thoroughly reviewed by the 3ID mental health team and the 3ID surgeon. As a result of this research, a training program designed for the 3ID was deemed necessary. The training program was designed to help maintain the fighting strength of the division. Any program initiated, however, must be practical and must reach the largest possible division audience.

Embodied in the program was the belief that even when the best evaluation means were available, the line medics and physician assistants would still, in most cases, see the earliest cases of combat stress reaction (CSR). However, if the CSR casualties were successfully treated, it was imperative that the commanders also be willing to accept back the treated soldiers.

THE TRAINING PROGRAM

The training program that developed was in two parts. The first part involved training the medical units, and the second part involved training the commanders. The issue of pragmatism was constantly kept in mind in the program development. The training program for the line medics, for example, had to be understandable, yet not be so simple as to gloss over important issues.

Because time for training is always limited, the program must be concise, and it must aim at developing important concepts. The program must also have a means of assessing impact. In other words, was the program as delivered effective in developing the key concepts? Finally, the program must have a means available for critical feedback that can incorporate and adjust to the participants' needs.

The training program that reflected the philosophy and goals deemed important took form slowly. Many adjustments were made from that inaugural training exercise, and the program as now described is the end result of many mistakes, changes, additions, and deletions.

Division Medical Personnel Course

The program for the participants begins at 0900 hours. The instructors arrive about 1 hour earlier to prepare the classroom. The presentation by the 3ID mental health team utilizes slide projectors, overhead projectors, chalkboards, and various handouts during the class. The required materials are listed below:

- 35mm slide projector
- viewing screen
- chalkboard
- handouts
- pencils
- patient triage cards
- overhead projector/overlays
- moulage kit
- protective mask
- load-bearing equipment

The 3ID mental health team has three officers, and it was among these three officers that the morning didactic session was divided. The morning started with the 3ID psychologist distributing a pretest evaluation to gauge the knowledge of the participants before instruction. The pretest evaluation covered some of the basics of CSR or "battle fatigue" treatment, identification, and history. A synopsis of the pretest is presented below:

1. Provide service member's (SM) identifying data (name, Social Security number, unit).
2. List previous CSR training.
3. Describe factors contributing to CSR.
4. Describe a CSR.
5. Estimate the number of CSRs in brigade unit.
6. List effective ways to treat CSR.
7. What percentage of CSR can be effectively treated?
8. Would you trust a returned CSR?

After the pretest evaluation was completed, the first phase of instruction began. This 1-hour discussion centered on the historical significance of psychiatric casualties. The purpose of this discussion was to provide a longitudinal view of CSR and its implications in war. Specific examples of psychiatric casualties in soldiers and units are explored.

Because one of the guiding principles in the conduct of this training program was repetition, an effort was made to examine key concepts from several vantage points. In the historical overview section for example, the principles of treatment were examined from their historical inception, through application, to current use in modern armies (principally the U.S. and Israeli armies). The examination of treatment principles in such a manner helps reinforce their validity and impresses on the listener the notion that these principles are "tried and true."

For example, during World War II, certain units experienced large numbers of CSR casualties.[1–3] The impact this had on operations can then be examined. This analysis can be developed over a considerable period of history, thereby lending credence to the concept that CSR casualties are important. Hopefully, at a point during the historical investigation, the listener will be prompted to ask himself what factors might make a unit or a soldier more vulnerable to become a CSR casualty. This question also can be approached from a historical viewpoint. Numerous lessons have been gleaned from a study of previous conflicts. Such factors as the combat intensity, wounded in action (WIA) and killed in action (KIA) rates, the type of unit, and characteristics in the service member can all influence the rate of occurrence of CSR. This information is important because it allows for potential modification of factors that might increase the rate of occurrence of CSR. Again, history's lesson is that the most cohesive units, those with the highest esprit de corps, will have the least problems.[2,4] Those factors that increase cohesion can then become part of the preventive psychiatric approach.

In summary, the first didactic hour focuses on the lessons of history with the explicit purpose of "legitimizing" the CSR problem through historical survey. This is one of the main teaching goals.

The second hour of didactic was presented by the division social worker and focused on the division's assets, limitations, and a different method that could potentially be employed in combat to address the CSR problem. In addition, this session focused on projected casualty generation figures, defining the scope of CSR in a statistical manner.

The assets of the division available to treat, manage, or otherwise respond to psychiatric battle casualties were explained from the standpoint of the available personnel. The division mental health team consists of three officers and six to eight enlisted personnel, who in Europe are geographically isolated from each other. Each officer has two or three enlisted personnel, depending on the community population that the team serves, that is, to staff a mental health center. The geographical fragmentation of the division mental health team is stressed as a limiting factor in the ability of the mental health team to pool its resources and develop a cogent training program.

On mobilization, the officers would support the forward support medical companies in the brigade support areas, with the 3ID psychiatrist providing supervision of the main support medical company in the division rear. This immediately poses a problem because one clearing company is left without a mental health professional. Another serious limiting factor of the European 3ID mental health team is the peacetime mission that emphasizes community mental health activities as a priority over the combat readiness mission. Varying with the professional degree, the division mental health team is almost totally ensconced in the deliverance of routine mental health services to active duty personnel, dependents, children, and civilians. In this case, the division mental health team either totally replaces or augments the medical command's or medical activity's supply resources. The division mental health team is so totally overwhelmed by these duties that primary consideration to a substantive preventive psychiatry program becomes difficult, thereby not allowing the division to benefit from the expertise of the division mental health team to aid in combat readiness. A shift in focus, allowing a higher priority of the training mission, is discussed as a remedy to this problem.

Estimates of projected CSR casualty figures are also discussed in a relatively detailed way. To make the statistics more relevant, the casualty figures are also estimated for division- and brigade-sized units. The point is made that these casualties represent recoverable manpower through the application of effective treatment. Evacuation procedures are also examined noting the correlation between high numbers of CSR casualties and the routine priority they are given in terms of evacuation. Numbers and types of evacuation vehicles are also discussed.

Various management approaches to handling the large numbers of CSR casualties are explored. One method is to have all CSR casualties evacuated for treatment to the medical companies' clearing stations. Here the officer and two or three enlisted personnel will handle all evacuations and area support. However, one medical company that will be acting as a central evacuation point will have no mental health officer, but rather only a behavioral science noncommissioned officer. (This shortfall should be corrected if the division is reinforced by teams from a corps-level combat stress control unit.)

The evacuation priority of "routine" given to psychiatric casualties also suggests, in the heavy casualty war scenario at least, that the projected WIA may limit the likelihood of large numbers of CSR casualties being evacuated, probably a desirable situation. The lowest echelon of identification of the CSR casualty may therefore also become the "treatment facility."

Further potential hindrances to CSR evacuation are explored. These might include chemical contamination of an evacuation route, the need for frequent moves by the "treatment facility," and vehicle maintenance problems.

By reviewing the evacuation issues, the automatic notion of many line personnel to evacuate "back" is short circuited. The conclusion generally drawn by the participants, then, is that many CSR patients will by necessity need to be treated at the lowest echelons of medical care, that is, the company medic and the battalion aide station (BAS). Again, the importance of the CSR problem is borne out, and again, the necessity for a training program becomes evident.

After presenting these two topics, the history and longitudinal scope of the CSR problem plus present capabilities and projected casualty figures, hopefully, the listener is by this time asking himself, "How can I recognize and treat psychiatric and CSR casualties?" The answer to this question then becomes the basis for the third and final didactic discussion. Pragmatism must be the key concept in presenting the medical aspects of psychiatry in the combat zone. Esoterics have little place here. The discussion must underline the importance of combat psychiatry and then offer guidelines for field management.

The division psychiatrist presents the topic on the medical aspects of combat psychiatry. In addition to the lecture, a medical briefing booklet was prepared and given to each participant. The booklet covered in more detail what the lecture provided. The medical briefing booklet becomes a permanent resource to which the medic can return to review treatment, diagnostic, and evacuation guidelines.

The booklet contains information on more specific areas than time allows in the morning session. The subjects include the psychiatric aspects of chemical warfare, substance abuse, a brief primer on the major psychiatric disorders, and CSR. The booklet is designed to be used in the class and later to be a resource. In fact, the primary purpose for preparing such a booklet is to give the participants a concentrated referral source. Differences in division locations and missions will mean that only general guidelines can be provided in a medical briefing booklet.

The table of contents for the 3ID's medical briefing booklet, which was titled "Psychiatry in the Combat Zone," also served as the outline for the morning medical discussion. Exhibit 12–1 details this outline.

The discussion of the medical aspects of combat psychiatry starts with a review of the approach of the former Soviet Union to combat stress. Topics center on the exploitation of surprise, use of propaganda, doctrine relating to "battlefield paralysis," and methods of protecting their soldiers from becoming combat psychiatric casualties.[5]

In summing up the potential threat, it is noted that adversaries may be prepared both to exploit the enemy human emotional factor and at the same time to defend themselves from becoming potential CSR casualties.

After presenting this brief overview philosophy, the lecture turns to the medical aspects of combat psychiatry. In trying to provide the most pragmatic approach to the issues of diagnosis and treatment, we repeatedly emphasized the time-honored medical approach. The listener must be left with a clear idea as to the variety of diagnoses that may be seen on the battlefield, in other words a differential diagnosis, and a means whereby the possibilities can be separated. To achieve this objective, the listener must learn what conditions may present themselves on the battlefield and then, through the use of a history and physical, separate them. Utilizing this principle throughout, the medical briefing starts with discussion of the psychiatric aspects of chemical warfare. In discussing chemical warfare from the psychiatric standpoint, we place particular emphasis on behavioral symptoms.[6,7] For example, the nerve agents are examined from the standpoint of tactical use, behavioral and physical symptom production, and treatment with atropine. This is not a general discussion but specific to include dosages of medications used in first aid.

EXHIBIT 12–1

PSYCHIATRY IN THE COMBAT ZONE MEDICAL BRIEFING BOOK OUTLINE

Section I	A Brief Synopsis of Philosophy of the former Soviet Army
Section II	The Psychiatric Aspects of Chemical Warfare
Section III	Combat Stress Reaction
Section IV	Substance Abuse
Section V	Major Psychiatric Disorders
Section VI	Appendix

a. WHO Chart
b. Conditions with Prominent Anxiety
c. The Acute Radiation Syndrome
d. Decision trees for differential diagnoses found in the *Diagnostic and Statistical Manual* of the American Psychiatric Association
e. A Simplified Overview of Combat Psychiatry
f. A Simplified Overview of Treatment Modalities
g. A Relaxation Program

In addition to discussing the hazards of exposure to chemical agents, we review other psychiatric difficulties encountered in a chemical environment. "Gas hysteria," a problem in World War I where symptoms developed without exposure to chemicals, is posed as a problem that may recur.[6,7] The need to obtain an adequate history and a thorough physical examination are thereby reinforced.

An anxious soldier not truly exposed to a chemical agent but thinking he was may inject himself inappropriately with atropine. The symptoms of atropine overdose are examined in detail. To reinforce the importance of gaining a history and doing a physical, we present a case example of an organically induced atropine psychosis. Without obtaining a good history and physical, the medic gives this "crazy person" chlorpromazine and evacuates him, a very common response from the uninitiated medics. The errors of such treatment in both producing a severe hypotension and the subsequent loss of the soldier's fighting strength are pointed out, as is the quick and effective treatment. Furthermore, chlorpromazine has strong atropine-like effects and may produce atropine psychosis when given to one already having atropine in his system.[8]

The psychological effects of prolonged confinement in mission-oriented protective posture (MOPP) gear are next examined, including possible symptoms.[9,10] For example, the increased respiratory effort needed to operate the protective mask may be misinterpreted as chemical exposure. To help differentiate these various problems, the medics are given guidance in history and physical assessment. For example, in taking a history of possible chemical exposure, questions that might be asked include the following:

- Was the unit exposed to chemicals, and if so, by what means and at what time?
- Where was the service member in relation to the other unit members?
- Did the service member have his MOPP gear on, and if so, for how long?
- What is the service member verbalizing as his problem?

The section on the psychiatric aspects of chemical warfare concludes with a short case example and its effective treatment.

Another medical problem that may be seen in the combat zone is the soldier with a substance abuse disorder. This is a large area of concern in peacetime, as indicated by the extensive military drug and alcohol abuse program.[11] A primary focus of discussion in the medical aspects of combat psychiatry is the clinical problem of acute drug usage and withdrawal and the differential diagnosis from chemical exposure, CSR, and other similar problems.

To aid the combat medic, we give a review of the symptoms of alcohol withdrawal.[8] The importance of gathering an alcohol history is emphasized because the symptoms of alcohol withdrawal may be similar to other disorders. Questions the medic might ask to help elicit the information are also provided as guidance.

In discussing treatment and evacuation guidelines, one needs to separate mild withdrawal from more serious conditions. Mild cases of alcohol withdrawal can be locally treated, reducing the need for evacuation and the subsequent loss of manpower. After describing the more serious withdrawal symptoms, we discuss their treatment. Other drugs of abuse presenting with withdrawal symptoms will also be seen. Some of the specific drugs and their effects can be discussed.

Phencyclidine (PCP) received separate consideration as a drug of abuse because of treatment difficulties.[8] A service member under the influence of PCP may be combative, negative, and hallucinating.[12] To the medic who does not have access to an adequate history, this service member will just look "crazy" and be "treated" with restraints and chlorpromazine. The pitfalls of this approach are examined to help reinforce the need for proper diagnosis and subsequent treatment and evacuation. The point should be emphasized that a drug and alcohol history, when routinely gathered, will spare evacuation, conserve manpower, and ultimately provide better battlefield medical care.

There will be, of course, a few major psychiatric disorders present in a wartime scenario. To bring this into perspective, a World Health Organization chart detailing the frequency of major psychiatric disorders is made relevant to a division-sized unit. Obviously, the entire field of psychiatry cannot be discussed. Instead, one method is again to rely on differential diagnosis and history. After having ruled out physical injury, chemical exposure, inappropriate atropine injection, and drug withdrawal, then consider a functional psychiatric disorder. For example, a service member presents with hallucinations and delusions and is incoherent, in short, "crazy." The medic should consider the differentials and obtain a history and physical examination including any history of previous psychiatric problems.

If no obvious diagnosis presents itself, a period of drug-free observation may be useful; however, if the condition is too severe, evacuation is appropriate. Particularly severe disorders such as suicidal behavior and psychosis are discussed in depth. The level of expertise of the audience must be gauged so that this material is presented in an understandable format. This is particularly true when discussing psychiatric terms such as psychosis, hallucinations, delusions, incoherence, and other terminology.

The final broad topic discussed in the medical aspects of combat psychiatry is CSR or "battle fatigue."CSR is discussed last because it should be assumed only after all other potentially dangerous, life-, limb-, or function-threatening diagnoses have been adequately ruled out.

The CSR is first defined as to what it is and what it is not. The point is made that a CSR is not "crazy" or even violent as a rule. It is useful to explain that a CSR is an exaggeration of the normal responses that might be seen in any very stressful situation. It is also useful to describe common normal responses to combat. The difference between a normal response to combat and a CSR can then be better understood. The CSR is presented, then, as an exaggeration of a normal response to combat. However, the CSR is no longer functional. In other words, the CSR's degree of psychophysiological response is severe enough to *temporarily* disable him in the performance of his duties as a soldier. The factors that might contribute to more stress in a combat scenario and increase the numbers of CSR patients are closely examined. The participants are instructed to preferably use the label "combat or battle fatigue" to convey the transient, benign nature of the disorder.

Such factors as combat intensity, WIA and KIA rates, the type of unit, the service member's previous battle experience, and the expectation regarding the anticipated outcome of the battle are studied from the standpoint of affecting the CSR rate. In addition, such factors as sleep deprivation, family concerns, and the individual's ability to handle stress in general are viewed as possibly tipping the balance in the direction of temporarily disabling symptoms.

After a definition of CSR has been given and factors influencing the CSR rate presented, there must be a very concrete description of how the CSR patient will present to the combat medic. A good way to present this information is with a chart that by statistics relates the symptoms seen in various previous conflicts. For example, in the 1982 Lebanon War, 56% of the Israeli CSR patients presented with anxiety, 38% as depressed, and 34% with fearful mood.[13,14] The presentation and discussion of symptoms will be followed by treatment and evacuation guidelines. The well-known treatment principles of the CSR patient are explained using proximity, immediacy, expectancy, and simplicity (PIES). Centrality, which is more of a management issue, is only briefly touched on here.

The relative safety of the medical unit, when combined with rest, food, and an expectation of return to battle, *is* the simple treatment. In addition, other treatments that can, and should, be used include work assignments, catharsis (debriefing), and a brief relaxation program that can be easily administered and "prescribed."

The important factor is to give the medic the tools to treat the CSR patient and thus short circuit the use of medicines or inappropriate evacuation. Finally, it is noted that the treatment is effective (relying on and reinforcing earlier material presented), and recidivism will be very low. However, for a small percentage of patients, the 48-hour period of restoration will not be successful, and evacuation to a reconditioning center should be considered. The 3-day to 2-week stay in a reconditioning center will still result in the return of the majority of CSR casualties to duty.

The morning session then ends with a summary that, in pictorial form, reviews the differential diagnoses and treatments. The medical briefing booklet that had been handed out earlier contains an appendix. The appendix has flowcharts that help organize a medic's differential diagnosis and treatment (Exhibit 12–2).

Of course, no flowchart is complete, and such a chart will never replace a careful evaluation, as is pointed out in the briefing. The afternoon field training exercise begins when volunteers are selected from the battalion aide stations to act as

EXHIBIT 12–2

DECISION TREE FOR COMBAT STRESS CASUALTY

1. Anxious, Irritable, Depressed, and Nonfunctional	
2. Psychological factors affecting physical conditions	2a. History of physical injury
3. Neurologic condition	3a. History of head or spinal cord injury
4. Withdrawal symptoms	4a. History of drug and/or alcohol use
5. Chemical symptoms Chemical hysteria	5a. Contact with chemical agent
6. Atropine overdose	6a. Anticholinergic symptom and/or use of Atropine
7. Radiation syndrome	7a. Exposure to nuclear environment
8. Biological contamination	8a. Exposure to biological agent
9. Psychiatric disorder	9a. Presence of major psychiatric symptoms (hallucinations, delusions, severe depression, suicidal)
10. Combat stress reaction	10a. Unable to temporarily function as a soldier secondary to combat stress

A soldier with symptoms (step 1) must be questioned about potential alternate causes (steps 2 through 9). The examining medic must rule out the alternates with negative responses to steps 2a through 9a before labeling the casualty as having a combat stress reaction (step 10) or as being a combat stress casualty (step 10a).

casualties, while part of the mental health team plays the role of psychiatric casualties. The remainder of the mental health staff (three people) act as trainers/supervisors to give both feedback and to create various scenarios during the actual running of the exercise.

A central casualty pool contains the physical, psychiatric, and CSR casualties. Through the use of color-coded patient cards (Exhibit 12–3), the 15 to 20 different patients are sorted and distributed to each battalion aide station. This method allows a regulated flow of patient types.

The color-coded cards give the medic information as to the medical/psychiatric history. The use of moulage kits adds realism for physical casualties. The mental health staff "acts" the psychiatric symptoms, thus also ensuring more realism.

Over a 1-hour period, 15 to 20 casualties of all types are sent from the casualty generation pool/ forward edge of the battle area to the company aidmen. The company aidmen are required to triage the casualties. Physical casualties needing bandages, splints, or stretchers are administered by the aidmen. Evacuation priorities are enforced; that is, psychiatric and CSR casualties are evacuated only after serious physical casualties. The aidmen are forced to confront and triage a wide variety of psychiatric and CSR casualties, thereby increasing their sensitivity to the magnitude of combat psychiatry.

EXHIBIT 12–3

SAMPLE PATIENT CARD

VITAL SIGNS: BP= 116/74; P= 74; R= 14;
Airway: clear
Hemorrhage: none

HISTORY: Over a period of several hours, the service member gradually withdrew and would not talk or follow any orders. The SM has refused all attempts to engage him, even refusing food and water. With great difficulty, the company aidman was able to evacuate the SM to the BAS.

PHYSICAL: Repeated attempts to question the SM were met with silence and a vacant stare. There is no evidence of neurologic abnormalities after a careful screen. There are no signs of, or history to suggest, drug abuse. SM has no history of exposure to CBR weapons.

After appropriate interventions, the aidmen will evacuate their casualties to the battalion aide station. Here, the physician assistant and his staff must diagnose, treat, and evacuate where appropriate.

To add further realism and to aid the training for "common soldiers' tasks," various scenarios are enacted. The trainer/supervisor will call a "gas alert," thereby requiring the donning of protective masks to both aidmen and to their patients. Patients will occasionally be evacuated with a protective mask, demonstrating the importance of facial cues and verbal communication in diagnosis. Physician assistants may also be "eliminated," forcing the battalion aide stations to operate without their services. Various other scenarios can be enacted including the decisions that must be made when the battalion aide station gets the order to move out.

The battalion aide station is required to fill out patient cards describing diagnosis and treatment. These cards are used later for feedback.

After completion of the training exercise, the participants return to the classroom. At this point, feedback is given, both positive and negative, as to unit performance. All the trainers/supervisors have their viewpoints. This is followed by a discussion of specific patients that were portrayed during the exercise and what might be considered as diagnostic, therapeutic, and evacuation guidelines.

A general discussion period follows that ends with the posttest examination being given. The posttest is used to gauge the immediate effectiveness of the training program and also to reinforce key points. Finally, a critique sheet is distributed that allows the soldiers to comment on the training program and give feedback on possible improvements. This has been a valuable tool for making meaningful modifications. The day-long program ends with each successful participant receiving a certificate of training.

Division Commanders' Course

As important as the training is for medical personnel, the command personnel must also understand what combat psychiatry is and how proper diagnosis, treatment, and evacuation will affect their fighting force. Commanders can also be told of preventive measures that may help reduce their losses.

The commanders' course is best initiated by first securing command support at the highest level available. Obtaining this support will generally entail a briefing that details the importance and need for commanders' attendance at such a course. This briefing is best directed at the division commanding general at a meeting arranged by the division surgeon. Another valuable addition is to obtain an introductory letter signed by the division commanding general emphasizing the need for the course and its attendance by commanders. This letter then becomes an integral part of the material that is disseminated before the commanders' briefings. Having now received command support, mental health personnel can begin the second phase of the training program.

Part 2 of the combat psychiatry training program is again divided into three parts, reflecting the desire to allow all three officers to utilize their expertise in training. The three parts of the briefing include an historical review of combat psychiatry, a medical review, and a section dealing with preventive measures.

The historical review is a 30 to 45 minute presentation designed primarily to demonstrate to commanders the importance of combat psychiatry. This is best done by exploring, through history, the impact that CSR casualties have had on tactical operations. This is also illustrated with actual case vignettes. It becomes necessary to touch on the issue of readiness. The theme developed is that an unprepared army is a vulnerable army. Examples supporting this notion, such as experiences in World War I, World War II, and Israel, are fully explained. During this initial briefing, a very powerful concept that can be discussed is the casualty generation figures. Here the commander actually sees what impact losses because of CSR will have on his unit. At this point, the need for a training program to help decrease these losses becomes more apparent. The Israeli Defence Force experience before and after the institution of such a training program is discussed last to demonstrate how effective such training can be in returning effective soldiers to the commander. At the end of the first presentation, the commanders should have a better appreciation of the tactical importance of the CSR casualty and of a preventive training program.

The middle presentation is an abbreviated medical overview, similar to that in part 1. Key concepts that should be developed include the social approach to the CSR, a brief overview of the scope of combat psychiatry, what the CSR casualty will look like, how the CSR casualty will be treated, and the effectiveness of this treatment. It is also important to describe the part 1 training program to the commanders so that they can appreciate both our concern and our approach to the issue of "readiness." The medical section concentrates less on specifics of diagnosis, treatment, and evacuation but instead leans toward issues of effectiveness of treatment, present preparedness, and the commander's vital role in the entire process. The point is made that without the commander's involvement, the whole program is less effective than it could be.

The final presentation revolves around preventive measures that commanders need to understand and, as appropriate, apply. Those factors that influence the rate of CSR casualties can be discussed. For example, the WIA/KIA rate, the expectation regarding the outcome of the battle, the service member's previous combat experience, and the combat intensity are just a few of the factors that are covered in this presentation. Unit cohesion, because of its particular importance in decreasing the rate of CSR casualties, receives special attention. Factors that might tend to produce more group cohesion such as regular combat training, physical training, and effective leadership are offered to the commanders for their consideration. The ability of the leader to influence the cognitive appraisal of the service member is emphasized.[15] Although effective leadership is a well-known principle for promoting more unit cohesion and subsequently less CSR casualties, this presentation does not offer guidelines for effective leadership because commanders receive this information elsewhere. The need for enforced periods of sleep is also discussed.

In the commanders' briefing, the use of research instruments to gauge the level of knowledge tends to be more politically sensitive than with the medics. If such an instrument is to be used, this should be thoroughly explained both when initially seeking approval to start the training program and later with the commanders themselves. A critique sheet, however, tends to be a less-sensitive issue and normally would represent the conclusion of the commanders' briefing. The critique sheet is designed to allow for feedback on the presentation as well as to elicit commanders' ideas for improving the program. Modifications can then be made to provide for more sensitive training.

Material and Methods

In collecting the data, a questionnaire was used. The questionnaire was distributed in the pretest mode to all participants. This information is considered the baseline because it reflects knowledge before training. The posttest was the same questionnaire. It was completed after the training. This information would represent short and intermediate memory retention of key training principles. Fifteen months after the medics had completed the combat psychiatry training program a retest gauged the degree of learning loss.

In the commanders' training program, the same questions distributed to the medics were again used. This allowed correlation of data. There was no posttest given because of time constraints.

The multiple choice questions dealt with basic principles of combat psychiatry. The questions were designed to elicit the respondents' knowledge in such areas as detection, description, treatment, and probabilities of occurrence. The questions were constructed to allow prejudices and misinformation to be revealed. This was done to test the proposition that such prejudices might exist. The choices to each question were designed to allow appropriate and inappropriate responses to be discerned and later tabulated.

The pretest and posttest responses were collected in 1983. There were 202 questionnaires obtained from the division medical personnel. The units tested included the major elements of the division. These units are separated geographically by as much as 100 miles.

Fifteen months after training, a reexamination of original respondents was conducted. This sample netted 16 questionnaires or 8% of the original group. Personnel losses accounted for the small size of this sample. Statistics are included for information and not for statistical inferences.

One hundred and seventy-eight commanders who received their training in 1985 contributed the most current data in this study. The combat arms were the main unit-type represented.

Responses to each question were tabulated and then converted to a percentile figure. The percentages of appropriate and inappropriate responses were compared in the pretest, posttest, retest, and commander's program. The pretest knowledge was the standard to which subsequent shifts after training were compared.

Results

In responding to the question "What are important things that cause a CSR?" the medics' top percentile choices on the pretest included: drug and alcohol abuse, 74%; previous difficulties adjusting in life, 68%; the KIA and WIA rate, 50%; and battle intensity, 46%. After the medical training, the data shifted to battle intensity, 82%; the KIA and WIA rate, 80%; experience in combat, 76%; drug and alcohol abuse, 74%; and lack of sleep, 60%. The 15-month retest data included lack of sleep, 88%; battle intensity, 82%; the KIA and WIA rate, 81%; experience in combat, 76%; and few friends in the unit, 44%. The commanders' selections included the KIA and WIA rate, 82%; lack of sleep, 71%; battle intensity, 66%; experience in combat, 60%; and poor unit morale, 49%.

Reviewing the percentages of inappropriate responses is also important because it can have a direct negative effect on decision making. For presumed etiologies of CSRs, the medics' pretest included weak personality, 42%; the way he was brought up, 14%; and previous difficulties adjusting in life, 68%. The commanders on this question chose a weak personality, 29%; the way he was brought up, 26%; and previous difficulties adjusting in life, 37%.

In describing "How a CSR would most likely act," the pretest medical responses included scared, 89%; jumpy, 78%; nervous, 71%; in a daze, 71%; and normal, 64%. The posttest responses were nervous, 81%; quiet, 74%; dazed, 72%; withdrawn, 71%; and scared, 61%. The 15-month retest responses were nervous, 88%; quiet, 75%; withdrawn, 75%; scared, 69% and dazed, 69%. The commanders answering to this question listed their responses as nervous, 68%; withdrawn, 54%; jumpy, 51%; dazed, 51%; and scared, 48%.

Inappropriate pretest responses included crazy, 18%; nuts, 20%; freaked out, 18%; haywire, 12%; wild, 19%; and screaming, 22%. These same data after training were crazy, 4%; nuts, 5%; freaked out, 11%; haywire, 2%; wild, 1%; and screaming, 6%. Inappropriate responses chosen by commanders were crazy, 16%; nuts, 11%; freaked out, 27%; haywire, 14%; and screaming, 24%.

In selecting the most appropriate treatments, the generally accepted principles were considered. These principles were letting the service member know he will return to duty; treating him close to the battlefield; assigning him duties; resting; returning to his unit; and talking gently. The latter is an attempt to elicit and subsequently incorporate an empathic approach.

The medics' pretest choices were restrain him, 69%; make him shape up, 44%; assign duties as he recovers, 43%; rest, 41%; and treat far away from the battlefield, 38%. The posttest choices were talk gently to the service member, 94%; treat close to the battlefield, 91%; rest, 89%; and expect his return,

81%. The medics' retest responses were talk gently to the service member, 94%; rest, 94%; treat close to the battlefield, 88%; expect his return, 81%; and assign duties as he recovers, 69%. The commanders' choices were send to a doctor, 60%; rest, 57%; talk gently, 43%; treat like a WIA, 43%; and send to hospital, 40%.

How soon could a successfully treated CSR return to duty? The pretest medical responses indicated that 47% felt 1 week was needed. An additional 22% felt 1 month of treatment was required. Forty-four percent of the commanders felt 1 month of treatment was necessary before a soldier could be returned to duty. Twenty-one percent selected 1 week of required treatment. The medics' posttest responses shifted to the more generally accepted time periods. Seventy-two percent selected 3 days. The medics' retests revealed that 46% selected 3 days, and 20% selected 1 day.

A reflection of the underlying philosophy regarding successful treatment is suggested by asking what percentage of CSRs could be returned to active duty. The medics' pretest indicated that 37% of the respondents felt that 60% of the CSRs could be returned. Thirty-six percent of the medics felt only 40% could be returned. The posttest results shifted as 74% of the respondents chose 80% as the likely return rate. In the retest, 70% of the medics felt that a return rate of 80% or better was possible. Fifty-two percent of the commanders chose return rates of 60% or less.

Discussion

The division medical personnel will be the first echelon that most CSRs will contact. Proper triage is mandatory to preserve the fighting strength. The general level of knowledge demonstrated by the medics' pretest was consistent with their lack of training in this area. If such unchallenged knowledge is taken into combat, the speculative results would be an intolerable mismanagement of CSRs. Although the relative inability to determine the etiology of the CSR could be excused, the identification and treatment cannot be. It was in these areas that the baseline knowledge of the medics was most deficient. A CSR was viewed as a scared, jumpy, crazy person or, as selected by a majority, even normal. Such responses do little to determine a CSR with an aim towards treatment. Even more important were the treatment choices selected. The general view of treating a CSR was consistent with their view of the CSR being unmanageable. The cluster of responses indicated that restraining the service member, making him shape up, and treating him away from the battlefield were considered most appropriate choices. Again, consistent with the perceived untreatability of a CSR, the medics felt that at least 1 week, and in a sizable minority 1 month, was needed for successful treatment.

The commanders were more likely to appreciate the factors that contributed to the CSR rate. There was, however, a wide range of responses to the appearance of the CSR. The predominant view, however, was still one of an agitated, jumpy, wild individual. The commanders' main treatment options were to evacuate the service members. The selected evacuation to mental health specialists or a hospital could suggest either a desire to eliminate from their ranks the CSR or the commander's philosophy of using his combat service support elements.

The commanders were even more pessimistic regarding successful treatment. Forty-four percent of commanders indicated that a 1-month treatment program would be needed before a CSR could return to duty.

The medics' posttest was designed to measure the shift, from baseline, of acquired knowledge. In every tested area, the posttest medics demonstrated that the responses concerning etiology, diagnosis, and treatment were more appropriate. This knowledge taken into combat could favorably alter an otherwise unrestricted flow of CSRs out of combat units. As a result of this training program, emotional first aid would more likely be rendered in or near a service member's unit.

Fifteen months after training, the medics could still identify appropriate precipitating factors, length of treatment needed, and, most important, proper treatment interventions. A loss of knowledge was noted only in certain diagnostic areas. A minority of retested respondents returned to a view of the CSR as a crazy, wild individual.

The training program had a positive effect on the identification and treatment of the CSR. This was maintained in the 15-month retest. By implication, such training will lead to better battlefield care. The training program should be followed up by sustainment training, including the presence of division mental health personnel (and supporting combat stress control unit teams) in field training exercises. This is especially important at the high stress exercises conducted at the National Training Center, Joint Readiness Training Center, and Combat Maneuver Training Center.

SUMMARY

The uncorrected myths and biases surrounding the CSR are not consistent with either good medical care or good leadership. As this study demonstrates, such myths and biases are prevalent. This study also concludes that effective training can have a definite impact. A well-briefed cadre of medics and commanders can only add to the readiness posture of the military.

All medical personnel in the military should attend a concentrated combat psychiatry training program. Commanders should attend a shorter, yet intensive, program. The issues in each program will be tailored to reflect the differing needs of the two groups. The goal of both training programs, however, should be the same—the preservation of manpower.

REFERENCES

1. Abraham P. Training for battleshock. *J R Army Med Corps*. 1982; 128(1):18–27.
2. Schneider RJ, Luscomb RL. Battle stress reaction and the United States Army. *Milit Med*. 1984;149:66–69.
3. Ingraham LH, Manning FJ. Psychiatric battle casualties: The missing column in a war without replacements. *Milit Rev*. 1980;60(8):18–29.
4. Jones DR. The Macy Reports: Combat fatigue in World War II fliers. *Aviat Space Environ Med*. 1987;58(8):807–811.
5. Donnelly C. The Soviet attitude to stress in battle. *J R Army Med Corps*. 1982;128(2):72–78.
6. Dick CJ. Soviet chemical warfare capabilities. *Int Defense Review*. 1981;1:31–38.
7. Cadigan FC. Battle shock: The chemical dimension. *J R Army Med Corps*. 1982;128(2):89–92.
8. Kaplan H, Sadock B. *Comprehensive Textbook of Psychiatry*. Baltimore, MD: Williams and Wilkins; 1985.
9. Brooks FR, Ebner DG, Xenakis SN, Balson PM. Psychological reactions during chemical warfare training. *Milit Med*. 1983;148(3):232–235.
10. Ritchie EC. Treatment of gas mask phobia. *Milit Med*. 1992;157(2):104.
11. US Department of the Army. *Alcohol and Drug Abuse Prevention and Control Program*. Washington, DC: DA; 1988. Army Regulation 600–85.
12. Kaplan HI, Sadock BJ. *Pocket Handbook of Clinical Psychiatry*. Baltimore: Williams and Wilkins; 1990.
13. Noy S. Division-based psychiatry in intensive war situations: Suggestions for improvement. *J R Army Med Corps*. 1982;128(2):105–116.
14. Soloman Z, Weisenberg M, Schwarzwald J, et al. Post-traumatic stress disorder among frontline soldiers with combat stress reaction: The 1982 Israeli experience. *Am J Psychiatry*. 1987;144(4):448–454.
15. Gal R, Jones FD. Psychological aspects of combat stress: A model derived from Israeli and other combat experiences. In: Jones FD, Sparacino LR, Wilcox VL, Rothberg JM, eds. *War Psychiatry*. Part 1. In: *Textbook of Military Medicine*. Washington, DC: Office of The Surgeon General, US Department of the Army and Borden Institute; in press: Chap 6.

Chapter 13

FROM COMBAT TO COMMUNITY PSYCHIATRY

FRANKLIN D. JONES, M.D., F.A.P.A.*

*Colonel (ret), Medical Corps, U.S. Army; Clinical Professor, Uniformed Services University of the Health Sciences; Past President and Secretary and current Honorary President of the Military Section, World Psychiatric Association

INTRODUCTION

Experiences from World War I onward have resulted in the identification of a wide range of psychiatric problems among soldiers in combat and in near-combat situations. In this chapter, I will discuss the applicability of principles derived from the treatment of combat-involved psychiatric casualties to psychiatric casualties that arise in peacetime situations.

The first psychiatric problems described[1] were anxiety-depressive, conversion, and dissociative types of psychiatric casualties in combat troops. These disorders, which range from simple fear to severe anxiety and depression, represent continuing problems. In high-intensity combat, another group of ineffective personnel will consist of soldiers exposed to sustained sleep loss, high-volume and high-intensity sound trauma, prolonged autonomic discharge, and other vicissitudes of unremitting combat. The U.S. Army Medical Department must also prepare for comparable casualties from toxic warfare agents and agents used to counter them. Another large group of ineffective soldiers are often found in support roles. These rear-echelon casualties with disorders, including sexual problems, alcohol and drug abuse, and antisocial acts, became the largest percentage of all U.S. casualties in the closing years of the Vietnam conflict.[2]

Study of psychiatric casualties reported in mass casualty incidents and in the Arab-Israeli wars[3] and the nature of modern warfare present the reasonable expectation that in addition to the above casualties, there will be casualties similar to those in disasters ("disaster fatigue"): temporarily dazed, immobilized responses in as many as one-half to two-thirds of unprepared soldiers and some hyperactive, panicky responses.

In wars as different in setting and culture as those of World War I and World War II,[1,4–6] the Korean conflict,[7–9] the Nigerian Civil War,[10] and the Arab-Israeli wars,[11,12] application of the principles of combat psychiatry,[13] usually described as "forward treatment," has minimized numbers and morbidity of psychiatric casualties while failure to treat has been uniformly deleterious.[14]

This chapter will describe how the principles of combat psychiatry developed during World War I and rediscovered during World War II were applied to noncombat settings toward the end of and during the decades following World War II. It will also address the applicability of these principles in treating certain civilian patients, including acute stress-induced conditions. These principles can also be utilized in the treatment of psychological burnout syndrome from inadequate social support as described in chapter 3 of this volume. Interventions utilizing these principles in disasters, terrorism, and hostage situations and refugee situations are also described in chapters 14 through 17 of this volume.

MILITARY VS CIVILIAN PSYCHIATRIC PRACTICES

The military approach to psychiatric casualties is quite different (for good reasons) from that of traditional office-based psychiatric practice; however, it may be quite similar to some community programs that are founded on principles independently discovered in military and civilian settings. The basic understanding of pathology, treatment practices, and theoretical considerations are the same in civilian and military practice. It is in application that the variance may be greatest.

Some of the reasons for the differences are based on the population involved. The military population is a healthy one. Chronic and debilitating diseases have been eliminated to a considerable degree by selection and disposition of those who are severely unhealthy both mentally and physically. The population also is relatively young and still predominantly male. A moderate degree of intelligence is assured, and outside of combat, the military culture supports good health. However, probably the most important reason for differences is that psychiatry in the military setting functions in terms of the needs of the service; that is, military psychiatry is unique because the mission of the military is unique.[15]

The military community devolves from the military mission. Unlike the army before World War II, the new military is largely married with children.[16]

This is to ensure the presence and morale of the soldier, that is, an enhanced recruitment device. The military family community tends to take on many aspects of the military organization. There is usually a formal and/or informal hierarchical structure. Residential communities are represented, sometimes with an elected "mayor," to pursue their complaints or interests. Wives' clubs often organize around issues of interest to them and can be quite influential, obtaining day care services for children, for example.

The Combat Psychiatric Casualty

The combat psychiatric casualty is a soldier whose instincts of self-preservation (or fears of death and being maimed) have temporarily overcome his loyalties to his fellow soldiers and his military mission. At first blush, this conflict between the need to save his life and the need to save his place in his group would seem most unequal. The presence of poor group leadership, the presence of physiological impairment from fatigue, hunger, and thirst, and the presence of personal stress in the soldier (for example, from family concerns) are all known to swing the balance toward becoming a casualty. The forces that bind a soldier to his unit, however, are by no means insignificant. Crane[17] was aware of the sustaining power of unit cohesion:

> There was a consciousness always of the presence of his comrades about him. He felt the subtle battle brotherhood, more potent even than the cause for which they were fighting. It was a mysterious fraternity born of the smoke and danger of death.[17(p31)]

Marshall,[18] after observing the 1956 Arab-Israeli War, put it more bluntly:

> When fire sweeps the field, be it in Sinai, Pork Chop Hill or along the Normandy Coast, nothing keeps a man from running except a sense of honor, of bound obligation to people right around him, of showing fear in their sight which might eternally disgrace him.[18(p304)]

The soldier who has succumbed to the forces to depart the battle will begin to develop severe guilt feelings and loss of self-esteem for having abandoned his buddies. Psychiatric symptoms develop defensively to salvage self-esteem and to assuage guilt. They present an honorable method of escaping combat. Unless interrupted, they will consolidate and increase because at some level the soldier is all too aware of his defection from duty. The further the soldier is from return to his unit, the stronger the symptoms become as he must more strongly justify his defection.

The Civilian Psychiatric Casualty

Obviously, it will be rare that the civilian psychiatric casualty has been exposed to the kind of conflict experienced by a combat soldier. Examples of persons exposed to hazardous occupations do come to mind—police, firefighters, and pilots—but these do not involve legal or psychological stigmas as with soldiers if they quit their jobs.

The better analogy is the marriage partner, teacher, therapist (as in professional burnout syndrome), parent, supervisor, or other person who has responsibilities to a group or another person and who becomes demoralized in discharging those responsibilities. Many such persons will be given labels such as adjustment reaction or depression or anxiety neurosis depending on presenting symptoms and therapeutic school. The principles derived from combat psychiatry are less effective than medications for "organic" mental illnesses such as schizophrenia and biological depressions but are important in treating conditions emanating primarily from psychological antecedents, usually generated by crisis situations. These principles, however, can be usefully applied adjunctively, even in treating organic conditions, particularly in terms of social support.

The similarity between military and civilian psychiatric casualties lies in the acceptance of a medical label as the solution to one's problems of living and one's inability to cope with them. This is not limited to psychiatric patients; in fact, it may be more common in other conditions; low back syndrome, headaches, irritable bowel syndrome, and others come to mind as ailments prone to result from one's efforts to escape from the daily fray of work and family. Such physical conditions do not carry the psychiatric stigma, making them even more desirable as avenues of escape. As will become clear, such persons are not usually malingering or consciously ineffective. Rather, for them the short-term rewards of the invalid or medical label outweigh the long-term rewards of mastery of their life situations.

PRINCIPLES OF PSYCHIATRIC TREATMENT

The basic principles of forward treatment involve treating the combat psychiatric casualty in a safe place as close to the battle scene as possible; as soon as possible; with simple treatment such as rest, food, and, if available, a warm shower; and most important, with an explicit statement that he is not ill and is expected to return to work with his comrades. The fifth principle of centrality was found to be important in the Vietnam conflict.[2] By centrality is meant the provision of sending all out-of-combat zone evacuations through a central screening center so that skilled personnel can prevent inappropriate evacuations. These principles are tailored to optimizing the return to duty of psychiatric combat casualties.

DEVELOPMENT OF COMMUNITY PSYCHIATRIC SERVICES

The development of community psychiatric services grew from a confluence of approaches in civilian settings with periodic injections of military experience. The late 19th century psychoanalytic writings of Freud,[19,20] emphasizing infantile sexuality, aggression, and trauma, logically called for evaluation of early childhood experiences in the genesis of adult psychopathology. Freud's disaffected follower, Adler, rejected the emphasis on childhood sexuality and emphasized family interactions in personality development. In Vienna in 1919, Adler founded the first child guidance clinic.[21]

A Viennese school teacher, Aichorn, worked with delinquent children and established two reformatories, the first in 1918 and the second in 1920. Aware of his work, Anna Freud persuaded him to undergo psychoanalysis to assist his understanding of why his highly successful programs worked. After completing psychoanalysis, Aichorn published *Wayward Youth* in 1925 in Europe and in 1935 in the United States.[22] Basically, he described a therapeutic community led by a warm, loving, father figure with whom the adolescents could identify.[21] Residential treatment facilities such as Boy's Town and Boy's Ranch have incorporated this model of firm discipline combined with warm acceptance of youth in a setting maximizing individual responsibility and autonomy.[23]

In the United States, Meyer[24] was teaching a holistic approach to the psychiatric patient that he termed psychobiology. In 1902, Meyer married Mary Potter Brooks, who became highly interested in his work. In 1904, she began visiting the families of his patients to learn about their backgrounds, thus becoming one of the first American social workers.[21] Commenting on his wife's work, Meyer stated, "We thus obtained help in a broader social understanding of our problem and a reaching out to the sources of sickness, the family and the community."[24(p22)] In 1927, Meyer was elected president of the American Psychiatric Association, and during the first third of the 20th century, he was considered the dean of American psychiatrists. He taught that people fell ill because of faulty reaction patterns that could be treated by reeducation and social therapies.[21] His students were the chiefs of most of the important American psychiatric training programs and state hospitals from the 1920s to the 1940s.

In 1907, Meyer met Beers, a graduate of Yale University who had suffered several severe psychotic episodes and received treatment that could only be called atrocious although life-saving. Beers later described his experiences in *The Mind That Found Itself* (1908)[25] which was highly influential in stimulating reform of mental institutions. Beers established the National Committee for Mental Hygiene in Connecticut in 1908. Among the 12 founding members were Meyer and William James. In 1912, Salmon was appointed director. By 1919, the International Committee for Mental Hygiene had been formed.[21]

When World War I broke out in Europe, Salmon was commissioned to go to France and Britain to learn what they were doing to treat psychiatric casualties of combat. Salmon's report, which became the primer for American psychiatrists when the United States entered the war, was published by the National Committee for Mental Hygiene.[4] Salmon was appointed chief psychiatrist for the American Expeditionary Forces.[1] Psychiatrists returning from World War I brought with them an understanding of Salmon's principles for treatment of acute, stress-induced malfunction; however, the psychoanalytic approach involving lengthy analysis was gaining prominence, and these insights were lost.[26] As in psychoanalytic theory, Salmon conceived a combat stress casualty as suffering from a mental conflict between the instinct for self-preservation (Freud's id) and the demands of military conformity (Freud's superego); however, rather than analysis of childhood antecedents, Salmon proposed simple, direct interventions.

In 1909, Healy was commissioned by a Chicago philanthropist, Dummer, to study the work on the causes and prevention of delinquency. Healy found only two clinics that were even giving children psychological testing, much less organized programs. Dummer then underwrote a research clinic, the Juvenile Psychopathic Institute, founded in 1909, under Healy's direction. After a 6-year study, in 1915, Healy[27] published *The Individual Delinquent: A Textbook of Diagnosis and Prognosis*, an exposé of the social and economic roots of delinquency that discounted the prevalent theories of defective mentality or genes, that is, degeneracy.

In 1912, the Boston Psychopathic Hospital was organized under Southard, who with Janett, introduced the psychiatric social worker into the child guidance team. In 1922, the National Committee for Mental Hygiene inaugurated a 5–year program for fellowships at child guidance centers, and in 1924, the American Orthopsychiatric Association was established to bring together disciplines in child guidance programs.[21] Child guidance centers were the forerunners of community mental health centers. By 1946, there were 285 psychiatric clinics exclusively for children in the United States, and another 350 served children and adults.[28]

While progress was being made in establishing child guidance clinics in the community, military psychiatry after World War I languished with minimal resources and no organized community programs. After World War II broke out in Europe and as the possibility of U.S. involvement increased, psychiatrists were recruited to screen out soldiers who might break down in combat, a program that was a dismal failure.[29] The community mental health approach in the military did not begin until the United States became involved in the war.

Community Mental Health in the U.S. Army

Halloran and Farrell[30] and Cohen[31] established mental hygiene consultation programs at replacement and training centers within the first years of U.S. entry into World War II. Initially, these programs furnished a kind of orientation and "pep talk" for soldiers being sent overseas. Later as the success in decreasing psychiatric casualties through such strengthening of morale became recognized, they spread to other settings and, by the end of the war, were an integral part of the mental health program of the U.S. Army. During the war, 35 mental hygiene consultation services (MHCSs) were established and, by the end of the war, many were practicing preventive psychiatry based on military experiences.[32]

With the end of World War II, the pioneer MHCS efforts were rapidly reduced, and by 1949, there were only two MHCS units left on army posts. After the outbreak of the Korean conflict in 1950, the MHCS concept was rapidly revived and implemented, with these services being established at all major posts.[33] The MHCS was described in Army Regulation 40–216, *Neuropsychiatry and Mental Health*, in 1958. By the mid-1960s, the army had 40 MHCS units.[34] Today, these facilities are called community mental health services (CMHS) or activities (CMHA), and almost every significant army post has one.

Bushard[15] chronicled the empirical development of army community psychiatric services during the decade following the Korean conflict. Cold War tensions had resulted in the continued need for drafted soldiers, many of whom preferred to be civilians. The early psychiatric services were little other than struggling outpatient clinics that were totally overwhelmed by the problems presented to them of large numbers of disaffected troops. Applying the usual psychiatric treatment techniques growing out of psychoanalytic theory in this situation produced results that were frequently discouraging. The usual conclusion was that in view of the disparity between large referral load and limited psychotherapeutic talent available, little could be offered. Considering the large caseload and the brief period of the patient's stay on post, traditional psychotherapy was not feasible. Dire predictions about the future of individuals examined were frequently offered.

After several years, a review of the situation by Bushard[15] led to several consistent observations:

- Extensive and intensive work-ups did not really contribute a great deal of helpful information. As far as the therapeutic result was concerned, frequently, a brief interview would have been as valuable as the thorough study conducted.
- Psychiatric and psychological data did not reliably predict future performance. Although indepth examinations frequently revealed highly disturbed and distressed individuals, prognostications based on these findings were not a reliable basis for predicting either actual job performance or

the future of the symptomatology. Information derived from actual observation of the patient at work and study of the actual nature of, rather than his verbalizations about, his relations with others were a far more valid basis for predicting the outcome of his problem. Army mental health professionals tended to over emphasize pathology and over predict failure.[35] It was observed that persons with more serious psychiatric disease, such as schizophrenia, frequently continued to function in the field without coming to psychiatric attention.

- The immediate determinants of the psychological reaction were usually clearly evident. For example, a soldier got a "Dear John" letter from his girlfriend and cut his wrist.
- The disability would be described by the soldier as of a more global nature than one ordinarily encounters. The number of things the patient "could not do" seemed to pervade a wider segment of his function than one was accustomed to find in other practice. Anxiety, anger, and other affective responses appeared to be related more clearly to the problems involved in mastery of the immediate situation than to infantile and oedipal experiences. There was an almost universal and nearly magical conviction that escape from the reality of the situation was the answer. Rarely did one encounter the attitude that success or mastery was the desired endpoint, as it might be, for example, in marriage, career, and parenthood. It was not seen as an important aspect of growing up.
- There was a predominant use of the mechanism of rationalization. A patient might explain his discomfort on the basis of intolerance of military profanity, on rejection of the use of force in human relations, or on the basis of concern for sick parents. These were usually recognized as transparent devices. In the absence of such rationalization, there was frequently a willingness to admit to weakness and unpatriotism and being simply no good as an explanation for giving up. Such persons were influenced very little by competitiveness and group spirit.
- Even when it was available, traditional psychotherapy had little impact. The psychotherapeutic interpretation, however clever, was lost; the urge of the patient toward health, if that involved staying in the military, was minimal. To address one's efforts to the classical psychiatric syndromes was simply not feasible and had little value. If this were done, the mass of the referral load went untreated and the patient would often be abandoned either to punitive measures or, conversely, to environmental manipulation that would tend to produce continuation of the symptom.

Concurrence and Commitment

Eventually a view of the soldier emerged in which he is seen as part of an interactional set with his environment. The dynamics involved relate not so much to oedipal traumas and disturbed biochemistry as to disturbed homeostasis in the soldier's social ecology. Figure 13–1 shows the stresses that tend to precipitate psychiatric casualties and the supports that tend to prevent or terminate illness. Depending on the balance achieved, one may see increased or decreased rates of ineffectiveness as measured by absent without leave, venereal disease, sick call, and disciplinary action rates.

Bushard used the concepts of concurrence and commitment to explain both the soldier's problems in adapting and their solution:

> By concurrence we mean that aspect of internal psychological operations which looks to the incoming sense data for evidence that one's behavioral negotiations with the environment are leading to goal achievement, instinctual gratification and successful social interaction.[15(p436)]

It is easy to translate this concept into behavioral terms involving positive social reinforcement; in fact, research projects for treating delinquent soldiers used such translation.[35–37]

The soldier would seek concurrence as he looked for the support of his chaplain, his inspector general, his family, his legislators, or anyone else who might agree that the proper solution of his discomfort was a specific change such as return to his home. Seeking support from more official sources, he had usually either abandoned his immediate colleagues or failed to obtain a comfort-giving concurrence from them.

If the soldier did allow himself to see his sameness with those about him as opposed to his difference, he would begin to sense a diminution in anxiety level, an increased capacity to function, and a waning of his conception that he could not succeed and that escape was essential. He might continue to have his problems, but functionally, he was approaching a level of mastery.

In the concept of commitment, Bushard attempted to describe

> that emotional and behavioral set by which the individual addresses himself to the mastery of the problem at hand. It involves his maintaining his attention to it at an intensity that results in the mobilization of his physical and psychological resources in the direction of achieving this goal as opposed to or differentiated from others.[15(p437)]

The inductee who had failed to make provision for the needs of his dependents and who did not find some source of pleasure and relaxation within the military had little likelihood to succeed. Failing to commit himself through a realistic appraisal of the situation, he became distracted, worried, and preoccupied or found life so dull that in no way could he conceive of success in any undertaking.

Life is full of examples of lack of commitment. It is absent in the student who watches television rather than doing homework, in the worker who does not get enough sleep, and in the adolescent who quits school altogether. Failure of commitment in other situations such as work, schools, and family responsibilities is a frequent finding in people who fail to commit themselves to military service as an accepted responsibility.

Commitment and Concurrence Example: Burnout Syndrome

Psychological burnout syndrome frequently afflicts persons who are exposed to repeated or continuous psychological stress. This includes occupations such as teachers, police, fire fighters, air traffic controllers, nurses, and mental health workers among others.[38–42] While time away from the job (reminiscent of the rest from combat utilized in the Vietnam conflict)[2] may be helpful, real prevention requires intervention at the small group level. The potentially afflicted person must feel the concur-

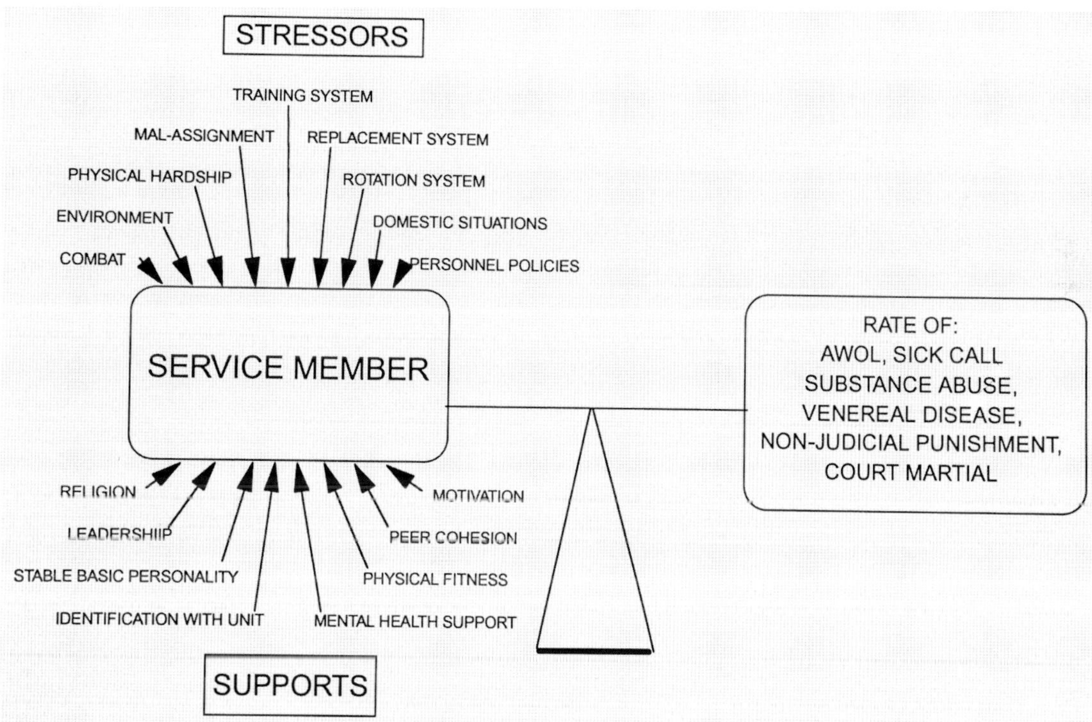

Fig. 13–1. Factors in mental disorders in the military. This figure demonstrates the stresses that tend to precipitate psychiatric casualties in the military and the supports that tend to prevent or terminate illness. Depending on the balance achieved, one may see increased or decreased rates of ineffectiveness as measured by absent without leave (AWOL), venereal disease, sick call, and disciplinary action rates.

rence of his support group. This social reinforcement toward mastery of efforts will then strengthen his commitment to the job and create further social reinforcement. When effective, this interaction should increase productivity and group morale. Group discussions and exercise, recreation, and eating meals together can be effective tools in producing a sense of group belonging and cohesion.

The Japanese management system employing group decisions even involving the lowest manual worker has elements of concurrence and commitment. It is, thus, not surprising that psychological burnout, even among those engaged in repetitive, boring tasks, is relatively rare.[43–45]

Applicability of Principles to Noncombat Settings

The practice of military psychiatry in combat and garrison settings can be shown to have a number of similarities, particularly when one is handling acute adjustment disorders. These practices can be seen to include various elements of the centrality, proximity and immediacy, simplicity, and expectancy elements of treating combat psychiatric casualties. These elements will be discussed separately.

Centrality

Centrality is an important aspect not only of battlefield psychiatry but also of preventive psychiatry. In the combat setting, it refers to having a casualty evaluated before departure from the combat zone, but in a noncombat setting, it is better seen as an aspect of what Glass[46] has referred to as related echelon psychiatry. Related echelon psychiatry is traced back to Salmon's[4] provision of a first echelon division psychiatrist supported by a second echelon small (150 bed) neurological hospital and third echelon special base hospital. The comparability with a community mental health center and the hospital to which it refers patients should be obvious. The two must closely coordinate their efforts to ensure that the patient is not lost to follow-up care. A further refinement increasingly found in mental health settings is the provision of partial hospitalization or interposition of an echelon between outpatient and inpatient status.

Proximity and Immediacy

In initially treating the disaffected soldier, it is as important to know what his unit is, who is his commander, and how long he has been in the service as to know who he is, where he came from, and what his specific symptoms are. This kind of information can only be obtained by an intense familiarity with the supported community. Hospitalization is avoided if at all possible, and attempts are made to prevent the patient from being taken for any significant period from actual, if impaired, participation in his work. He is seen immediately on the day of referral; delay tends to consolidate the problem. Physical separation of the patient from the scene of his difficulties will cause him to indulge in the hope of not having to return, which usually increases his symptom in a manner making return to work less possible with the increasing distance in time or space between him and his group (loss of immediacy and proximity).

Simplicity

This crisis-generated patient seldom requires more than simple supportive psychotherapy. This psychotherapy usually involves some degree of catharsis and a great deal of clarification. Other significant members may be brought in for consultation if they are supervisors or for additional support if they are peers or relatives.

Expectancy

These maneuvers alone will begin to create the expectancy that the patient will continue performing; however, other procedures will enhance this expectancy. The soldier is kept in uniform, a part of his healthy identity. Interviewing is restricted to the situation. Lengthy inquiries into childhood vicissitudes moves the emphasis from the present that can be overcome or influenced, to the distant past that cannot. Most efforts are directed at keeping the patient in the fray where his own innate adaptive talent may come to his aid. This talent is indicated more nonverbally by returning him rapidly to work than in any verbal manner. Psychiatric labels are avoided if possible. If a diagnosis must be made, it is kept bland (adjustment disorder, for example) to keep the patient from being treated as, and learning to respond as, a patient rather than a person. Follow-up is of extreme importance and should be at the working level rather than at the clinic. Here it is possible to assess the manner of the patient's effort, the degree of his success, and the limitations that are insuperable. By one's working with the supervisor, work restrictions or other changes may be recommended and job limitations implemented. Medication is usually not indicated and gives the wrong message if given electively.

When adaptation to the work or social unit is impossible, the therapist may recommend changes. This recommendation is seen as a therapeutic environmental manipulation and should be under circumstances and by means that encourage the least possible persistence of chronic symptomatology, yet does not encourage others to follow suit. All of this approach is directed at resolving anxiety through implementing the patient's use of his own skills, the treating of anxiety as a normal phenomenon rather than as a pathological one, and the dealing with it in such a way as to imply that success is possible.

This approach appears to meet Caplan and Caplan's definition of community psychiatry:

> Community psychiatry denotes the body of knowledge, theories, methods, and skills in research and service required by psychiatrists who participate in organized community programs for the promotion of mental health and the prevention, treatment and rehabilitation of the mental disorders in a population. It *supplements* the clinical knowledge and skills which equip the psychiatrist to diagnose and treat his individual patients.[47(p1499)]

Current Situation

The military currently has a CMHS at most significant military posts and division psychiatrists assigned to almost all combat-ready divisions. A regimental system assigns physicians, including psychiatrists, to specific field units in the event of deployment. Unfortunately, there may be little contact with the field unit until deployment.[48,49]

The mental hygiene consultation model has proved quite successful. In 1951, just before the wide-scale use of these methods, the rate of admissions for all psychiatric disease was 24 per 1,000 troops per year. By 1965 and roughly since, the rate dropped to 5 per 1,000 troops per year. The number of outpatient visits in 1951 was 107 per 1,000 per year and, in 1965, 305 per 1,000 per year.[33,50]

In civilian settings, crisis intervention walk-in centers are prevalent in decentralized, community settings (immediacy and proximity). There is an emphasis on current environmental factors to assist the patient in coping with work and home (expectancy), and remote childhood dynamics are usually deemphasized (simplicity).[47] Many state hospital programs require entrance via community mental health clinics and maintain close liaison with them (centrality).[34] Many businesses have employee assistance programs. The Department of Veterans Affairs eventually established store front Vietnam Vet Centers to provide a community-based, nonhospital setting for helping veterans with posttraumatic stress disorders and other problems of adjustment. Recently, "Vietnam" was removed from the title because the centers were authorized to assist veterans of Operations Urgent Fury (Grenada), Just Cause (Panama), and Desert Storm (Persian Gulf).

SUMMARY AND CONCLUSION

The concept of community psychiatry has undergone a slow evolution during the past 100 years. Major contributions to the movement came from the child guidance programs and psychiatric experiences in the two world wars. The major drawback to this approach has been the failure to allocate adequate financial resources despite the general recognition that keeping the individual as a productive community member is far less expensive than maintaining him in a state hospital. The military has continued to exert leadership in this area, probably because the soldier is guaranteed free access to medical care. Even in the military, however, the community mental health team has been somewhat fragmented by professional jurisdictional issues (independent social work, psychology, and psychiatry services), resulting in duplication of services and failures to refer appropriately. This issue is awaiting the efforts of an enlightened command to reinstate the integrated community mental hygiene services of the decades after World War II.

REFERENCES

1. Bailey P, Williams FE, Komora PO. In: *Neuropsychiatry in the United States.* Vol 10. In: *The Medical Department of the United States Army in the World War.* Washington, DC: GPO; 1929.

2. Jones FD, Johnson AW. Medical and psychiatric treatment policy and practice in Vietnam. *J Soc Issues.* 1975;31(4):49–65.

3. Glass AJ, Drayer CS, Cameron DC, Woodward WD. Psychological first aid in community disasters. *JAMA.* 1954;156:36–41.

4. Salmon TW. *The Care and Treatment of Mental Diseases and War Neuroses ("Shell Shock") in the British Army.* New York: War Work Committee of the National Committee for Mental Hygiene, Inc.; 1917.

5. Glass AJ. Lessons learned. In: *Zone of Interior.* Vol 1. In: Glass AJ, Bernucci R, eds. *Neuropsychiatry in World War II.* Washington, DC: GPO; 1966: 735–759.

6. Glass AJ. Lessons learned. In: *Overseas Theaters.* Vol 2. In: Glass AJ, ed. *Neuropsychiatry in World War II.* Washington, DC: GPO; 1973: 989–1027.

7. Glass AJ. Psychiatry in the Korean campaign. *US Armed Forces Med J.* 1954;4(parts 1 and 2):1387–1401, 1563–1583.

8. Glass AJ. Psychotherapy in the combat zone. *Am J Psychiatry.* 1954;110:725–731.

9. Peterson DB. The psychiatric operation, army forces Far East, 1950–1953. *Am J Psychiatry.* 1955;112:23–38.

10. Kalunta A. Experiences of a non-military psychiatrist during the 1966–1970 Nigerian Civil War—affected area of "Biafra." In: Belenky GL, ed. *Contemporary Studies in Combat Psychiatry.* New York: Greenwood Press; 1987: 133–141.

11. Noy S. 1987. Combat psychiatry: The American and Israeli experience. In: Belenky GL, ed. *Contemporary Studies in Combat Psychiatry.* New York: Greenwood Press; 1987: 69–86.

12. Solomon Z, Benbenishty R. The role of proximity, immediacy, and expectancy in frontline treatment of combat stress reaction among Israelis in the Lebanon War. *Am J Psychiatry.* 1986;143(5):613–617.

13. Jones FD, Crocq L, Adelaja O, et al. Psychiatric casualties in modern warfare: I, Evolution of treatment. In: Pichot P, Berner P, Wolf R, Thau K, eds. *Psychiatry: The State of the Art.* Vol 6. New York: Plenum; 1985: 459–464.

14. Belenky GL, Tyner CF, Sodetz FJ. *Israeli Battle Shock Casualties: 1973 and 1982.* Washington, DC: Walter Reed Army Institute of Research; 1983. Report WRAIR NP–83–4.

15. Bushard BL. The US Army's mental hygiene consultation service. In: *Symposium on Preventive and Social Psychiatry.* Walter Reed Army Institute of Research (WRAIR). Washington, DC: GPO; 1957: 431–443.

16. *Military Family Demographics: Profile of the Military Family.* Arlington, Va: Military Family Clearinghouse; 1992.

17. Crane S. *The Red Badge of Courage.* New York: Appleton; 1985.

18. Marshall SLA. Combat leadership. In: Rioch, DMcK, ed. *Symposium on Preventive and Social Psychiatry.* Washington DC: GPO; 1957: 303–307.

19. Freud S. The war neuroses (1919). In: *An Infantile Neurosis and Other Works (1917–1919).* Vol 17. In: Strachey J, ed. *Complete Psychological Works of Sigmund Freud.* London: Hogarth Press; 1955: 205–215.

20. Freud S. Beyond the pleasure principle (1920). In: *Beyond the Pleasure Principle, Group Psychology and Other Works (1920–1922).* Vol 18. In: Strachey J, ed. *Complete Psychological Works of Sigmund Freud.* London: Hogarth Press; 1955: 3–64.

21. Alexander FG, Selesnick ST. *The History of Psychiatry: An Evaluation of Psychiatric Thought and Practice from Prehistoric Times to the Present.* New York: Harper and Row; 1966.

22. Aichorn A. *Wayward Youth.* New York: Viking Press; 1935.

23. Howells WD. *A Boy's Town, Described for "Harper's Young People."* Westport, Conn: Greenwood Press, 1970.

24. Meyer A. A historical sketch in outlook of psychiatry and social work. *Hosp Soc Serv Q.* 1922;5:22–24.

25. Beers C. *The Mind That Found Itself.* 1908. The National Committee for Mental Hygiene. New York: The Country Life Press; 1938.

26. American Psychiatric Association. *One Hundred Years of American Psychiatry: 1844–1944.* Hall JK, Zilboorg G, Bunker HA, eds. New York: Columbia University Press; 1944.

27. Healy W. *The Individual Delinquent: A Textbook of Diagnosis and Prognosis.* Boston: Little, Brown and Company; 1915.

28. Deutsch A. The mental hygiene movement. In: *The Mentally Ill in America.* 2nd ed. New York: Columbia University Press; 1949: 300–331.

29. Glass AJ. Lessons learned. In: *Zone of the Interior.* Vol 1. In: Glass AJ, Bernucci RJ, eds. *Neuropsychiatry in World War II.* Washington, DC: Office of The Surgeon General, US Department of the Army; 1966: 735–759.

30. Halloran RD, Farrell MJ. The function of neuropsychiatry in the Army. *Am J Psychiatry.* 1943;100:14–20.

31. Cohen RR. Mental hygiene for the trainee. *Am J Psychiatry.* 1943;100:62–71.

32. Perkins ME. *Preventive Medicine in World War II.* Vol 3. U.S. Army Medical Department. Washington, DC: GPO; 1955.

33. Allerton WS, Peterson DB. Preventive psychiatry: The Army's mental hygiene consultation service. *Am J Psychiatry.* 1957;113:788–795.

34. Hausman W, Rioch DMcK. Military psychiatry: A prototype of social and preventive psychiatry in the United States. *Arch Gen Psychiatry.* 1967;16:727–739.

35. Wichlacz CR, Jones FD, Stayer SJ. Psychiatric predictions and recommendations: A longitudinal study of character and behavior disorders. *Milit Med.* 1972;137:54–58.

36. Jones FD, Stayer SJ, Wichlacz CR, Thomes LJ, Livingstone BL. Contingency management of hospital-diagnosed character and behavior disordered soldiers. *J Behav Ther Exp Psychiatry.* 1977;8:333.

37. Poirier JG, Jones FD. A group operant approach to drug dependence in the military that failed: Retrospect. *Milit Med.* 1977:141:366–369.

38. Bartz C, Maloney JP. Burnout among intensive care nurses. *Res Nurs Health.* 1986;9:147–153.

39. McCranie EW, Brandsma JM. Personality antecedents of burnout among middle-aged physicians. *Behav Med.* 1988;14(1):30–36.

40. Neale AV. Work stress in emergency medical technicians. *J Occup Med.* 1991;33(9):991–997.

41. Savicki V, Cooley A. The relationship of work environment and client contact to burnout in mental health professionals. *J Counsel Dev.* 1987;65(5):249–252.

42. Pines A, Kafry D. Occupational tedium in the social services. *Soc Work.* 1978;23:499–507.

43. Cole RE. Work redesign in Japan: An evaluation. In: Grusky O, Miller GA, eds. *The Sociology of Organizations: Basic Studies.* 2nd ed. New York: Free Press; 1970; 495–529.

44. Cole RE. *Work, Mobility, and Participation: A Comparative Study of American and Japanese Industry.* Berkeley, Calif: University of California Press; 1979.

45. Hatvany N, Pucik V. Japanese management practices and productivity. *Organizational Dynamics*. 1981;Spring:5–21.

46. Glass AJ. Psychiatry at the division level. *Med Bull US Army Med Dept*. 1949:9:45–73.

47. Caplan G, Caplan RB. Developments of community psychiatry concepts in the United States. In: Freedman AN, Kaplan HI, eds. *Comprehensive Textbook of Psychiatry*. Baltimore: Williams and Williams; 1967: 1499–1516.

48. Jones FD. Personal Communication, 1992.

49. Stokes J. Personal Communication, 1994.

51. Tiffany WJ, Allerton WS. Army Psychiatry in the mid-60's. *Am J Psychiatry*. 1967;123:810–819.

Chapter 14

MILITARY PSYCHIATRY AND DISASTERS

FRANKLIN D. JONES, M.D., F.A.P.A.,* PINCHAS HARRIS, M.D.,† RONALD J. KOSHES, M.D.,‡ AND YENG HOI FONG, M.D.§

*Colonel (ret), Medical Corps, U.S. Army; Clinical Professor, Uniformed Services University of the Health Sciences, Bethesda, Maryland, Past President and Secretary and currently Honorary President of the Military Section, World Psychiatric Association

†Director of Rehabilitation Services, Herzliya Medical Center—Hafia, Israel; formerly Medical Officer, Israeli Defence Forces

‡Medical Director, Adult Services Administration, Commission on Mental Health Services, Department of Human Services, District of Columbia, Washington 20032; Guest Scientist, Department of Military Psychiatry, Walter Reed Army Institute of Research, Washington, D.C.; Clinical Assistant Professor of Psychiatry, Uniformed Services University of the Health Sciences, Bethesda, Maryland; President, Society of American Military Psychiatrists

§Former Chief Psychiatrist, Singapore Armed Forces

INTRODUCTION

The authors have experienced combat and see a relation between the mass casualties and other aspects of combat and civilian disasters.[1,2] In addition to the various similarities between disasters and combat, understanding the dynamics of these situations and the modes of treatment are of great importance to the military psychiatrist. The military is generally called in to assist in large-scale disasters, as was seen in the destruction and population disruption occasioned in Florida and along the Gulf Coast by Hurricane Andrew in 1992 and the floods in the Midwest in 1993. An attempt to develop criteria for military medical interventions in the United States and foreign countries sustaining disasters would be helpful.[3] Such a review should include not only criteria for intervention but also arrays of personnel and equipment for such interventions. It is, therefore, the intent of this chapter to acquaint the military mental health worker and physician with these problems and, in doing so, to enable him to give appropriate medical and/or psychiatric aid when called to assist in similar settings.

Since World War II, sporadic articles[4–8] have appeared in the psychiatric literature discussing various aspects of military psychiatry and disasters. Most of these articles were written in the 1950s when the fear of future atomic war was at its highest and the need for preparation was at least being considered. One common conclusion by most of the writers was that there existed a lack of knowledge in psychiatric circles and that there was the need to learn and prepare in time. This is essentially the conclusion of this chapter.

Disaster is a state of massive collective stress caused by an external calamity over which neither the affected individual nor the society has control.

Disasters can be grouped into two categories:

- Natural disasters. Earthquakes, floods, hurricanes, and so forth
- Manmade disasters. War, fires, accidents, (industrial and transportation), and so forth

Disasters may also be grouped according to the onset, as follows:

- With warning. Floods, hurricanes, and so forth
- Acute, without warning. Fires, accidents, and so forth
- Chronic. War, warlike conditions, drought, and so forth

Disasters can also be subgrouped by their effect on property, income, involvement of a whole family or only one member, with massive casualties or with minimal physical casualties, and so on.

There is a lack of scientifically based data on the effects of disasters on human behavior. The reason for this lack stems mainly from lack of experimental studies by simulation methods. Experimentation is sharply limited by the fact that extreme stress, such as in disaster situations, cannot be reproduced in controlled, laboratory studies. Systematic studies of disaster victims by interviews or by questionnaires have the disadvantage of being performed some time after the disaster and thus depend on the recollections of the victim. Highest stress levels are associated with disasters with sudden, unanticipated onsets; disasters in which victims are unfamiliar with and unprepared for impact; disasters where victims are exposed to life-threatening situations and/or witness the death of others; disasters that impact on a large segment of local populations when accompanied by widespread property damage; and disasters that are followed by continued threat of recurrence.[9]

There has long been debate on whether to understand the psychological dysfunction that follows a disaster as arising from the disruption in the community or in the individual. Research in disaster has not helped in clarifying this point because the criteria for studying psychopathology have been inconsistently applied.[10] In fact, it is generally agreed that distress is often a normal reaction to abnormal circumstances, rather than a manifestation of character pathology.[11]

DISASTER PHASES

Few field studies have been reported during the period of the disaster itself. However, the most notable of these was by Tyhurst,[12] from which he was able to define a pattern of three overlapping phases and describe human behavior in the various phases. Glass[7] extended Tyhurst's classification, and in accord with his model, we base our suggestions for psychiatric intervention.

Glass describes the five phases of disaster as follows:

1. Preimpact or threat period
2. Warning period
3. Impact period
4. Recoil period
5. Postimpact period

Each of these periods has its specific psychological and social phenomena; however, it must be remembered that there is an overlapping of phases and that not all disasters present five distinct periods.

Preimpact or Threat Period

The preimpact or threat period is everyday life, the time when we discuss the possibilities and probabilities of future disaster. At this time, whenever we assume that there is a high probability of disaster, preplanning and training should commence. Preplanning and appropriate training in a period of calm may produce, however, higher levels of tension and worry in society. Individuals tend to overcome anxiety in this situation by the mechanisms of denial: "it cannot happen to me"; and fatalism: if disaster occurs, no preplanning will change the outcome.

These attitudes cause apathy and disinterest toward the problem and, in the majority of cases, prevent defined planning; in addition, in some cases, plans are kept secret and, in the event of disaster, remain secret.

It can be argued that discussion of disasters causes increased anxiety in individuals. This is true but only in the minority of cases, and this anxiety can be overcome by proper explanation and realistic attitudes. In communities that have previous experience with disaster, attitudes toward preplanning differ. Feelings of denial and fatalism can change to overreaction, especially shortly after a disaster.

The tasks of mental health workers in the preimpact stage include becoming part of the planning team. Mental health workers can assist the team by presenting information on the psychological phenomena during disasters and methods to minimize undesirable reactions. In addition, by educating the planners about attitudes of denial, fatalism, and increased anxiety as normal behavior patterns in the preimpact period, they can encourage appropriate preventive measures.

Preplanning and training cannot stop an earthquake or hurricane, but they are definitely the best methods of preventing ineffective behavior in times of disaster and thus in assisting survival of the victims of such disasters.

Warning Period

The warning period is the period when disaster is imminent. The period may be minimal, a question of minutes or usually hours and, in unusual cases, days.

There has been much controversy in scientific literature[10,11] on the need to inform potential victims about impending disaster. This controversy is basically due to a misunderstanding of human behaviors. Some writers[10,11] believed that mispresented information could cause panic-like behavior and so aggravate the already extremely stressful situation.

Panic can be defined as an acute fear reaction marked by loss of self-control—uncontrolled physical flight or nonrational and nonsocial behavior. Panic occurs most commonly when an individual or a group has the feeling that it will quickly become too late to escape the impending threat and a feeling of entrapment occurs. The most common disasters in which panic occurs are in fires or similar situations when the route of escape is threatened. Flight is always directed toward a believed way of escape. When no escape route exists, panic does not occur. Strange as it may seem, panic, which prepares the body for maximal effort, can be in some cases the most effective way of escape for the individual.[13]

There is a tendency toward overemphasis of panic in the literature on disaster.[10,11] This reaction is relatively uncommon compared with other modes of behavior seen in disasters. It must be remembered that panic only occurs when threat to life is real and not before the disaster happens.

The current informed consensus[10,11] is that when disaster is imminent, accurate and clear information should be communicated to the probable participants. Information should be given in simple understandable language and should be repeated at regular intervals. When given an accurate picture, as bad as it may be, the individual can prepare for the oncoming event. Adverse reactions to such warnings are rare, and the common belief that they will occur is unfounded.[10,11]

Behavior patterns during this period are usually overactivity, denial, and fatalism, all of which are noneffective although some persons perform effectively by concentrating on protective action. Some potentially useful actions, such as stockpiling food, gasoline, and other emergency supplies, can be carried to the extreme of selfish hoarding. This activity is one of the important behavior patterns that effective mental health and stress control intervention can help individuals and leadership modulate to keep in the communally adaptive range.

The effect of preplanning and training in such periods is obvious, with the majority of participants performing effectively. Previous experience of disasters by individuals allows them to participate in taking effective precautionary action.

The duration of this period can last days in extreme cases. There is no disruption of social structure, families tend to stay closely together, and there can be some group forming among individuals involved in the imminent danger.

Psychiatric assistance in this stage may seem impractical. Often, there will be no time for such aid, and the mental health team will have arrived after the onset of the disaster. However, military or civilian psychiatric and mental health personnel who are onsite during the warning period must, of course, be concerned with safeguarding their own survival as well as with preparing for their postdisaster roles. They may also have direct responsibility for safeguarding and/or evacuating psychiatric patients in inpatient and community-based programs. Those mental health personnel who are consultants to the civil or military leadership must continue to monitor and advise regarding crucial stress control measures, such as information dissemination, rumor control, effective staff operation, sleep planning, and individual and group stress management techniques.

Mental health and stress control teams that are peripheral to the anticipated disaster area may be called on to provide disaster relief. These teams should monitor the news, review their contingency plans, advise their highest headquarters of their state of readiness, and place their personnel on a higher state of alert. In the U.S. Army, these mental health teams include medical combat stress control detachments and companies (in the active component and the U.S. Army Reserve) and the neuropsychiatric wards and consultation services of active, U.S. Army Reserve, and National Guard combat support, field, and general hospitals. The U.S. Navy provides special psychiatric rapid intervention teams (SPRINTs) from its major hospitals for deployment to disaster areas. The U.S. Air Force could provide similar teams from its 50-bed air transportable hospitals. The Veterans Administration has provided debriefing teams of mental health personnel. Mental health and combat stress control personnel must *always* think proactively. They must drill at thinking ahead and defining their own contributions and never let themselves lapse into a purely reactive or passive mode.

Impact Period

The impact period occurs when the threat becomes a reality and disaster has struck. Duration of impact varies from seconds to hours depending on the type of disaster. We usually include in this phase the immediate postimpact stage before relief and rescue operations begin. Various models of psychopathology have been developed to understand the response of individuals to disasters. Warheit,[14] in a review of these models, stated that stressful events arise from and interact with the individual's biological constitution, the individual's psychological characteristics, the social structure (including interpersonal relationships), the culture, and the geophysical environment.

Psychological phenomena of this period (for acute, violent disasters such as earthquakes, tornadoes, explosions, and fires) have been grouped into three main categories by Tyhurst[12] as follows:

1. About 12 to 25 percent of those involved present *effective behavior* even though they are somewhat tense and excited. Many in the effective group are people who have training and experience in reacting to emergencies—the police, fire, emergency medical, and combat-trained military personnel. While not completely protected against dysfunctional stress reactions, these groups are able to apply their well-drilled team skills to the work that needs to be done. Sound preparation and training can bring more of the general population into this group.
2. Roughly 60 to 75 percent will be *dazed, stunned, and bewildered*. These individuals show lack of emotion, lack of decision, lack of activity, and automatic behavior in which they continue to apply "normal" habit patterns to the very abnormal situation (such as huddling or straightening up one corner of a completely destroyed room). This psychological state has been called the disaster syndrome, disaster shock, or disaster fatigue.[5] These people (like the mildly battle-fatigued soldier in combat) can often be "refocused" and turned into helpers if the effective per-

sonnel take them in hand, give them strong reassurance and positive expectations, and lead them in simple, group work tasks.

3. The remaining 10 to 25 percent may present highly agitated, uncontrolled behavior characterized by *hysterical reactions*, *severe affective disorders*, and even *psychotic-like states*. These psychological phenomena can be misinterpreted as states of panic. These disruptive cases need to be brought under control and calmed for their own safety and to prevent the agitated behavior from spreading to the larger group of disaster-fatigued people.

Social structure in this period is disrupted depending, of course, on type of disaster. Emergency social systems can be put into effect if such preparation has been made; if not, the immediate response is unorganized. Aid from outside the afflicted community has not yet arrived. Local leadership may begin to emerge in this period. During this phase, the family unit is of great importance with most people acting to keep this unit intact.

In this period of disruption of social structure and fight for survival, military mental health and stress control teams that find themselves fighting for life at the center of the disaster must, of course, be most concerned with their own survival. They should have been prepared by their training to be members of the effective group. They should continue to monitor and advise the effective group on stress control measures while assisting with acute survival and trauma life support activities. They may take primary responsibility for calming and shepherding the acutely agitated survivors while mentoring the effective group in how to mobilize the disaster fatigue group into helpers during the crisis. Mental health and combat stress control teams outside the life-and-death impact area continue to provide consultation, monitor the situation, and prepare for their roles in the recoil phase.

Recoil Period

The recoil period is the time when the primary stress has passed, and rescue teams and volunteers begin pouring into the disaster area. During this period, the afflicted community must rebuild and adjust to a new, although temporary, way of life. Secondary stresses, sometimes severe, may occur in this phase, depending on the type of disaster, for example, severe weather conditions after an earthquake. Earthquakes and hurricanes frequently leave large populations without shelter, food, or potable water and in danger of plagues from inadequate hygiene. They may cause disruption of natural gas lines with risks of fire and explosions. This period lasts until constructive return to the previous lifestyle begins; it can last days, weeks, or months depending on the type of disaster and on the individual himself.

Age-Specific Reactions

Mental health workers should be aware that not all people will react similarly in the aftermath of disaster. In fact, there are age-specific symptoms that occur in different age groups, as follows:[15]

- Preschool reactions: Crying, thumb-sucking, loss of bowel or bladder control, fear of being left alone, fear of strangers, irritability, confusion, and immobility
- Latency age reactions: Headaches, other physical complaints, depression, fears about weather, safety, confusion, inability to concentrate, poor school performance, fighting, and withdrawal from peers
- Preadolescent and adolescent reactions: Headaches, other physical complaints, depression, confusion, poor school performance, aggressive behaviors, withdrawal and isolation, and changes in peer group and friends
- Adult reactions: Psychosomatic problems, such as ulcers and heart trouble; withdrawal; suspicion; irritability; anger; loss of appetite; sleep problems; and loss of interest in everyday activities
- Senior citizen reactions: Depression, withdrawal, apathy, agitation, anger, irritability, suspicion, disorientation, confusion, memory loss, accelerated physical decline, and increased somatic complaints

Behavior patterns noted in adults in this stage are as follows:[5]

- The effective type: This group of people consists of those who remained effective during the impact period and additional individuals who have overcome the disaster syndrome. Out of this group, the constructive leaders will emerge.
- The dependent type: This is the large majority of those afflicted. These are people

who in the previous period showed the typical disaster syndrome and also some who, during the impact, were highly agitated. This behavior is characterized by childlike dependency, talkativeness, emotional release, and search for safety. Some of these individuals also present the staring reaction (unresponsiveness and staring into the distance). This group is highly suggestible.

- The nonfunctional type: These are people who have not overcome the disaster syndrome and remain dazed and bewildered and those who previously were highly agitated and have not yet calmed down. This group consists of the minority of cases although it is these individuals to whom initial psychiatric first aid should be diverted, usually in the form of reassurance, positive expectancy, and task assignment.

Community Reactions

Perhaps the most useful concept of community disaster response was developed by Gist and Stolz[16] in their description of community adjustment following a major building collapse. They noted that community adjustment was enhanced by identifying and augmenting natural helping systems. This is in marked contrast to the "waiting model," which implies that mental health workers provide clinic-based treatment on request from self-referring patients.[17]

Social patterns in this stage are the result of interactions between the afflicted community and the official rescue teams. The normal reaction is for the involved community to reorganize its social structure with outside assistance; although in devastating disasters with massive physical casualties, survivors may be incapable of such tasks. There is a tendency for survivors to rely on their own resources at this stage.

There is a marked tendency of group formation among survivors at this time. These groups are usually unstable and can interfere with rescue operations if not headed by positive and constructive leaders. The family remains in this period the most stable effective unit.

Leadership in this phase is a crucial element. As noted before, the majority of survivors are extremely dependent. Good leadership helps shorten the recoil period and assists individuals to return to constructive activity. The best leaders are local predisaster leaders or leaders emerging from the stricken population. Only when the afflicted community shows no signs of social reorganization and leadership should a leader be appointed from outside the community. Tierney[18] noted that disaster creates a very high demand for a range of activities that exceeds the community's normal response capability. Tierney described four models for adaptation of community structures to meet the needs of disaster:

1. Type 1. Established organizations perform the same tasks for which they are responsible during nondisaster times, with basically the same organizational structure (hospital, electrical or water supply workers, waste management, and so on).
2. Type 2. Expanding organizations are small and comparatively inactive during nondisaster times but increase during the emergency and also become involved in activities different from their everyday, nondisaster tasks. Military mental health organizations, the Red Cross, and the Salvation Army are examples.
3. Type 3. Extending organizations retain their predisaster structure but engage in disaster-related tasks that are new for those organizations. Examples include community service organizations that mobilize to assist disaster victims and business enterprises that provide needed resources and personnel.
4. Type 4. Emergent groups comprise private citizens who work together in pursuit of collective goals relevant to actual or potential disasters, but whose organization has not yet become institutionalized. Emergent groups develop in part out of the shared belief that there are disaster-related needs that are not being met by community responders. Such groups devise new structures that address these needs, engaging in tasks that are nonroutine for their members. An example might be groups pursuing a joint lawsuit.

Highest stress levels are associated with evacuations in which families are separated or in which there is a lack of consensus on the decision to evacuate. Emergency shelter stays that are protracted or the center of interpersonal conflict, evacuations that are poorly managed or expose victims to continuing environmental threats, temporary housing that is perceived as dangerous or inadequate, failure to establish stable temporary housing, temporary housing or relocation programs that socially isolate victims from their old communities and neighborhoods, and exclusion of victims from, or their failure to qualify for, formal aid programs are all factors that exacerbate stress during the rescue effort.[9]

Application of Principles of Combat Psychiatry

It is in the recoil period that mental health assistance can be of the most importance. The basic principles of combat psychiatry should be applied in this situation, and these principles are as follows:

- Primary emphasis on proactive interventions. Promote positive coping behaviors, and prevent stress-induced dysfunction by consultation-liaison and education.
- Brevity. Keep treatment and interventions as brief as possible.
- Immediacy. Treat those in need as soon as possible.
- Centrality. Maintain only one policy of psychiatric treatment.
- Expectancy. Reassure those in distress that their reaction is normal, they will overcome it, and they will return to their previous selves.
- Proximity. Treat those in distress near the site of disaster. This principle seems to be as important in times of disaster as in combat.
- Simplicity. Keep treatment as simple as possible; avoid any attempts at psychotherapy, and only in extreme cases, use medications.

It must be stressed that the most effective treatment, as in combat, is fulfillment of physiological needs of food, fluid intake, rest, and clothing. These basic needs not only help strengthen the individual physically but also psychologically and can assist in preventing future psychological suffering.

The mental health team, being part of the medical team, assists initially in treating the seriously physically wounded, an important reason for including psychiatrists and nurses in the team. Stress control interventions are provided to the patients, their families, and the care givers in a few words concurrently with the life- and limb-saving support or during brief breaks from the triage activity. Nonmedically trained mental health personnel can triage the stress casualties who have no physical wounds. They can direct other nonmedical helpers to remove the stress casualties from the stimuli of physical trauma and begin the process of reassurance and replenishment in accordance with the principle of immediacy. While all sufficiently trained members of the mental health team should give priority to assisting with salvage of life and limb, it is contrary to doctrine to defer mental health intervention until all the physical casualties can be evaluated. A directive from The Surgeon General, dated 8 September 1918, pointed out the folly of the division surgeon who had set his World War I division psychiatrist to sewing up minor wounds while several hundred psychiatric (mild war neurosis) casualties flowed past to the rear and were lost to combat duties. Furthermore, if the stress casualties are not taken in hand (especially the agitated ones), they can burden, disrupt, and even endanger the rescue operation. Psychological disturbances are quite common among physical casualties of disasters, in contrast to what is seen among wounded combat casualties.

The following guidelines are proposed for mental health workers who are involved in disaster management and planning:[2]

- Provide for ongoing mental health services in times of crisis at locations that can best serve the population effected. Consult with disaster relief coordinators to determine the best location for services. Involve planners in decisions like this to empower leaders during loss of control.
- Practice "aggressively being there."
- Ensure access to all financial and service aid programs. Consult with administrators of these programs to propose locating services as close to the site of the disaster as possible, while assuring absolute safety.
- Provide ongoing consultation to leaders of the disaster relief effort to inform them of mental health needs.
- Keep families and other social units together.
- Allow for ventilation of fears and frustrations. With children, allow for ventilation of fears and frustrations through play.
- Establish regular communication with areas outside the disaster area.
- Ensure that the disaster relief effort concentrates on food, clothing, water, sanitation, and shelter as the basic needs of people in crisis.

The following specific interventions during the various disaster phases are useful in reducing the amount of stress experienced by both victims and disaster relief workers.[19]

- During the preimpact period (alarm) and impact period phases, provide workers with as much factual information as possible about what they will find at the scene. Provide this information via radio communications or in a quick briefing as new personnel arrive at the scene. This forewarning can help personnel gear up emotionally for what they may find. Try to get information for workers about the location and well-being of their family members.
- During the recoil and immediate postimpact periods, remember that early identification and intervention in stress reactions is the key in preventing worker burnout. Review lists of stress symptoms; remember that multiple symptoms in each category indicate that worker effectiveness is diminishing. Use mental health assistance in field operations if plans have been made to do so. Mental health staff can observe workers functioning, can support workers, and can give advice to command officers about workers, fatigue levels, stress reactions, and need for breaks. Check in with workers by asking, "How are you doing?" Assess whether verbal response and worker's appearance and level of functioning match; that is, workers may say they are doing fine but may be exhibiting multiple stress symptoms. Try to rotate workers among low-stress assignments (such as staging areas), moderate-stress assignments, and high-stress tasks. Limit workers' time in high-stress assignments (such as triage or morgue) to approximately 1 hour at a time, if at all possible. Provide breaks, rotation to less stressful assignments, and personal support. Ask workers to take breaks if effectiveness is diminishing; order them to do so if necessary. Point out that the worker's ability to function is diminishing because of fatigue, and that you need him functioning at his full potential to assist with the operation. Allow workers to return to the scene if they rest and their functioning improves. On breaks, try to provide workers with bathroom facilities, a place to sit or calm down away from the scene, quiet time alone, food and beverages, shelter from weather, dry clothes, and an opportunity to talk about their feelings. Coworkers, chaplains, or mental health staff are to assist.

The main task of the mental health team is in a consultative capacity and not in treating individuals except in cases of extreme psychological impairment. Consultation should be given to the following groups:

- The medical teams in rescue crews, to assist in the diagnosing and treatment of psychological disorders.
- The local professionals, physicians, social workers, and teachers, in explaining the various behavior patterns and how to assist in overcoming them. It is also important to reassure local professionals and, by doing so, reinforce them. To avoid possible misunderstanding, explain that outside psychiatric aid has no intentions of replacing professionals of the afflicted community.
- Casualties among the rescue teams. Members of rescue teams themselves can be under extreme physical and psychological stress. Members of the mental health team should be aware of the appearance of abnormal behavior patterns among these individuals and advise on the changing of crews and rest for the afflicted ones.
- Psychiatric casualties. These casualties are seen in the previously described nonfunctional type of behavior. The highly agitated individuals are in need of appropriate sedation, while the dazed and bewildered need more intensive reassurance and simple occupational therapy. It is only with this relatively small group that individual treatment should be attempted by the mental health team.

Following the disaster, the following steps are important in returning both the victims and the mental health workers to a state of normalcy.[19]

- Arrange debriefings for all workers involved in the disaster.
- If dealing with military personnel, give line personnel an opportunity to participate in a critique of the event. Often, a critique is limited to officers and supervisors, but line staff participation can assure that workers are recognized for their contributions to

the operation. In addition, their viewpoints are valid and provide valuable input toward improving operations the next time around.

- The organization can help workers and their families to set up meetings to provide them with information about the event, as well as education about normal stress reactions in workers and the potential effects of such stress on the family.
- Formal recognition by the organization of a worker's participation in a disaster operation can mean a great deal. A letter in the individual's personnel file or a certificate of appreciation for contributions to an unusual and important job lets the worker know that his participation meant something. Workers who remained at the office or station "minding the store" during the disaster should also receive recognition; their contribution was essential, and leaving them out might precipitate guilt.
- Managers and supervisors should plan for the letdown their staff may experience. Discuss stress reactions in a staff meeting, and emphasize that they do not imply weakness or incompetence; it is similar to being wounded in action.
- If workers' reactions are severe or last longer than 6 weeks, encourage them to use professional assistance. Again, this does not imply weakness; it simply means that the event was so traumatic that it had a profound effect on the individual.

Postimpact Period

The postimpact period is the period of rehabilitation or building a new life. There is no limitation on the duration of this period, and it can last for the rest of the individual's life. During this period, outside assistance has stopped, and the afflicted community relies on its own reconstructed social structure.

In the initial postimpact period, reactions of guilt, grief, and depression are predominant, changing later to anger and resentment. Anger is commonly directed against some authority that can be blamed for the cause or outcome of the disaster. It is quite common at this time to see cases of scapegoating, especially if information is inaccurate.

Later on, as the disaster becomes part of the past, there can be increased physical illness and psychosomatic illness among survivors, together with the appearance of post-traumatic stress disorders. Some writers[9,14] believe that there is no increase in psychiatric morbidity as a result of disaster; this belief is apparently true of psychotic ailments but doubtful in regard to less extreme pathology.

The altered social phenomena in a community that has experienced disaster are usually seen in changed attitudes concerning economic and cultural values. At least in the immediate postimpact period, positive group forming is seen with the common trying experience producing a more tightly knit community although the stable family is the greatest asset in overcoming the stresses of this period.

Psychiatric treatment during this phase should rely on local professionals. It is important that they should be acquainted with the psychological sequelae of disasters on the individual.

SUMMARY AND CONCLUSION

We have briefly described some psychological and social aspects of disaster. Disasters affect communities and individuals as groups, we have mainly addressed the effects of disasters on communities, and this approach can be somewhat misleading because individuals exposed to more severe psychological trauma may sustain long-lasting consequences, such as post-traumatic stress disorder, while their cohorts are less affected. Thus, humans exposed to trauma respond as individuals as well as groups.

We mentioned the importance of preplanning and training in the first two stages of disaster. Even though there are no scientific data on this subject, it is our strong belief that thought and preparation are of major importance in all phases of disaster.

Preplanning and training are not just topics of importance for individuals and communities but are also important for those who are expected to assist in times of disaster. Mental health teams do not form on the spot; their formation takes time, and the time for this is before such disturbances occur.

A mental health team should consist of at least five mental health professionals, with a psychiatrist heading the team. This number of professionals should enable the team to cope with the problems discussed previously. The team is part of the medical setup with all its members being able to deliver physical first aid in case of need.

In times of mass disruption, rescue systems must be kept as simple as possible. It is much easier to work with one large medical team with one leader than with a number of teams, each in charge of different problems. We have stated the need for psychiatric personnel to be capable of administering physical first aid, but we must also stress the necessity that the medical teams have an understanding of the psychological and social phenomena of disaster.

The mental health team can consist of members from all mental health care professions—psychiatrists, psychologists, psychiatric social workers, and psychiatric nurses. We do not believe that there is any special composition needed to make up the team. But we do believe that the team must be composed before the disaster and that it must operate with one agreed on policy.

Disasters produce psychological suffering among survivors, but with appropriate interventions, some of the later effects of postdisaster disturbances can be avoided. It is essential that mental health circles become interested in and prepared for disaster situations.

REFERENCES

1. Jones FD. Combat psychiatry in modern warfare. In: Adelaja O, Jones FD, eds. *War and Its Aftermath*. John West Publishers of Nigeria; 1983: 63–77.

2. Jones FD, Harris P, Fong YH. Military psychiatry and civilian disturbances: Disasters, terrorism, hostage and refugee situations. In: Pichot P, Berner P, Wolf R, Thau K, eds. *Psychiatry: The State of the Art*. New York: Plenum Press; 1985: 465–470.

3. Luz GA, Hooper RR, DePauw JW, Legters LJ, Gaydos JC. The role of military medicine in military civic action. *Milit Med*. 1993;158(6):362–366.

4. Caldwell JM, Ranson SW, Sacks JG. Group panic and other mass disruptive reactions. *US Armed Forces Med J*. 1951;2(4):541–567.

5. Drayer CS, Cameron DC, Glass AJ, Woodward WD, Woods OT. *Disaster Fatigue*. Washington, DC: American Psychiatric Association; 1956.

6. Glass AJ. Management of mass psychiatric casualties. *Milit Med*. 1956;118(4):335–342.

7. Glass AJ. Psychological aspects of disaster. *JAMA*. 1959;171(2):222–225.

8. Glass AJ. Psychologic considerations in atomic warfare. *US Armed Forces Med J*. 1964;7(5):625–639.

9. Bolin R. Response to natural disasters. In: Lystad M, ed. *Mental Health Response to Mass Emergencies: Theory and Practice*. New York: Brunner/Mazel; 1988: 22–51.

10. Lystad M. Perspectives on human response to mass emergencies. In: Lystad M, ed. *Mental Health Response to Mass Emergencies: Theory and Practice*. New York: Brunner/Mazel; 1988: xvii–xliii.

11. Gist R, Lubin B. Ecological and community perspectives on disaster intervention. In: Gist R, Lubin B, eds. *Psychological Aspects of Disaster*. New York: John Wiley and Sons; 1989: 1–8.

12. Tyhurst JS. Individual reactions to community disaster: The natural history of psychiatric phenomena. *Am J Psychiatry*. 1951;107:764–769.

13. Nesse RM. Panic disorder: An evolutionary view. *Psychiatric Ann*. 1988;18:478–483.

14. Warheit GJ. Disasters and their mental health consequences: Issues, findings and future trends. In: Lystad M, ed. *Mental Health Response to Mass Emergencies: Theory and Practice*. New York: Brunner/Mazel; 1988: 3–21.

15. Lystad M. Innovating mental health services for disaster victims. *Child Today*. 1985;14(1):13–17.

16. Gist R, Stolz SB. Mental health promotion and the media: Community response to the Kansas city hotel disaster. *Am Psychol*. 1982;37:1136–1139.

17. Rappaport J, Chinsky JM. Models for delivery of services from a historical and conceptual perspective. *Prof Psychol*. 1974;5:42–50.

18. Tierney KJ. The social and community contexts of disaster. In: Gist R, Lubin B, eds. *Psychological Aspects of Disaster*. New York: John Wiley and Sons; 1989: 11–39.

19. Division of Education and Service Systems Liaison, Emergency Services Branch, National Institute of Mental Health. *Prevention and Control of Stress Among Emergency Workers: A Pamphlet for Team Managers*. Rockville, Md: DHHS; 1988.

Chapter 15

MILITARY PSYCHIATRY AND REFUGEES

FRANKLIN D. JONES, M.D., F.A.P.A.,* PINCHAS HARRIS, M.D.,† MANUEL FEBO, M.D.,‡ AND PEDRO J. CRUZ, M.D.§

*Colonel (ret), Medical Corps, U.S. Army; Clinical Professor, Uniformed Services University of the Health Sciences; Past President and Secretary and Current Honorary President of the Military Section, World Psychiatric Association
†Director of Rehabilitation Services, Herzliya Medical Center—Haifa, Israel; formerly Medical Officer, Israeli Defence Forces
‡Colonel (ret), Medical Corps, U.S. Army; formerly Psychiatry Consultant to The Surgeon General, U.S. Army; formerly Chief, Inpatient Psychiatry, Walter Reed Army Medical Center, Washington, D.C.
§Chief, Department of Psychiatry, Caguas Regional Hospital, Caguas, Puerto Rico

INTRODUCTION

The 20th century may be described as the century of the uprooted or homeless man.[1] Since the beginning of the century and especially since World War II, there have been millions of displaced persons in various parts of the world at the same time. As of April 1991, there were nearly 15 million refugees worldwide, mostly women and children. More than 2 million are "boat people" escaped from repressive regimes or civil war in Southeast Asia, and 1.6 million of these were resettled in 30 countries since 1975.[2] The 1991 to 1992 dissolution of Yugoslavia and ethnic fighting have added several more millions to these figures.[3,4] The recent tribal fighting in Rwanda has added over 200,000 refugees fleeing to neighboring countries.[5]

Much has been written in the scientific literature[1] on the various aspects of the refugee problem, but relatively little has appeared in the psychiatric literature until recently. Psychiatrists have usually been interested in psychiatric morbidity of the resettled refugees, while only a few papers have been devoted to psychiatric phenomena encountered in the initial stages of refugee resettlement.[6]

An area of particular interest for psychiatrists is treating the post-traumatic stress disorders that refugees may suffer as a result of exposure to mass violence and torture. A few studies[7,8,9] have indicated that psychiatric interventions may be helpful in reducing depression and anxiety symptoms in these refugee populations.

The military is called to assist when the influx of refugees is so great that civilian organizations have difficulties in coping with all of the initial problems.[10,11] Such a state has developed numerous times in the United States. In 1975, the large number of Vietnam refugees who arrived in California were assisted by the navy.[12] In 1979 and 1980, the influx of Cubans who arrived in Florida required the army to assist in various aspects.[13] In 1992 and 1993, an influx of Haitian refugees was threatened and only aborted by a navy blockade of Haiti.[14] Naval action was also required to stem an influx of refugees from China.[15] Most of these recent refugees are seeking to better their economic situation, a chronic cause of illegal aliens from Latin America and developing nations.[16]

Another such situation requiring military assistance occurred in the summer of 1992 when Hurricane Andrew devastated areas of southern Florida and Louisiana, the costliest natural disaster in U.S. history up to that time. The military was required to maintain order and set up refugee camps.[17] Finally, large-scale flooding in the midwest United States resulted in massive numbers of refugees in 1993.[18]

Under current policy and law, military assistance is only temporary and only in the initial stages until civilian organizations can take over completely. We shall describe, therefore, psychiatric and psychological phenomena that can be seen in the early stages of resettlement, after first defining different categories of displaced persons.

TYPES OF DISPLACEMENT

Refugees

The most common type of displacement of modern times is the refugee. In this situation, the individual is forced to leave his previous home and does not expect to be able to return home in the future. Refugee situations occur as a result of war (for example, Afghanistan, Iran, Iraq, Yugoslavia, and Central America) or as a result of political changes that force specific communities and racial, ethnic, religious, or political groups to leave their homes and countries (for example, Vietnam, Cambodia, Laos, Haiti, Bulgaria, and Rwanda). It is refugees that we discuss in detail later. Refugee status may also be transient as occurred with Hurricane Andrew and the 1993 Midwest flooding in the United States. In this chapter, we will use the term *refugee* to refer to someone who has left his country of origin, unless otherwise stated.

Migrants

A migrant is someone who voluntarily decides to leave his homeland, looking for a new life in a new country. The individual in this situation has the possibility of returning to his previous country so that there need not be a total discontinuation with the past. Even though this is a self-initiated process controlled by international agreements, the receiving country can be faced by large numbers of immigrants. This situation rarely needs assistance from military sources because the influx is regulated and the immigrant is required to have a sponsor.

Voluntary Exiles

Voluntary exiles are people who, by voluntarily leaving their homeland, know that they cannot return, that is, unless there is a radical political change in their country of origin. This type of displacement is encountered when people leave totalitarian regimes of their own accord. This group is the smallest of all types of displacement and rarely causes strain on immigration authorities of the accepting countries although there are some instances of mass voluntary departure of individuals from their homeland. The influx of Cubans to the United States in 1979 and 1980[19] and the Jewish flight from the former Soviet Union[20] can be seen as examples. In addition, the 1992 flight of ethnic groups from Yugoslavia sparked riots in Germany where they were viewed as competitors for scarce jobs and welfare resources.[21] Some phenomena in the various stages of resettlement are common to all types, the main sufferer being the refugee who had no control over his flight.

SOCIAL IMPLICATIONS

Three social conditions are common to almost all refugees: statelessness, homelessness, and powerlessness.

By being forced to leave his country, either by reason of war or politics, a refugee becomes stateless. He loses his status of citizenship and thus loses the rights and the protection each citizen receives from his country. Being evicted from his home, a refugee becomes homeless. He loses his economic stability, gives up previous personal and cultural ties, and becomes a stranger in a new society.

A refugee is generally a person who has no home, who has no power or control over his flight or fate, and who is in the hands of others for survival and later resettlement. When the individual overcomes these obstacles, he ceases to be a refugee.

PSYCHOLOGICAL IMPLICATIONS

The clinical picture encountered among refugees is extremely varied both in individual responses and in changes within the individual over time. To understand these phenomena, we suggest the following phases of responses be considered in what shall be called the refugee syndrome. Our suggestion is based in part on what Tyhurst[22] calls the social displacement syndrome. The phases are initial phase, phase of preentry, phase of entry, period of psychological arrival, and period of resettlement.

Initial Phase

The initial phase is the period in which the individual becomes a refugee. He has been evicted from his home and surroundings. The refugee in this stage usually has terrifying or threatening experiences caused by war, disaster situations, or captivity and jailing because of political reasons. This period is characterized by various degrees of physical discomfort such as hunger, physical illness or injury, torture, and so forth.

The initial phase terminates when the individual has successfully managed to arrive in a new surrounding that does not impose any specific danger to him. The suffering in this phase can definitely impair the resettlement of the refugee.

The psychological phenomenon seen in this stage can be defined as "survival." The individual wants to live, and he does everything in his power, consciously and unconsciously, to remain alive.

Phase of Preentry

In the phase of preentry, the refugee has arrived at a safe place, but as yet he does not know where he is going to settle or which country is going to allow him to enter. This phase is mainly seen when there is a mass influx of refugees to a country that cannot or that is unwilling to resettle all of the refugees. The period can last for years, with the refugee being in an internment camp without being able to begin the process of resettlement.

This period can also be a period of selection, when one country agrees to accept a certain number of refugees for resettlement. The obvious choice for selection are the young, the healthy, the skilled, and the more educated, while the others await some other solution.

Psychological phenomena encountered in this period are comparable with those experienced during phases of disaster, namely the recoil period.[10] Responses consist of three main behavior patterns: (1) effectiveness, (2) dependency, and (3) noneffectiveness. Generally, preexisting personality type and occupational role determine which behavior pattern a refugee will exhibit. Firefighters, police, and medical workers, for example, tend to be effective. Dependent and histrionic personalities tend to be noneffective.

The clinical picture here is complicated by the unknown future, the feeling of insecurity, and sometimes the fear of being repatriated to the country of origin. Group cohesion is of great value in this stage in combatting these fears. Individuals tend to coalesce into groups according to cultural background, with the emergence of leaders as in times of disaster. Mental health intervention at this stage is similar to that for combat stress casualties—restoration of physiological deficits and restoration of morale.[23]

Phase of Entry

The phase of entry is the initial period when the refugee arrives in the country in which he is to resettle. The harrowing experiences of the past are behind him, and theoretically, at least, the refugee can begin rebuilding his life. Strangely, the refugee shows more concern over the immediate past than the present or future during this period. His interest in the present is directed mainly toward fulfillment of basic physiological needs such as food, sleep, shelter, and so forth. Concern about the future seems lulled.[24]

Psychological characteristics common to this phase are usually a sense of well-being, in some euphoria; increased psychomotor activity, usually nonconstructive; dependency, more so than in the previous stage of preentry; and finally feelings of unreality and confusion, described by some refugees as being "as if it were a dream."[10] The first two characteristics apply usually to those who were previously effective, while the fourth characteristic is often found in those who were noneffective. The third characteristic of increased dependency usually occurs in those who had been dependent during preentry. This initial period can last for 2 months after entry, and it is during this phase that we see the influence of the group and leadership diminishing.[10]

Period of Psychological Arrival

The period of psychological arrival is the time when the refugee awakens from his "daze" and begins to realize the difficulties of building a new life. The period can last up to 1 year after arrival in the new country; it is an extremely trying period for both the refugee and for the authorities assisting in resettlement.[10]

It is difficult to categorize the quite varied psychological phenomena of this phase, but the more common characteristics are feelings of insecurity, isolation, resentment, unhappiness, guilt, inadequacy, and so forth. We believe it is more appropriate to define the psychological reactions in terms of the clinical entities most commonly encountered:[1,24,25]

- Somatic ailments. Refugees frequently complain of various physical discomforts. Their complaints are usually of pain, with a tendency to shift complaints from one system to another.
- Anxiety and depression. Anxiety is more common among the younger refugees, while depression is found more often among the older ones.
- Paranoid reactions. Paranoid trends and varying degrees of suspiciousness are quite common among refugees. True paranoid psychoses, however, usually appear at a later stage.

During this period, the individual has to make significant readjustments in major ways of life; to learn a new language, new culture, and new professional skills; to adapt to a new social and economic status; and so on. It is the individual's personal attempt to build a new life. There is very little group reinforcement at this time, and it is quite common to see severe strains in previous interpersonal relationships.[1,24,25]

Period of Resettlement

In the period of resettlement, by definition, the individual has ceased to be a refugee; he has attained residency or citizenship, a home, and power. This period lasts for the rest of the refugee's life, and although resettlement can be complete, most refugees suffer to some extent from events of their past.[24–27]

Psychiatric literature[24–27] reveals much interest in this stage, with a number of studies showing higher psychiatric morbidity among resettled refugees than that found in the equivalent population in the same area and, in some cases, compared with psychiatric morbidity of the country of origin of the refugee. Depression and post-traumatic stress disorders are common, especially if torture occurred.[22] Apparently, an individual cannot sever his original ties to his homeland; longing for his past home or nostalgia remains with the refugee for the rest of his life.

MILITARY ASSISTANCE: THE CUBAN MARIEL BOAT PEOPLE

In the spring of 1980, Fidel Castro allowed the emigration of approximately 125,000 Cubans. Unlike the 1 million earlier Cuban refugees who had been predominantly from middle-class backgrounds, these refugees were mainly from lower social economic classes and included many elderly, many mentally ill, and some criminals. Most of the emigres were housed in four military camps with miliary and civilian assistance including military psychiatric personnel. In the ensuing months, problems of chronic mental illness, rioting, and stress-induced emotional problems as well as general medical problems were managed. Lessons learned included the need for a clear authority structure with security measures; the need for segregation by culture, class, and family; and the need for personnel familiar with the culture. The growing number of Hispanic refugees due to the conflicts in Central America makes the most important lesson, the need for preplanning, vital.[19]

Burkle stated that one of the unfortunate "phenomena of the 70's is the instant refugee camp."[28(p800)] The "Freedom Flotilla" in May 1980 introduced the same phenomena in the 1980s, with the migration of approximately 125,000 Cuban people to the United States and the establishment of four refugee camps in Florida, Arkansas, Pennsylvania, and Wisconsin. We will describe the psychosocial aspects of one of these camps, Fort Chaffee, Arkansas, and although it is not representative of all the camps, it describes some elements common to them. This information is derived from the assignment of one of the authors (Pedro Cruz) as psychiatrist for the refugee camp at Fort Chaffee. It is based on his observations and clinical experiences while he was there.

Psychological Phases

Prerefugee Camp

As retold by many of the Cuban refugees, life under the Communist regime of Castro brought many dramatic changes to the Cuban people. Castro's announcement of his embracing Communist doctrine led to the realization of a new form of government resulting in a wave of migration that started in the 1960s and continues sporadically more than 30 years later. The motivating factor was primarily political, and the Cuban society was depleted of its upper class, middle class professional, semiprofessional, managerial, and business elements. Those who remained were the uneducated, unskilled, and lower socioeconomic strata.[19]

The new government provided a political structure that demanded unquestioning loyalty to the state and the sacrifice of traditional institutions and values (the family, friendship, religion, ownership of land and businesses, and military structures). The extended family, one of the strongholds of Cuban society, was torn apart, and a new entity was born—the nuclear family—committed to survival and void of strong family ties with an increasing sense of isolation because neighbors and family were encouraged to report on one another for possible disloyal activities. With promises that the government would provide everything and the barren reality of the situation, covert black-market activities flourished, bringing new dangers to individuals and their families as well as adding to the existing feelings of isolation.[19]

Refugee Camp

As increasing numbers of refugees overwhelmed resources in southern Florida, the U.S. government set up four refugee camps, including the one at Fort Chaffee, Arkansas. Refugee camps were not a new experience to the nearby Arkansas community. During the mid 1970s, it was the temporary home for thousands of Vietnamese refugees and provided a good source of income to an economically depressed area. The local population had viewed its past experience as a positive one and viewed the advent of the new camp primarily as an economic blessing. As the news coverage revealed that these Cubans were different from the Vietnamese in every aspect and that Castro had emptied Cuban jails and mental hospitals, the economic dream threatened to become a horrifying nightmare. Rumors of rape, murder, and pillage were born in the local populace, fed by the national press, confirmed by a few isolated incidents, and probably immortalized in the mind of the American public.[29]

Refugee camps were also not new to many of the personnel of the federal and volunteer agencies involved in the management and administration of the resettlement camp. Like the local populace, many had been involved with the Vietnamese refugees and many remembered the experience as a positive one. Like the local populace, many did not know that Asians and Hispanics could be diametrically opposite in cultural, psychological, and behavioral aspects.

Plans had been made by personnel lacking knowledge of these differences to operationally set up the camp as it had been set up for the Vietnamese. Planners believed that any Hispanic or Spanish surnamed individual would be competent to deal with the cultural issues of this group of refugees, as was the view of the local populace. This did not account for whether the Hispanic was from the Caribbean, Central America, or South America or whether the Hispanic was a first, second, or third generation Hispanic-American. This apparent lack of a clearly organized and centralized authority structure in the initial phase of establishing the camp contributed to the confusion inherent to a chaotic and stressful event.

Entry Phase at Fort Chaffee

During the month of May 1980, approximately 19,000 Cuban refugees were flown to Fort Chaffee from Florida. It is located in the western part of Arkansas. The entry process to the United States consists of a medical evaluation, issuance of a temporary identification card and number, a series of interviews by federal agencies that can lead to a Washington clearance for entry, and issuance of an immigration card and work permit. Release into the general population takes place once a sponsor for the refugee has been found.

The refugees were housed in World War II barracks by random assignments of both families and unaccompanied individuals to the same buildings—a practice utilized during the Vietnamese operation. Meals were served in military dining facilities, and clothing was provided by relief agencies. The medical services were primarily of two types: (1) various triage and treatment facilities through the compound for providing initial screening and referral to (2) central emergency service for triaging and provision of both inpatient and outpatient medical care set up in tents by the field hospital.

As refugees and camp personnel increased their daily contacts and interactions, there emerged a series of psychosocial phenomena that can be divided into three phases. The initial phase—entry phase—lasted about 2 weeks and was characterized by a period of euphoria shared by both the refugees and camp personnel. On the part of the Marielitos (a term for refugees from Cuba derived from their departure port, El Mariel), it was based on having the perilous boat trip over and reaching the land that promised freedom and a better life; on the part of the camp staff, it was based on feelings of satisfaction from helping people. Accompanying this euphoria was a hyperactivity throughout camp as people celebrated their good fortune and searched for families and friends. Confusion for the camp staff was also a hallmark of this period because the central authority was not able to provide the daily decisions on issues concerning the increasing influx of refugees, the lack of adherence to procedural guidelines by agencies, and refugees switching assigned quarters without informing the authorities. The psychiatric casualties were few and consisted mainly of adjustment reactions to the relocation because some people were separated from their families or feared being sent to places other than Florida.

A second phase—the reactive phase—was of 1 month's duration and was characterized by fear, insecurities, and regression to behavioral patterns that were more characteristic of their homeland. With the surfacing of the criminal element, violent behavior, black-market activities, gang formation, and the manufacturing of homemade weapons occurred. As the families who shared the buildings were beginning to be threatened and victimized, they reacted in a similar fashion of manufacturing weapons and forming groups for individual and family protection. The confusion for the camp staff further increased as this unexpected group emerged and there was no provision of personnel or security measures.

As the news of the prisoner element hit the local news, there were local demonstrations against the refugees that created a panic reaction in the refugees and resulted in the riot of 1 June 1980. The army's response was to bring in 1,500 troops to control the riot and maintain a sense of order. Under a new administration, steps were taken to segregate the unaccompanied refugees (those not traveling with family) in their own barracks.

Psychiatric casualties were surfacing in large numbers during this period primarily as adjustment reactions due to the stress of camp. In addition, the chronic psychiatrically ill began to surface because they were beginning to run out of medication or the levels of the medication in their systems were diminishing. Another behavior peculiar to this phase was the hoarding of food (perhaps a carryover from their homeland experience) although it was obvious that there was enough food for everyone. An epidemic of food poisoning ensued because of spoiled hoarded food, and a special ward was opened to treat the many dehydrated patients.

The third phase—the depressive phase—that lasted the remaining time of the camp was characterized by resignation, depression, a feeling of hopelessness, and acting out behavior. During this phase, the camp staff had organized themselves under a clear line of authority with role definition among the existing agencies, and the issue of personal safety for everyone was resolved. Many of the refugees were leaving, and those left behind were becoming irritable, depressed, and angry at the lengthy process of leaving camp. Some wished to return to Cuba and referred to the Americans as no better than Castro's police force. Others resigned themselves to the situation and waited for the resolution of their problems. Psychiatric casualties were more on the depressive spectrum with suicidal ideation or gestures. A pattern of self-mutilation surfaced as the remaining population dwindled to unaccompanied males, many of whom had been released directly from jail to El Mariel. The depressive illnesses were directly related to the waiting time in camp and a feeling that the promised land was not what they had been led to believe.

Patient Data Profile

The psychiatric team providing services consisted of a psychiatrist, a psychiatric nurse, and two behavioral science specialists—all military personnel. Around-the-clock emergency services, coordination of transfers to community facilities, outpatient follow-up, and later an inpatient service were provided by the team. A total of 465 people were referred from mid-May to mid-August, with a total of 993 patient contacts. Of the 465 referrals, 41 (9%) patients required hospitalization in the camp inpatient facility or the community facility for the more severe cases. A review of 200 of the outpatient records revealed that the majority of the patients (93%) were referred from medical sources because of "nervousness" or "depression." These patients also had a previous psychiatric history (78.0%), and a substantial percentage (20.0%) had a previous history of incarceration. Evaluation revealed that these patients were undergoing an adjustment disorder, and they received outpatient treatment with medication. These data are presented in Tables 15–1 and 15–2.

The population evaluated can be subdivided into three subgroups: (1) those with prior psychiatric histories but no prison experience (120 cases); (2) those with histories of imprisonment (40 cases), and (3) those who had no histories of either (40 cases). All of the three groups were predominantly

TABLE 15–1

PSYCHIATRIC PATIENT PROFILE (N=200) DEMOGRAPHICS

	Category	No.	(%)
Age (yr)			
	0–17	15	(7.5)
	18–25	73	(36.5)
	26–35	71	(35.5}
	36–45	28	(14.0)
	46–55	11	(5.5)
	56–65	2	(1.0)
Sex			
	Male	150	(75.0)
	Female	50	(25.0)
Marital Status			
	Single	50	(25.0)
	Married	29	(14.5)
	Unknown	121	(60.5)
Legal Status (history of incarceration)			
	Present	40	(20.0)
	Absent	53	(26.5)
	Unknown	107	(53.5)
Referral Source			
	Medical	186	(93.0)
	Agencies	14	(7.0)

in the age range of 18 to 36 years, were predominantly males, and were medically referred. In the psychiatric group, the disorders were primarily chronic in nature with psychotic disorders (28.3%) being the most common, followed by affective disorders (26.6%), anxiety disorders (15.8%), and disorders of impulse (15.0%). In the prison group, 77.5% of the patients had previous psychiatric histories, with disorders of impulse (37.5%) being the predominant entity, followed by psychotic disorders (25.0%), anxiety disorders (25.0%), and affective disorders (12.5%).

TABLE 15–2

PSYCHIATRIC PATIENT PROFILE (N=200) PSYCHIATRIC ISSUES

Category		No.		(%)
Previous Psychiatric History				
Present		156		(78.0)
Inpatient	79		(39.5)	
Outpatient	77		(38.5)	
Medication History		139		(69.5)
Presenting Complaints				
Nervousness		49		(24.5)
Depression		34		(17.0)
Insomnia		24		(12.0)
Evaluation		23		(11.5)
Medication		17		(8.5)
Suicide gesture		11		(5.5)
Anxious and depressed		6		(3.0)
Self-mutilation		5		(2.5)
Suicidal ideation		4		(2.0)
Sexual dysfunction		4		(2.0)
Diagnosis (Axis I only)				
Adjustment disorder		79		(39.5)
Schizophrenic disorder		28		(14.0)
Affective disorder		24		(12.0)
No diagnosis		21		(10.5)
Impulse disorder		17		(8.5)
V codes		7		(3.5)
Deferred		6		(3.0)
Anxiety disorder		6		(3.0)
Somatoform disorder		6		(3.0)
Psychosis/other		3		(1.5)
Psychosexual disorder		3		(1.5)
Disposition				
Medications and outpatient		118		(59.0)
Hospitalization		29		(14.5)
No follow-up		26		(13.0)

The impulse disorders in both groups were characterized by episodic outbursts of anger, violence towards self and others, and an inability to remember these outbursts. Eleven of the prisoners (27.5%) reported their symptoms to have first manifested themselves while incarcerated. In addition, eight (20.0%) of these reported being in jail for political reasons. In the psychiatric group, 55.8% of the patients had been hospitalized at least once, while 30.0% of the prisoners had also received inpatient services; 44.2% and 60.0%, respectively, had received outpatient services. In the psychiatric and prison group, the primary reason for referral was nervousness, while the third group was referred for evaluation to rule out a psychiatric condition.

The incidence of suicide gestures was highest in the group that had negative histories for psychiatric problems or incarceration, 10.0% (4/40), followed by the prison group, 7.5% (3/40), and the psychiatric group, 3.3% (4/120). The prison group showed the highest incidence of self-mutilation, 7.5% (3/40), followed by the nonpsychiatric nonprison group, 2.5% (1/40), and the psychiatric group, 0.8% (1/120).

In all three groups, the most frequently diagnosed condition was an adjustment disorder. Surprisingly, the nonpsychiatric nonprison group showed the highest number of hospitalizations, 25.0% (10/40), followed by 13.3% (16/120) in the psychiatric group and 7.5% (3/40) in the prison group. The relatively low hospitalization rate compared with the nonpsychiatric nonprison group related to the fact that a large percentage of the psychiatric group were stabilized on psychotropic medications; the nonpsychiatric nonprison group included many adolescents, some of whom were hospitalized for their own protection (fear of rape or physical violence).

Discussion

Current literature on mass migratory events emphasizes a multidimensional approach when trying to study the psychosocial factors and psychiatric morbidity of immigrants.[10,11,19,22,24–28,30,31] The interplay of cultural, social, psychological make-up, the presence or absence of psychiatric illness, and the stressors of the migratory event all contribute to the manifestation of clinical psychiatric entities.

One of the striking phenomena encountered with the Cuban refugee group in Arkansas was, despite contrary rumors, the low psychiatric morbidity (2.9%) in a population that was thought to be high in the number of mentally ill individuals. Several factors account for this figure: this population was confined in a similar situation before leaving Cuba, which served as a premigratory conditioning for the events to come, many of the refugee population came as intact families with built-in support systems, the expectation of being absorbed into well-established Cuban communities in this country, and the rapid release of the majority of the refugees into the general population.

The number of psychiatric cases identified were primarily the manifestations of disorders in predisposed individuals or exacerbation of established disorders where the stress of the migration and the conditions of the camp were the precipitating causes. The most common reasons for referral were "nervousness" and "depression," which were the presenting complaints in 44.5% of patients and similar to the findings of Nguyen[26,30] in his studies of the Southeast Asian population in Canada. Whereas Nguyen's group fell into the diagnostic categories of affective disorders (39.0%), psychotic disorders (20.0%), and anxiety disorders (18.0%), the Cuban group fell into diagnostic categories of adjustment disorders (39.5%), psychotic disorders (15.5%), and depressive disorders (12.0%). The difference was that the Cuban group was in its initial phase of arrival in the country, while the Asian group had resettled into the general population.[26]

The subgroup of patients with a history of incarceration is similar to the group described by Bach-Y-Rita[32,33] in the study of 62 prisoners with histories of habitual violence and self-mutilation and who were very impulsive and "would warrant the diagnosis of explosive personality or impulsive character disorder."[33(p1015)] Bach-Y-Rita also points out that neurological impairment was a contributing factor and has to be kept in mind when these patients are being evaluated.

Several authors[10,19,26] have described psychosocial phenomena associated with displacement of masses of people in terms of group dynamics. Nguyen[26] lists three stages in the adjustment of an Asian population in Canada. Harris et al[10] have coined the term *the refugee syndrome* and ascribe five phases in the adaptive process. Both reports describe euphoria, hyperactivity, anxiety, and depression as some of the psychological manifestations in the initial phase of resettlement. These manifestations were also evident in the Cuban experience and give support that the phenomena transcend the cultural boundaries of refugee groups. Unique to the Cuban group, however, was the hyperactivity accompanying the initial euphoria, which later on was transformed and associated with the threat of physical violence posed by the prison population, lack of organizational effectiveness, and the hostile reactions of the local populace. The hyperactivity culminated in the riot responsible for the provision of measures of safety and the segregation of unaccompanied refugees.

The Hispanic component of the camp personnel needs to be addressed in its role in the provision of medical and psychiatric services to the refugee population. Many of the personnel were of Mexican-American extraction and of second- or third-generation Hispanic-American families. For all practical purposes, these individuals were Americans with Spanish surnames and had lost the language, cultural, and other characteristics unique to the Latin-American people. Although the situation was of an acute nature and these differences generally did not matter, in the gathering of information for medical and psychiatric purposes, the language factor is definitely critical.

SUMMARY AND CONCLUSION

The acceptance of emigres has been an element in the history of the United States, and one can assume that it will also be part of the future. The Mariel Cuban experience was a recapitulation of events experienced by other refugee groups, and it reemphasized the importance of the multiplicity of factors contributing to the psychosocial profile of migrant groups. Cultural variables, provision of basic needs (especially individual safety), clear authority structure, segregation of refugees according to social parameters unique to the migrant group, and education of the general populace are critical in the preplanning phase of resettlement operations to reduce the psychiatric morbidity of these groups.

Understanding the various periods of the refugee syndrome is of utmost importance to the mental health worker who can be called to assist in such situations. Military assistance in these matters is an extraordinary basis; therefore, the advisory role of the mental health worker is to be emphasized more than the role of the therapist.

The possibility of military assistance in refugee situations is usually limited to three of the previously described phases. Military aid may definitely be involved in the initial phase as it was for (1) the Shiite refugees in southern Iraq (where U.S. troops watched them being massacred by the Republican Guard, forbidden to intervene until they had run or crawled to U.S. checkpoints, at which point, U.S. personnel could begin giving emergency medical life support, food, and so on); (2) the Kurds in northern Iraq in Operation Provide Comfort; (3) disaster relief operations such as those in Nicaragua, Armenia, and so on after earthquakes while U.S. personnel helped to dig the survivors out of the rubble; and (4) United Nations observers and peacekeeping units in Bosnia, Croatia, Cambodia, and so on that the United States may join. In the initial phase, the mental health and combat stress control personnel must be sensitive to the psychological reactions and trauma of the victims as well as to their physiological needs. Intervention will be at a system level rather than one-on-one because of the pressure of workload. Cultural factors and differences must also be recognized and adjusted to. The principal mental health and combat stress control role in this phase will be to sustain and debrief the rescuers and caregivers so that the latter can continue to give psychologically sensitive care. Suggestions for psychiatric assistance are directed, therefore, to the periods of preentry, entry, and psychological arrival.

The principles of combat psychiatry that apply to most situations of acute and chronic stress need little modification in dealing with the refugee. Rapid interventions and simple, supportive treatments, such as providing shelter, nutrition, and rest, are critical. A positive expectancy of normal functioning and eventual social stability must be maintained. This can be assisted by activities such as learning the new native language and teaching cultural mores and job skills when time allows. The principle of centrality is embodied in a single authority with the power to enforce rules and ensure protection.

During the preentry period, the mental health worker should educate authorities and medical teams about the future difficulties ahead for the refugee. This period can also be utilized for the education of the refugee to assist him during following periods. It must be stressed that the period of preentry can be one of inactivity and boredom, possibly lasting for years. The longer this situation lasts, the more difficult it will be to readjust in the future. Accordingly, the mental health worker should emphasize the need for constructive activity among refugees. These activities may involve learning languages and skills.

The refugees who may need direct psychiatric treatment will be found in the ineffective group. It is advisable for these patients to be treated by the regular medical teams if they are available, with advice from the assisting mental health worker, and only in extreme cases should they be treated initially by the assisting mental health worker.

It is possible at entry time for the assisting mental health worker to gain an impression of well-being among refugees. This impression is accurate to some extent, but it is definitely temporary. Even though this period lasts only for about 2 months, it is our belief that the shorter the period, the easier it will be for the refugee to face the following period.

Decreasing morbidity during this period can be achieved by creating constructive activities such as learning a language or job skills. This may be a difficult task among refugees who have had lengthy periods of inactivity. Gradual exposure to the new surroundings is suggested to avoid the overwhelming effect of new impressions and experiences, a kind of sensory overload. It is important that the refugee's basic physiological needs be met to relieve him of this worry, which can be a convenient excuse for inactivity. Other ways to decrease morbidity include assuring the free flow of accurate news and information to the refugees and the suppression of rumors and fostering self-help programs to build and maintain hygiene and sanitary facilities, recreational and educational activities, and traditional and occupational skills. (Occupational therapists are members of the mental health team.) A knowledge of the cultures of the refugees is essential to providing accurate mental health consultation or direct intervention. Potential sources for this information are the civil affairs staff and especially the special operations and civil affairs units that are expert in this region of the world.

As stated above, this is the period when the influence of the group diminishes, a process that can be slowed if proper attention is given. The mental health worker must stress these points to the receiving authorities. He himself can assist only minimally in direct interventions, but he can explain the future outcome of mistreatment during this phase. The mental health worker's role as a therapist should be directed to treating the more confused refugees. Our suggestion is to give extremely brief psychotherapy and attempt to avoid drug therapy that can complicate the situation even more.

In the period of psychological arrival, the mental health worker's assistance as a therapist can be of great importance; however, it is our strong belief that the mental health worker should mainly advise local medical teams in the treatment of the troubled refugee, and only in the more severe cases act as a therapist.

The following three points should be stressed to treating physicians:

1. They must become aware of psychological disturbances among patients, especially those who often present changing and unexplained physical symptoms.
2. They must give reassurance and reinforcement to those who appear anxious or depressed. Brief psychotherapy is of greater value than any type of medication.
3. Kindness and understanding must be shown to those who show signs of suspiciousness and paranoid trends. Overt sympathy is to be avoided because it tends to aggravate these feelings.

The influence of the group in this period is minimal, and the refugee's attempt at readjustment is as an individual. Simple and brief "group therapy" could be of aid in helping the refugee to understand his personal hardships and interpersonal difficulties. This method could also assist in the reformation of constructive grouping, which is of prime importance for individuals in extreme stress. The mental health worker's influence and assistance in this field could be his greatest contribution in helping refugees in this trying period.

We have described some of the psychological and social phenomena seen in the refugee syndrome. Our intention was to outline points of importance that can be of guidance to mental health professionals who might be called to assist in refugee situations. It is our belief that appropriate advice and help can lessen the suffering of the refugee in three of the periods of the syndrome and, by doing so, assist him in rebuilding a healthier and happier life.

REFERENCES

1. Rumbaut RG. Mental health and the refugee experience: A comparative study of Southeast Asian refugees. In: Owan TC, ed. *Southeast Asian Mental Health: Treatment, Prevention, Services, Training, and Research.* Washington, DC: DHHS; 1985: 433–486. Publication No. (ADM) 85–1399.

2. Holman RL. Spain honors U.N. agency (United Nations High Commission for Refugees). *Wall Street Journal.* 29 April 1991: A10.

3. US Congress. Senate Committee on Armed Services. Current military operations: Hearings before the Committee on Armed Services, US Senate, 103rd Congress, 1st Session, 6 August, 4, 7, 12–13 October 1993. Washington, DC: GPO; 1994.

4. Gunby P. Changing of the medical guard in Croatia. *JAMA.* 1994;271(2):894.

5. Richburg KH. Instant city of misery in a lush land: Rwandan refugees crowd into Tanzanian border camp. *Washington Post.* 4 May 1994: A1, A31.

6. Owan TC, ed. *Southeast Asian Mental Health: Treatment, Prevention, Services, Training, and Research.* Washington, DC: DHHS; 1985. Publication No. (ADM) 85–1399.

7. Mollica RF, Wyshak G, Lavelle J, Truong T, Tor S, Yang T. Assessing symptom change in southeast Asian refugee survivors of mass violence and torture. *Am J Psychiatry.* 1990;147(1):83–88.

8. Goldfield AE, Mollica RF, Pesavento BH, et al. The physical and psychological sequelae of torture: Symptomatology and diagnosis. *JAMA.* 1988;259:2725–2729.

9. Bosoglu M, Marks I. Torture: Research needed into how to help those who have been tortured. *Br Med J.* 1988;297:1423–1424.

10. Harris P, Jones FD, Fong Y. Applications of military psychiatry in civilian disturbances: Disasters, terrorism, hostage and refugee situations. In: Pichot P, Berner P, Wolf R, Thau K, eds. *Psychiatry: The State of the Art.* Vol 6. New York: Plenum; 1985: 465–470.

11. Jones FD. How to treat refugees' special problems. *Behav Today*. 1986;17(25):4–5.

12. Rahe RH, Genender E. Adaptation to and recovery from captivity stress. *Milit Med*. 1983;148(7):577–585.

13. Cruz P, Febo M, Jones FD. Cuban refugee camps: Psychological perspectives. 1986. Syllabus.

14. Pine A. US moves to stifle Haitian exodus. *Los Angeles Times*. 16 January 1993. Vol 112:A12.

15. Kamen A. US seizes illegal aliens from China. *Washington Post*. 5 September 1991. Vol 108:A5.

16. Fritz S, Mann J. House votes to suspend deporting illegal aliens of 3 nations. *Los Angeles Times*. 26 October 1989. Vol 108:A13.

17. Healy M, Stolberg S. Hurricane relief blows in winds of change for military. *Los Angeles Times*. 11 September 1992. Vol 111:A24.

18. Parrett C, Melcher NB, James RW. *Flood Discharges in the Upper Mississippi River Basin, 1993*. Washington, DC: GPO; 1993.

19. Rumbaut RD, Rumbaut RG. The family in exile: Cuban expatriates in the United States. *Am J Psychiatry*. 1976;133(4):395–399.

20. US Congress. Staff Report. *Soviet Jews Arriving in Israel: The Humanitarian Needs*. Washington, DC: GPO; 1992.

21. Vogel S. German anti-foreigner riots in 4th night. *Washington Post*. 26 August 1992. Vol 115:A7.

22. Tyhurst L. Displacement and migration: A study in social psychiatry. *Am J Psychiatry*. 1951;101:561–568.

23. Jones FD, Johnson AW. Medical and psychiatric treatment policy and practice in Vietnam. *J Soc Issues*. 1975;31(4):49–65.

24. Cohen JD. Psychological adaptation and dysfunction among refugees. *Int Migration Rev*. 1981;15(1):255–275.

25. Burwill PW. Immigration and mental disease. *Aust N Z J Psychiatry*. 1973;7:155–162.

26. Nguyen SD. The psycho-social adjustment and the mental health needs of Southeast Asian refugees. *Can J Psychiatric Nurs*. 1984;(April/May/June):6–8.

27. Valdes T, Baxter J. The social readjustment rating questionnaire: A study of Cuban exiles. *J Psychosom Res*. 1976;20:231–236.

28. Burkle FM. Coping with stress under conditions of disaster and refugee care. *Milit Med*. 1983;148(10):800–803.

29. *New York Times*. Cuba denies accord with US on criminals (says it did not agree to accept 1,500 Cuban prisoners from the US). *New York Times*. 10 October 1993. Vol 143:12(N), 24(L).

30. Nguyen SD. Mental health services for refugees and immigrants. *Psychiatr J Univ Ottawa*. 1984;9(2):85–91.

31. Pedersen S. Psychopathological reactions to extreme social displacement (refugee neurosis). *Psychoanal Rev*. 1949;33:344–354.

32. Bach-y-Rita G. Habitual violence and self-mutilation. *Am J Psychiatry*. 1974;131(9):1018–1020.

33. Bach-y-Rita G, Veno A. Habitual violence: A profile of 62 men. *Am J Psychiatry*. 1974;131(9):1015–1017.

Chapter 16

MILITARY PSYCHIATRY AND TERRORISM

FRANKLIN D. JONES, M.D., F.A.P.A.* AND YENG HOI FONG, M.D.†

*Colonel (ret), Medical Corps, U.S. Army; Clinical Professor, Uniformed Services University of the Health Sciences; Past President and Secretary and Current Honorary President of the Military Section, World Psychiatric Association

†Former Chief Psychiatrist, Singapore Armed Forces

INTRODUCTION

The related topics of terrorism and hostage negotiations have not been comprehensively reviewed in the psychiatric literature, but recent years have borne witness to a continuous stream of terrorist incidents with hostage taking in numerous countries. This trend has shown no signs of abating, and a number of law enforcement agencies have expressed their anxiety about a possible extension of terrorist activities in frequency, increasing violence, and the use of high technology, possibly nuclear, weapons. It can be argued that the Iraqi missile attacks on Israel during the Persian Gulf War were an attempt to utilize terrorist tactics to influence the course of the war by provoking Israeli retaliation and inflaming Arab sentiments.[1]

With the dissolution of the former Soviet Union and the end of great power rivalries, numerous ethnic rivalries have emerged. This has resulted in mutual terrorist acts, civil wars, and the large-scale Persian Gulf War. Individual terrorist acts have changed political strategies. For example, the marine barracks bombing in Beirut of American peacekeepers resulted in the removal of the U.S. presence and ability to influence events in Lebanon, the escalation of its civil war, and a change of government in Lebanon.[2]

More recently in Somalia, a rescue mission aimed at saving starving Somalis was converted into a police action when a disaffected warlord arranged for the ambushing and killing of more than 20 United Nations (UN) forces. A major mission of UN forces became not only protecting helping personnel but also attempting to capture and punish the warlord.[3]

Official responses to any terrorist incident have, in general, initially been made by civilian law enforcement agencies; however, there have been occasions in the past in which it was deemed necessary to enlist the assistance of military tactical teams to bring terrorist acts to a conclusion. Military personnel, bases, and military family housing areas may be the target of terrorist attack. Military mental health teams, such as the Navy special psychiatric rapid intervention teams (SPRINTs) and the army's 7th Medical Command stress management teams from Heidelberg, Germany, provide expert mental health support after terrorist attacks. For example, the stress management teams from the 7th Medical Command, Heidelberg, Germany, responded to numerous terrorist actions in the mid-1980s. The team included psychiatrists, social work officers, chaplains, psychiatric nurses, psychologists, and enlisted specialists. They deployed to the *Achille Lauro*, a civilian cruise ship that had been hijacked in the Mediterranean, and to Karachi, Pakistan, for a TWA airliner highjacking. The mental health professional working within the police force or the army, therefore, cannot afford to remain uninformed or incapable of rendering assistance when terrorist incidents occur.

Terrorism, as defined by the U.S. Army, is the calculated use of violence or the threat of violence to attain goals, political, religious, or ideological in nature.[5] This is done through intimidation, coercion, or instilling fear. Terrorism involves a criminal act that is often symbolic in nature and intended to influence an audience beyond the immediate victim. A terrorist group, therefore, is any organization that uses terrorism in a systematic way to achieve its goals.[4] The following definitions have been derived from a task force report by the National Advisory Committee on Criminal Justice Standards and Goals.[5] Terrorism acts may be classified according to the motivation and aims of the perpetrators of terrorist violence and whether the activities are carried across national boundaries. There are several subcategories of terrorism. *Political terrorism* is violent, criminal behavior designed primarily to generate fear in the community, or a substantial segment of it, for political purposes. *Nonpolitical terrorism* involves acts of violence inflicted by organized crime, teenage groups, or pathological groups or cults. *Quasi-terrorism* is characterized by activities incidental to the commission of crimes of violence that are similar in form and execution to true terrorism but lacking in a basic ideology, for example, taking of hostages in a bank robbery to secure a means of escape. *International and transnational terrorism* involves acts of terrorism inflicted within other countries, and these acts are further classified as international terrorism when perpetrated by individuals or groups controlled by a foreign state, or transnational when carried out by essentially autonomous, nonstate actors. Terrorism, therefore, is separated from discrete instances of murder for political or social motives of politicians or community leaders by individuals or small groups; that is, political assassinations.

The increasing cooperation between former Soviet republics and western democracies is diminishing the financial resources and safe havens available for terrorists. However, the relative success of transnational terrorists in the past decade has been viewed with increasing alarm by the world community because the failure of countries to agree even on the basic issue of differentiating terrorism and national liberation movements has often prevented effective collective action. Under such conditions, it remains for persons involved in management of terrorist incidents to anticipate them and continually to expand their knowledge and expertise.

MODERN TERRORISM AND FUTURE TRENDS

Basically, the use of terrorist methods occurs when there is an imbalance of power between two antagonists. It is a weapon wielded by the few or weak against the many or strong, and the terrorist's real strength lies in his own ruthlessness, recklessness, or, in the case of a psychotic terrorist, the extent of his mental derangement. In considering a response to terrorism, one needs to know just how far the terrorist will go to attain his objectives. One of the attendant dangers that law enforcement agencies face may be the need to match violence with violence without becoming brutalized and without damaging the population to be protected.

It is important to understand the essentially psychological nature of terrorist objectives. Not only do the terrorists want to flaunt the powerlessness of the authorities to prevent their attacks, they also want to provoke the defending authorities into taking repressive countermeasures that will turn the local population and world opinion (through the media) against the authorities. The terrorists maximize the ambiguity by deliberately hiding among and looking like the people the government or military is supposed to protect. They use ambushes, booby traps, and women and children as auxiliaries and combatants. The extreme ambiguity is deliberately intended to warp the minds of the defenders and make them distrust the local population and consider them unworthy of protection. The high ambiguity elicits misconduct stress behaviors, including excessive force and brutality, alcohol and drug abuse (as compensatory tension relievers that further disinhibit the defenders), insubordination, and commission of atrocities. The mental health team should play a major role in helping command to protect the soldiers against this threat. These issues are discussed in Field Manual 22–51[6] and in the *Combat Stress Control in Operations Other Than War* draft white paper.[7]

Modern society with its dependence on sophisticated services and institutions to provide for its basic needs has rendered itself, as a whole, more vulnerable to terrorist attacks. Modern terrorism has been assisted by developments facilitating international travel and mass communications. Terrorists have been able to travel freely and widely, train with and utilize an assortment of sophisticated weapons, and have used mass media to publicize their activities. Attempts to curb the increasing power wielded by the modern terrorist have to be counterbalanced by an awareness of the need for constraint to avoid infringing the civil rights of, and thus alienation of, the very people who are in need of protection.

Terrorism in its various forms has changed over the years. Some nations have recognized the potential of terrorism and have used the terrorist as the spearhead of a developing theory and practice of surrogate warfare. Governments, unwilling to risk the consequences of conventional warfare to realign the balance of power or to achieve political aims, have been subsidizing, training, and deploying such groups to create terror for carefully designed coercive purposes.[8] The probable trend is for increases in such sponsored forms of terrorism. In addition, there is an increasing likelihood that terrorists will employ sophisticated modern weapons and means of destruction to back their demands as resistance to terrorism stiffens, including the potential use of nuclear devices.

A minor form of terrorism but often having significant financial repercussions is the increasing proliferation of computer viruses. Important military and scientific databases have been adversely affected by such viruses. Unfortunately, military psychiatrists can offer little in this area other than developing perpetrator personality profiles that often reveal a highly intelligent, narcissistic young adult with an extensive computer "hacker" background.[9]

PSYCHOPATHOLOGY OF TERRORISM

Terrorism per se has no ideology, and it merely draws on ideologies of varying vintages or adopts a convenient political umbrella for guidance and rationalization. There appears to be a peculiarly addictive quality to terrorism, and an individual terrorist or terrorist group may change ideology apparently simply to continue perpetrating violence.[10]

Beneath a veneer of ideology, the political terrorist's motivation can usually be seen to be extremely personal. For example, many terrorists are quite paranoid, and the terrorist acts are rationalized expressions of projected hostility. True terrorist behavior often shows an extreme callousness and disregard for the victim and his feelings, thus an antisocial component.[10]

An understanding of the psychopathology of the terrorist is necessary when responding to his act. In addition, an assessment of the mental state, thought processes, and personality of the terrorist will help toward formulating adequate responses in assessing a terrorist threat. It is in this assessment that the behavioral scientist can be of assistance.

There is considerable evidence[10] that contagion and imitation are significant factors in the incidence of terrorist activities, just as suicide, arson, rioting, and other destructive activities seem to be influenced by the same factors. Hijacking of commercial aircraft is a good example. Hijacking has continued to remain a popular terrorist act in spite of the uncertain meeting of terrorist demands in many instances.

What of the terrorist himself? Often, one is tempted to think of him as insane or suffering from a characterological disorder, but this thought is probably too sweeping a generalization. There is, however, strong evidence of the paranoid tendency to hold onto overvalued ideas (even if mutable) on some political or social issue, which has often subsequently led to the perpetration of terroristic acts.

It has been said[10] that few terrorists will push their demands to the extent that they may have to end up paying with their own lives. Events have so far shown[11] this to be generally true, but it would be a mistake to conduct negotiations on this premise. For example, a suicidal fanatic drove a truck loaded with explosives into the marine barracks in Beirut.[11]

CONSEQUENCES OF TERRORISM

The very nature and intent of terrorism are such that apart from the act itself and the principal actors involved, fear and the impression of power vested in the terrorist are communicated to a large population and the whole society. This brings into relief the impotence of the civil authority and leaves the authority with the choice of ignominiously accepting the terrorist demands or else resorting to drastic counteraction in which innocent lives may be lost—a loss for which the authorities can still be blamed.

One terrorist acting alone is sufficient to induce severe psychological stress in a large number of people, but continuous terrorist activity may produce severe long-lasting effects on a society. Such a situation can substantially impair the quality of life in a community, insidiously alter the day-to-day habits of its people, and interfere with the free exchanges and interactions previously possible between people.[10]

Attitudes of the population may change with people becoming suspicious and intolerant. Regard for the authorities may decline, and the authorities may, in efforts to redeem themselves, resort to actions that may further alienate the population they support. This sequence of events is by no means the rule; there are countries that have absorbed the effects of repeated terrorist attacks without having to change the basic tenets of their governments and without subjecting their populations to progressively dictatorial rule. The United Kingdom stands as an example of a nation little changed by repeated Irish Republican Army atrocities, while Ulster (Northern Ireland) has been devastated by opposing terrorist groups.[12]

In terrorist incidents involving mass casualties, a situation similar to the aftermath of a disaster may ensue. It may take months or years for the society to find its equilibrium again.[13]

THE PSYCHIATRIST AND THE RESPONSE TO TERRORISM

Involvement of the psychiatrist or other mental health professional in an antiterrorist response means a significant departure from his normal role. From being a clinician delivering healthcare to patients, he becomes part of a law enforcement team to probe the psychopathology of a terrorist or terrorist group, to assist in threat evaluation, and to give advice as necessary during negotiations. This role requires a complete change of perspective in the usual practice of psychiatry.

As a rule, it would not be expected that psychiatrists or other mental health professionals would take a central and dramatic role in a terrorist and/or hostage-holding incident except in cases in which the psychiatrist has had previous professional involvement with the terrorist or when negotiations have reached the stage at which further rapport with the terrorist is thought to be possible via the psychiatrist. In spite of the desirability of such rapport, the psychiatrist must remain sensitive to the personalities and dynamics of the situation and guard against an undue identification with the interests of the terrorist. When asked to comment, the psychiatrist should refrain from replying in technical jargon that may prove incomprehensible or objectionable to police or military personnel. The advice should be offered in concise and practical terms.

Two main considerations render the participation of the psychiatrist in terrorist incidents necessary. First, such incidents put participants and law enforcement personnel under severe stress. Second, before a response can be planned, responding personnel must have an understanding of human behavior under stress and of the motivation and behavior patterns of psychotics or antisocial people or normal but stressed terrorists in a terrorist incident. The participatory roles therefore suggested for the psychiatrist are discussed below.

Police and Military Training

The psychiatrist may help in curriculum design and provide lectures involving topics such as the psychopathology of terrorist violence, reactions to stress, methods of coping under the stress of terrorist acts, captor-hostage relationships, threat evaluation, and negotiation techniques. The psychiatrist himself should have gone through such training courses to gain insight into problems for which he might be asked to find solutions.

Threat Analysis

In this instance, the psychiatrist is part of a multidisciplinary team drawn together to assess the credibility and seriousness of a threat of impending violence. His contribution will be related to the field of forensic psychiatry and profiling of the suspect.

Negotiations With Suspects

The psychiatrist generally cannot be assumed to be better qualified as a negotiator in a hostage-holding incident than a law enforcement officer, and, except for the circumstances listed earlier, it would be more appropriate for the psychiatrist to function mainly as an adviser to the main negotiator. Unlike the reality of most psychiatrists, the negotiator generally should be an articulate person of junior rank with a bland, unflappable personality. His junior rank allows him to defer decisions and buy time. Strong personalities tend to alienate hostage takers.

During the course of the negotiations, the psychiatrist should be on hand to detect any untoward effects that long, drawn-out negotiations may have on the negotiators and advise on remedial action. He may also prescribe medications for stress reactions or somatic disorders in hostages and possibly antipsychotic medications for hostage takers. A subsequent role that he can play is to assist in the postoperational review of the negotiations and to prevent post-traumatic stress sequelae among the surviving victims, rescuers, caregivers, and families.

In this context, it may be helpful to conduct formal debriefings of the surviving victims, rescuers, caregivers (eg, medical personnel) and, when feasible, families of victims. These are best done within days of the event, after everyone has rested. This debriefing can follow the civilian[14] critical incident stress debriefing model, the Marshall historical group debriefing model,[15] or several other variations.

Overall Postoperational Review Process

For the psychiatrist, valuable lessons may be learned from the incident regarding terrorist patterns of behavior and their impact on the victims and law enforcement personnel. He will also have an opportunity to assess the efficacy of his evaluation techniques and the success of his psychological management tactics. He may also be called on to comment on the performance of personnel placed under stress and to work out measures for improving his performance.[16]

Research on Terrorist Violence

The public media attention to terrorist activities continues to be provoked by terrorist abuses, indicating the need for mental health professionals to undertake further inquiries into this highly emotional subject. Research into this topic may improve techniques for threat evaluation and the conducting of hostage negotiations, serve to clarify the role of the psychiatrist as an adviser in the team, and help devise interventions for hostages who suffer posttraumatic reactions or persistent symptoms from their ordeals.

Other areas of involvement that require exploration are the acute and ongoing psychological needs and supports for the victims and the negotiating team. For example, one way of enhancing a victims' self-control during a hostage-holding incident is to provide advance consideration of the prospect of victimization. Ensuring his continued survival may depend on an appropriate behavior pattern based on understanding the psychological relationship between a captor and a victim.[17–19] A particularly vulnerable group of potential victims are diplomatic mission personnel, and following the Iranian hostages situation, many U.S. diplomats received ongoing training in this area.

THE AFTERMATH OF A TERRORIST INCIDENT

The conclusion of a terrorist incident may not mean the real ending of the affair for the psychiatrist. With the apprehension of the terrorist, the psychiatrist will most probably be called on to testify in court as to the sanity of or other testimony about the prisoner. By the very nature of his act, the terrorist raises the suspicion of harboring a mental illness or serious personality disorder. Those diagnosed as psychopathic in particular produce ambiguity. The lay public and sometimes the judiciary are often prejudiced one way or another on hearing such a classification.[10] But in the final analysis, the sentencing of either a psychotic or psychopathic terrorist should follow the letter of the law with the provision that appropriate treatment be provided if it is needed.

SUMMARY AND CONCLUSION

In the roles outlined above, it becomes apparent that the psychiatrist plays an active, interventionist role quite different from traditional office practice but quite similar to that of the combat psychiatrist. Like the transient, situationally induced malfunctions of combat, the stress-induced responses of all participants in a terrorist event will respond to an expectancy of return to normalcy, particularly when physiological needs have been restored and a central policy of intervention has been utilized. The logistics of the situation generally determine the proximity to the arena of action, and proximity, therefore, characterizes interventions taken both in terrorist incidents and combat.

In this chapter, we have attempted to bring into focus the psychiatric aspects of one of the sociopolitical phenomena of today's world and have briefly outlined some areas in which the psychiatrist—especially one working within the armed forces—may find himself a participating member. There is still much to be learned. Terrorism is a constantly changing phenomenon in form and intensity, and accordingly, the response to it must remain in dynamic flux.

REFERENCES

1. Bleich A, Dycian A, Koslowsky M, Soloman Z, Wiener M. Psychiatric implication of missile attacks on a civilian population: Israeli lessons from the Persian Gulf War. *JAMA*. 1992;268(5):613–615.

2. Jenkins BM. *The Lessons of Beirut: Testimony Before the Long Commission.* Santa Monica, Calif: Rand Corporation; 1984.

3. Richburg KB. UN's Somalia quandary: Search for warlord said to limit military options. *Washington Post.* 8 August 1993, vol 116:A19.

4. U.S. Department of the Army. *The Army Combatting Terrorism Program.* Washington, DC: DA; 26 June 1992. Army Regulation 525–13.

5. National Advisory Committee on Criminal Justice Standards and Goals. *Disorders and Terrorism.* National Advisory Committee on Criminal Justice Standards and Goals. Washington, DC: GPO; 1976. Task Force Report. GPO stock no. 052–003–00224–8.

6. US Department of the Army. *Leader's Manual for Combat Stress Control.* Washington DC: DA; In press, 1994. Field Manual 22–51.

7. *Combat Stress Control in Operations Other Than War.* Draft white paper. Preliminary draft FM 8–51–1, CSC in 00TU.

8. Kaplan A. The ethics of terror. In: B Eichelman, DA Soskis, WH Reid, eds. *Terrorism: Interdisciplinary Perspectives.* Washington DC: American Psychiatric Press; 1983: 5–29.

9. Munge P. *Approaching Zero: The Extraordinary Underworld of Hackers, Phreakers, Virus Writers, and Keyboard Criminals.* New York: Random House; 1992.

10. Jenkins B. Research in terrorism: Areas of consensus, area of ignorance. In: B Eichelman, DA Soskis, WH Reid eds. *Terrorism: Interdisciplinary Perspectives.* Washington DC: American Psychiatric Press; 1983: 153–177.

11. Hammel EM. *The Root: The Marines in Beirut, August 1982–February 1984.* San Diego: Harcourt Brace Jovanovich; 1985.

12. Kelley K. *The Longest War: Northern Ireland and the IRA.* Westport, Conn: L. Hill, 1988.

13. Lyons HA. Psychiatric sequelae of the Belfast riots. *Br J Psychiatry.* 1971;118:265.

14. Mitchell JT. Demobilizations. *Life Net* (Newsletter of the American Critical Incidence Stress Foundation). 1991;2(1):8–9.

15. Marshall SLA. *Bringing Up the Rear: A Memoir.* San Rafael, Calif: Presidio Press; 1979.

16. Lancely F, DeSarno J. *Advanced Hostage Negotiation Course.* Quantico, Va: Federal Bureau of Investigation Academy; 1982.

17. Jenkins BM. *Hostage Survival: Some Preliminary Observations.* Rand Corporation. 1976. Typescript.

18. Cooper HHA. The terrorist and the victim. *Victimology.* 1976;1(2):229–239.

19. Jacobson SR. Individual and group responses to confinement in a skyjacked plane. *Am J Orthopsychiatry.* 1973;43(3):459–469.

Chapter 17

MILITARY PSYCHIATRY AND HOSTAGE NEGOTIATION

FRANKLIN D. JONES, M.D., F.A.P.A.*

*Colonel (ret), Medical Corps, U.S. Army; Clinical Professor, Uniformed Services University of the Health Sciences; Past President and Secretary and Current Honorary President of the Military Section, World Psychiatric Association

INTRODUCTION

The principles of treating combat stress casualties were derived empirically during World War I[1] although their anlage can be seen in the treatment of nostalgia developed by Larrey as quoted in Rosen[2] during the Napoleonic Wars. These principles for treating the acute, situational-induced symptoms of combat stress can be usefully applied to the handling of stress experienced by hostages. The role of the mental health worker in a hostage situation, however, is of broader scope than just treating the victims. This chapter will address that role during the various phases of hostage negotiation.

Hostage negotiation as a legitimate strategy for handling certain forms of criminal behavior is of relatively recent origin. Following the terrorist attack at the 1972 Munich Olympics, the New York Police Department (NYPD)[3] pioneered the development of the principles and techniques of hostage negotiation under the leadership of Harvey Schlossberg, Ph.D., a psychologist who had been an NYPD patrolman. His work was furthered by collaboration with another NYPD officer, Frank A. Bolz.[4,5] Since then, others ranging from psychiatrists[6] to labor negotiators[3] have added to the current consensus on how such situations should be handled. The first application of formal hostage-negotiation techniques developed by the NYPD occurred during the takeover of a sporting goods store by African-American Muslims in January 1973.[3] Since then, there have been numerous, almost always successful, negotiations.[3]

TYPES OF HOSTAGE SITUATIONS

There appear to be three main types of hostage situations that differ according to the personalities and intentions and, to some extent, the victims of the hostage taker. Because these differences are relevant to the negotiation, they will be addressed briefly.

Criminal

With the advent of the widespread usage of silent alarm warning systems in the United States, criminals caught in the criminal act have become a major source of hostage taking. The purpose of the hostage taker is to escape from the law and the victims are likely to be a cross-section of middle-class persons who work at or frequent banks or stores.[3] Another hostage situation involving criminals can occur during riots in prisons. In these situations, the hostage takers are likely to be multiple and include a range of criminal backgrounds; the hostages may include unlucky visitors in addition to prison guards or authorities against whom some prisoners may hold grudges.

The hostage-taker personality type is likely to be antisocial or inadequate and immature. The negotiator advantage is that such individuals are usually acting out of their own rational self-interest so that harm to the hostages may be less likely. Disadvantages in the case of the antisocial, in particular, are that he seldom develops positive feelings toward his captives, and he may have an extensive prior criminal record so that he feels he has nothing to lose by further violence. In addition, the antisocial, like some terrorists, usually has a callous disregard for his captives.[3,7]

The immature or inadequate criminal is more likely to develop positive feelings toward captives and is likely to be inept, giving hostages more chances to escape. Disadvantages of negotiating with the immature hostage taker are that his demands tend to be exorbitant, and his own ineptitude may lead to unintended violence.[3]

Domestic

The victims of the domestic hostage taker are usually relatives, often spouses and children; however, friends and suspected lovers may become captives.[5] Such hostage takers often suffer from severe mental illness rather than personality disorders, making them less amenable to rational discourse. In addition, in some cases, particularly those in which the captor is severely depressed, the hostage-taking incident often shades into a suicidal or homicidal/suicidal act.[3]

Often hostage takers in domestic situations are found to have schizophrenic and bipolar illnesses, especially when paranoid thinking is present. In such cases, imagined enemies, public officials, and innocent bystanders are frequent victims.[3]

Unlike the inadequate personality who makes exorbitant demands, the antisocial who makes moderate demands or the depressed person who usually makes no demands other than to be left alone, the paranoid schizophrenic makes strange demands. In January 1976, Miklos Petrovicks, a hostage taker later found to be mentally ill, was called "the birdseed bandit" because of his demands that tons of birdseed be distributed at banks in Los Angeles.[3]

Terrorist

There have been few terrorist hostage-taking incidents in the United States; however, many Americans stationed in other countries have been such victims. Only three groups, the Puerto Rican nationalists Fuerza Allianza Libertad Nacional (FALN), the Croatian nationalists, and the Cuban Freedom Fighters have been active in the United States. There have also been sporadic incidents such as the Symbionese Liberation Army abduction of Patricia Hearst,[8] the Hanafi Muslim takeover of federal government offices,[9] the Jewish Defense League activities,[10] and the 1993 World Trade Center bombing in New York City by Muslim fundamentalists.[11] Federal Bureau of Investigation (FBI) studies[7] have revealed a fairly standard organizational profile of terrorist groups. The leader is usually an ideologue, often of upper class or middle-class upbringing, usually considered to be honest and upright, although ruthless, and usually well-educated. The leader furnishes the ideological rationale for the terrorist activities. In the FALN, the leadership includes college professors and lawyers.[3,7]

Followers frequently use the group as a family substitute. They may be quite dedicated but have usually been "losers" in life with immature personalities, job instability, and sexual problems. The third element, which often plays a leadership role during incidents of violence, is primarily criminal, usually with antisocial tendencies. In the Symbionese Liberation Army, this figure was Cinque, a man with a long criminal record.[3,7]

The motives of the terrorist are usually quite different from those of the common criminal, such as a Mafia "enforcer," although the method is similar—coercion of others by inducing overwhelming fear (terror). The victim is an integral part of the attack and is often chosen for purposes of demonstrating the impotence of constituted authority. For this reason, the innocent are as likely, or even more likely because they are unprotected, to be victims as those in authority.[3,7]

PRINCIPLES OF HOSTAGE NEGOTIATION

Two assumptions make hostage negotiations differ from other forms of kidnapping: (1) confrontation is necessary; that is, the hostage taker is potentially within the control of the law enforcement agency with reasonably direct communication with him being possible; and (2) it is not in the criminal's interest to do violence to the hostage.

When hostages have been taken, one or more of several courses of action by law enforcement personnel are possible. These possibilities are listed below in decreasing order of preference:

- Contain, isolate, and negotiate.
- Contain, isolate, and demand surrender.
- Use chemical agents to flush out.
- Use sharpshooters to wound or kill.
- Assault the barricaded hostage taker.

Negotiation, the first alternative, will result in the safe release of hostages in 97% of cases.[3] The failure of this alternative can later allow escalation to the other more dangerous (for police and hostages) alternatives. In a study[3] of a number of incidents in which assault was the alternative chosen, 65 hostages and 355 law enforcement agents were involved. Assault resulted in the deaths of 3% of participants during negotiations, and 12% died during assaults. One problem with the use of sharpshooters is that the hostage taker may have or claim to have a bomb.[3]

Chemical agents produce risks of fires (for example, the Symbionese Liberation Army home was probably burned down from ignition by a tear gas grenade at a time when Patricia Hearst was still thought to be a hostage[3]), chemical pneumonia and respiratory problems among hostages, and risks the deaths of hostages because chemicals work too slowly to incapacitate the hostage taker before he has a chance to kill the hostages. In addition, in these times of specialization, some hostage takers may have gas masks. Similarly, a demand for surrender can push the hostage taker into violence directed at hostages.

Hostage reactions are similar to those of disaster victims, with three types described by Tyhurst.[12] These may be universal responses to sudden, unexpected, life-disrupting events:

1. *Effectives* may take independent action dangerous to the group.
2. *Ineffectives*, those who are hysterical or agitated, mainly pose a danger to themselves by irritating the hostage taker.
3. *Dependents* readily develop the Stockholm syndrome; they do what they are told to do.[3]

The Stockholm syndrome refers to the positive feelings that develop on the part of the hostages toward their captor which engender similar positive feelings by the captor toward his captives.[3] It is the task of the hostage negotiator to try to encourage development of the dependent category because experience has shown them to be most likely to survive. Interestingly, the effectives and ineffectives do best in the long run (if they survive); the Stockholm syndrome usually does not develop in them.[3]

THE NEGOTIATION

The hostage negotiator should be a relatively junior law enforcement officer who is in good physical health, is good with words, and is of rather placid temperament. If he is of higher rank, he may not be able to stall for time by claiming a need to consult with a superior; that is, he will have too much authority to make decisions. Also senior officials generally do not have the desired placid temperament; if they did, they would not have become senior officials.[3]

The basic approach of the negotiator is to stall for time until the fundamental human needs, both biological and psychological, will force the hostage taker to make concessions. The skillful use of time will also reduce anxiety and increase rationality in the hostage taker, which should reduce his expectations. Time will frequently produce rapport between the hostage taker and negotiator, thus increasing the negotiator's ability to influence the hostage taker. Finally, time will often allow the formation of the Stockholm syndrome.

An unfortunate but inevitable additional element of the Stockholm syndrome is the formation of negative feelings of the hostages toward law enforcement personnel. The negotiator, nevertheless, attempts to foster the Stockholm syndrome because it becomes a powerful factor in the survival of the hostages. The development of the Stockholm syndrome is a normal, survival-oriented adaptation to an abnormal situation. This tendency to cling to a person who has the power of life or death over one may have roots in the instinctual behavior of man's hominid ancestors,[13] and this same instinctual matrix may account for similar behavior on the part of battered spouses and children.[3,14]

The negotiator may foster this development by asking about hostages through the hostage taker and by furnishing bulk food that requires the captor and captives to work together in its preparation. Similarly, the hostage taker may be induced to become responsible for disbursement of medications to hostages who often have stress-induced medical problems. Because he can prescribe medications, the psychiatric consultant is of particular value in this situation.

Other than stalling for time during which biological and psychological variables can be manipulated, the negotiator has certain guidelines to follow with regard to handling demands, including those from the media. These guidelines take into account the police priorities (established by the NYPD) and are listed below.

1. Preserve the lives of the hostages, the public, police, and hostage taker.
2. Apprehend hostage taker.
3. Recover and protect property.

Experience[3,4] has shown in terms of the demands made by hostage takers that some items are negotiable and some are not. These demands are listed in Table 17–1.

Regarding hostage demands, the negotiator attempts to avoid giving anything without getting some concessions in return, avoids suggesting possible demands, avoids offering anything unless it is requested, avoids giving more than is requested, and avoids dismissing any demand as being trivial. In terms of the developing biological needs, food, water, and amenities (such as portable toilets, air conditioning, and so forth) become preeminent and should not be given away without gaining concessions despite one's humanitarian impulses.

Alcoholic beverages are frequently requested by criminal hostage takers and usually they should not be given unless it is known that the hostage taker's

TABLE 17–1

HOSTAGE TAKER DEMANDS

ITEM	NEGOTIABLE	SITUATIONAL	NONNEGOTIABLE
Food	X		
Water	X		
Amenities	X		
Money	X		
Alcohol		X	
Transportation		X	
Media Coverage		X	
Weapons			X
Exchange Hostages			X

Source: Adapted with permission from Lancely F, DeSarno J. *Advanced Hostage Negotiation Course.* Quantico, Va: FBI Academy; 11–22 January 1982.

response to alcohol is benign, such as falling asleep.[3] Transportation is usually demanded, and, if given, frequently creates problems in command (who is in charge local, military, federal, or airline officials), in communication (telephones and other systems may not be available), and in control (the captor may escape and continue to keep the hostages).[3]

If possible, demands for media coverage should only be met after the hostage taker has surrendered. Crowd control can become a very serious problem and can produce unnecessary loss of life. Media coverage can exacerbate this problem as well as create problems in the negotiation. For example, television reports showing heavily armed special weapons and tactics (SWAT) teams can deter a subject from surrendering.[3]

Although the hostage taker is not told so (he is stalled), weapons and exchange of hostages (with rare exceptions) are not negotiable demands. The reason for not giving weapons is obvious; however, the rationale for not exchanging hostages is not so obvious. For example, some countries may consider giving hostages in exchange for visiting dignitaries taken hostage to avoid involving friendly countries in a terrorist incident and also to use this exchange as a sign of good faith during the negotiations. The reasons for not exchanging, however, are persuasive and have to do with the willingness of the hostage taker to kill those under his control or himself.

The hostage taker may feel less guilt in killing a law enforcement official than an innocent bystander whom he has captured. Killing an authority may be more likely also in terms of the hostage taker's self-esteem; that is, more prestige is associated with killing a policeman or government official. The person demanded by the hostage taker may well be someone whom he wishes to kill but otherwise does not have the opportunity. Even if the person requested is a relative, especially a spouse, this person may be the desired victim or the deranged hostage taker may wish the person demanded to be present as an audience for his suicide. The presence of persons significant to the participants may, at minimum, increase the tension level and hinder one of the aims of the negotiation, decreasing tension and increasing rationality. The exchanged person can also increase the tension level if he is a trained law enforcement official because he will be viewed as a greater threat.

Finally, even if the exchanged person would not increase tension for reasons mentioned, he would still disrupt the nascent development of the Stockholm syndrome. Probably such exchanges should only be made in desperate circumstances in which the exchange is used as a ploy in anticipation of an assault operation.

MENTAL HEALTH PROFESSIONALS AND HOSTAGE NEGOTIATION

The military mental health professional is likely to be called on during hostage-negotiation procedures because of availability and presumed knowledge of crisis situations. It is important for the professional to be familiar with the basic principles of hostage negotiation outlined above and of the usages to which his expertise can best be put. It is also important for him to know how he should not be utilized. In a recent misuse of a mental health professional, a well-known Baltimore psychiatrist was asked by police to approach an airplane hijacker face-to-face and unprotected.[15] The mental health professional must remain in the consultant role except, perhaps, in the rare instance in which the hostage taker is his patient. The professional rarely has the knowledge of police resources and methodology or has the correct temperament for the hostage-negotiator role.[3]

In the consultant role, he can offer expert advice about the psychological and, if a psychiatrist, the medical aspects of the situation. He can usually help the negotiator to understand which of the personality types or illnesses are found in the hostage taker and possible responses that can be expected. For example, he can often advise of the need for immediate gratification and low frustration tolerance of the antisocial, the suspiciousness of innocent actions of the paranoid, and the degree of suicidal potential of the depressed hostage taker. He can also help arrange for appropriate treatment of a mentally ill hostage taker and occasionally may even begin that treatment during negotiations.

As an observer of the effects of stress and fatigue on the negotiator and other team members, he can warn of the loss of objectivity and need for replacement. In addition, the expertise of the negotiator is widely variable ranging from very sophisticated, trained negotiators to first-time rookies. He can aid the latter negotiator to understand the negotiation process and its expected course.

The mental health professional may also play a role during the negotiation in helping to relieve the distress of relatives of the participants, especially of the hostages. This role is primarily in terms of support, reassurance, and sometimes anxiolytic medication. In prolonged situations such as those that occurred in the capture of the USS *Pueblo* by North Korea[16] or the takeover of the U.S. Embassy in Iran, this can be a most important role.[17] Further, in such prolonged incarcerations, mental health personnel are important in planning the decompression (initial release) and follow-up handling of such hostages and families. Even after brief episodes, postincident help may be appropriate, particularly in ameliorating the unwanted aspects of the Stockholm syndrome.

The application of combat psychiatric principles[18] is most appropriate in handling the victims of a hostage taking. They begin with treating as proximally and quickly as possible (proximity and immediacy). With hostages, this treatment starts with a "decompression" period, immediately after release, allowing a respite from demands and responsibilities. This initial intervention is brief and involves physiological restoration through rest, sleep, and alimentation. Complicated psychodynamic formulations are avoided to make the point that the victim is not ill but had a normal reaction to the circumstances (principle of simplicity). This approach is especially important if the victim has guilt about "collaborating" with the hostage taker to save his own life and "survivor guilt" if deaths have occurred.

Critical incident stress debriefing[19] or historical group debriefing[20] to abreact, clarify, reconcile, and gain cognitive mastery over the traumatic memories may be useful. This debriefing can be done one-on-one with individual victims and, even better, in groups with multiple hostages. It is also worthwhile for the negotiator teams, SWAT teams, snipers, and medical caregivers, especially if the incident did not resolve happily.

These interventions should create an expectation that the individual is normal and will quickly return to normal functioning (principle of expectancy). The expectation of compensation, on the other hand, even if only in the form of special consideration, can undermine this approach and lead to disability.

The final principle of centrality, or echelon treatment, is important because the natural supports in the victim's environment are substituted for the mental health worker as soon as possible to avoid the development of a dependent relationship.

SUMMARY AND CONCLUSION

In summary, a body of knowledge exists concerning the personality types of hostage takers and the psychological responses of their victims. Mastery of this knowledge and application of principles derived from the treatment of combat psychiatric casualties will allow the mental health professional to play a variety of roles in the various phases of a hostage negotiation, drawing on his expertise in human behavior.

REFERENCES

1. Salmon TW. *The Care and Treatment of Mental Disease and War Neuroses ("Shell Shock") in the British Army.* New York: War Work Committee of the National Committee for Mental Hygiene, Inc.; 1917.

2. Rosen G. Nostalgia: A "forgotten" psychological disorder. *Psychol Med.* 1975;5:340–354.

3. Lancely F, DeSarno J. *Advanced Hostage Negotiation Course.* Quantico, Va: FBI Academy; 11–22 January 1982.

4. Bolz F, Jr. The hostage situation: Law enforcement options. In: Eichelman B, Soskis DA, Reid WH, eds. *Terrorism: Interdisciplinary Perspectives.* Washington, DC: American Psychiatric Association; 1983: 99–116.

5. Hassel C. Preparing law enforcement personnel for terrorist incidents. In: Eichelman B, Soskis DA, Reid WH, eds. *Terrorism: Interdisciplinary Perspectives.* Washington, DC: American Psychiatric Association; 1983. 117–128.

6. Ochberg F. Victims of terrorism: Psychiatric considerations. *Terrorism: An International Journal.* 1978;1(1):147–168.

7. Special Operations and Research Staff (SOARS), Federal Bureau of Investigation Academy. *Terrorist Organizational Profile: A Psychological Role Model.* Quantico, Va: SOARS, FBI Academy; 1982.

8. Payne L. *The Life and Death of the SLA.* New York: Ballantine Books; 1976.

9. National Advisory Committee on Criminal Justice Standards and Goals. *Disorders and Terrorism.* Washington, DC: GPO; 1976.

10. Dolgin JL. *Jewish Identity and the JDL.* Princeton, NJ: Princeton University Press; 1977.

11. Wright R, Ostrow RJ. Incident may signal new round of terrorist action (bombing of NYC's World Trade Center). *Los Angeles Times.* 28 February 1993, Vol 112:A1.

12. Tyhurst JS. Individual reactions to community disaster: The natural history of psychiatric phenomena. *Am J Psychiatry.* 1951;107:764–769.

13. Wilson EO. *Sociobiology: The New Synthesis.* Cambridge, Mass: Belknap Press of Harvard University Press; 1975.

14. Ochberg F. Hostage victims. In: Eichelman B, Soskis DA, Reid WH, eds. *Terrorism: Interdisciplinary Perspectives.* Washington, DC: American Psychiatric Association; 1983: 83–88.

15. Lion J. Personal Communication, March 1981.

16. Spaulding RC. The *Pueblo* incident: Medical problems reported during captivity and physical findings at the time of the crew's release. *Milit Med.* 1977;142(9):681–684.

17. Jones FD. Personal Communication. 1981.

18. Jones FD, Johnson AW. Medical and psychiatric treatment policy and practice in Vietnam. *J Soc Issues.* 1975;31(4):49–65.

19. Mitchell JT. Demobilizations. *Life Net* (Newsletter of the American Critical Incidence Stress Foundation). 1991;2(1):8–9.

20. Marshall SLA. *Bringing Up the Rear: A Memoir.* San Rafael, Calif: Presidio Press; 1979.

Chapter 18

PSYCHIATRIC EFFECTS OF DISASTER IN THE MILITARY COMMUNITY

PAUL T. BARTONE, PH.D.,* KATHLEEN M. WRIGHT, PH.D.,† AND ALAN RADKE, M.D.‡

*Major, Medical Service Corps, U.S. Army; Commander, U.S. Army Medical Research Unit—Europe; Headquarters and Headquarters Company, 7th MEDCOM, USAMRU–E, APO 09102–4428; Department of Military Psychiatry; Walter Reed Army Institute of Research, Washington, D.C.

†Department of Military Psychiatry; Walter Reed Army Institute of Research, Washington, D.C. 20307–5100

‡Medical Director, Willmar Regional Treatment Center, Willmar, Minnesota 56201; U.S. Army Reserve Psychiatrist and former Director, Psychiatric Education and Research, Walter Reed Army Medical Center, Washington, D.C.

INTRODUCTION

This chapter describes the characteristics of military communities and their responses to disasters. The Gander air disaster is explored in depth to exemplify the mental health approaches to handling such disasters and possible applications to combat stress.

Military Communities as *Gemeinschaft*

In the last several decades, many social and economic changes have occurred that seem to have predicted the end of the small, tightly knit community. It is now unusual for one's neighbors to also be one's friends or coworkers. Especially in metropolitan areas, people commute over longer and longer distances to get to work. Communities-of-place where people live, work, and socialize together are increasingly uncommon. Sarason[1] has described these and other social changes as resulting in a damaging loss of the psychological sense of community that is important to human well-being.

Sociologists have described in greater depth the changes that have led to a loss of the traditional sense of community, changes that primarily have to do with increased industrialization and the shift away from agrarian-based economies and lifestyles. Tonnies[2] provides the useful concepts of *gemeinschaft*, or communities involving implicit bonds, common values, and mutual dependency, and *gesellschaft*, communities where relationships are rule-bound, formalized, and explicit. Durkheim[3] made a similar distinction between an earlier form of community, *mechanical solidarity*, based on shared customs, beliefs, and face-to-face interactions, and the more recent *organic solidarity*, based on the interdependence of functionally distinct units in a society marked by specialization and division of labor. For Durkheim, more so than for Tonnies, the roots of the earlier, more basic form of community are thought to persist, providing an essential framework for social solidarity even as society changes and becomes more specialized.[4] For Tonnies, *gemeinschaft* communities are essentially a thing of the past because societies have grown larger and more industrialized.

Military communities in some ways provide an exception to this rule, still appearing as more *gemeinschaft* than *gesellschaft* in quality. Such communities encompass the families of military personnel assigned to a particular locale or post, as well as nonmilitary workers engaged in providing goods and services for military members and their families. Unlike most modern civilian communities, members of military communities are distinctively bound together by a common overall work mission and by a concentration of services, homes, and activities in a well-defined geographic space, the traditional military post.

Despite their unusual qualities, it would be naive to consider modern military communities as strictly *gemeinschaft*; they are marked by the same division of labor and formalized and highly individuated roles as pertain in modern nonmilitary communities. Still, the lines of *gemeinschaft* (or mechanical solidarity) are still quite strong in military communities. Unlike modern American nonmilitary communities, which increasingly appear as fragmented collections of strangers, American military posts are usually self-contained communities-of-place, with well-defined borders and clear rules of membership. Members of such communities usually reside on or near post, where they have military and community facilities to meet most of their needs (that is, schools, banks, commissary, child-care services, automobile service stations, restaurants, post office, bowling alley, and so forth). This is particularly true in overseas and rural posts. Consequently, there is more face-to-face contact among members of military communities.

Still, it is important to remember that military communities are not immutable, and they are not isolated from the larger communities in which they are embedded. Military families come and go; service members must move to new assignments every few years. Military communities also have various ties to surrounding civilian communities. The most apparent links are based on economic exchange. Many service members live in offpost housing, paying rent to local landlords and interacting with nonmilitary neighbors. Military family members often hold jobs in the civilian sector. Goods and services not available on post (for example, cars, furniture, certain banking services, and entertainment) are purchased from nearby civilian establishments. Thus, a significant amount of economic and social exchange occurs between military communities and their surrounding civilian communities. Members of a military community are members of other communities as well, with religious, political, social, and family ties that extend far beyond the post borders. The modern military community is united with larger, superordinate communities at the local, state, national, and world levels through the power of print and broadcast media, especially television. Still, the military community retains more *gemeinschaft* qualities of organization than, perhaps, any other large type of American community today. As will be discussed in the sections to follow, this aspect of social organization may have important consequences for how the military community responds to disaster.

Disaster and the Military Community

Even during peacetime, the military occupation entails unusual risks. Military communities routinely confront the loss of some community members through fatal training accidents and, somewhat less commonly, large-scale air disasters or terrorist attacks.[5] Such traumatic incidents require individuals and whole communities to adjust to sudden, unexpected, and sometimes massive loss. Through their actions before and after a disaster, military psychiatrists and mental health workers can influence the course of recovery in either a positive or negative direction. In December 1985, a U.S. Army transport plane crashed in Canada, killing all 248 soldiers on board. This military disaster provided an opportunity to explore responses to trauma in the military community and to observe the effects of various interventions.

THE GANDER AIR DISASTER

The Fatal Crash

On December 12, 1985, a jet chartered by the U.S. Army stopped at Gander, Newfoundland, to refuel. The flight was carrying 248 soldiers home to Fort Campbell, Kentucky, following 6 months of peacekeeping duty in the Sinai. This flight was the second of three flights transporting soldiers back to the United States. After refueling in somewhat icy conditions, the heavily loaded DC–8 departed for its final destination, Fort Campbell. Shortly after takeoff, the plane apparently stalled, lost altitude, and rolled sharply to the right. As it crashed into the heavily forested terrain, the aircraft disintegrated, and fuel tanks exploded, scattering bodies and debris over a wide area. Subsequent fires burned for over 14 hours, while a blizzard covered the crash site with snow and ice.[5]

Early Aftermath

At Fort Campbell, some of the families had already assembled at the airfield to welcome the soldiers home for the Christmas holiday. Word of the tragedy reached the Brigade Headquarters at Fort Campbell about 1 hour after the crash. During the next several hours, efforts to confirm the flight manifest were initiated while families were asked to assemble in the gymnasium. There, the Brigade Commander announced that while the report was still unconfirmed, the awaited plane had apparently crashed in Canada, leaving no survivors.[5]

U.S. officials worked together with Canadian authorities to organize crash-site search and recovery operations. Recovery of remains from the site was a long and gruesome process. The fire that followed the crash had melted snow on the ground, which later froze solid over bodies, body parts, and debris. It was necessary to erect heated tents to free remains from the ice. The smell of burnt and rotting flesh mixed with jet fuel was overpowering for many of the people working in these enclosures. Once recovered, bodies were flown to the mortuary at Dover Air Force Base in Delaware for autopsy and identification. This process continued for nearly 3 months and eventually involved over 120 professional workers and 400 volunteers.[5]

In addition to various support personnel, the army death toll included fully one-third of the infantry peace-keeping battalion. The Gander crash represents the largest single-incident loss to a battalion in U.S. Army history and the worst aviation disaster ever on Canadian soil. Approximately one-third of the dead were married and had maintained homes at Fort Campbell. Thirty-six children were left fatherless.[5]

In the first days following the crash, several memorial ceremonies were held at Fort Campbell, with specialized services provided for bereaved families and friends. The devastated battalion was reconstituted over the Christmas holidays and resumed normal training activities about 2 weeks after Christmas. It was nearly 3 months after the crash before the last set of remains was positively identified at Dover Air Force Base and returned to the family for burial.[5]

Disaster in Two Communities

Although not a "typical" community disaster—involving destruction of homes and disruption of essential services—the Gander crash was a human disaster for both the military communities of Dover Air Force Base and Fort Campbell. At Dover, the large number of bodies commanded the attention and resources of the entire community for over 2 months. Even those who were not directly involved in morgue operations were called on in a variety of ways to respond to the influx of outsiders and the special demands this placed on local supplies and services. Several major planned activities were postponed or canceled. Intensive media scrutiny ensured that the entire community was aware of the progress (or lack thereof) in body identifications. Children, teachers, parents, and clergy discussed the crash itself, the horrific condition of the bodies, the body identification process, the media, and other matters related to the tragedy.[5]

That the event was a major community disaster for Fort Campbell is also clear. Unlike many air disasters in which the victims are strangers from scattered locations, these soldiers all lived and worked together at Fort Campbell for nearly 2 years. Even for those not personal friends or relatives of the dead, there is still a close affinity and identification with them that derive from a shared occupation, lifestyle, and organizational commitment. Not just relatives, but the entire post community was shocked by the news and experienced a collective blow. In the hours and days immediately following the crash, all nonessential activities around the post ceased while attention focused on dealing with the crisis. Regular schedules were suspended, and a series of special responses were initiated. Planned community Christmas activities were canceled or radically modified. Quarantelli[6] defines community disaster as a collective, extreme stress situation disruptive to a community. By this definition, the Gander crash was undoubtedly a community disaster for Fort Campbell.[5]

We examine responses to the Gander crash at the two military posts most directly affected, Dover Air Force Base and Fort Campbell. We consider these communities as essentially *gemeinschaft* in quality, a perspective that we feel is very helpful in identifying effective intervention strategies to facilitate healthy community recovery from disaster. The data on which this report is based come from interviews and observations collected over the 6 months following the crash. During the first 4 weeks, members of the research team observed events and reactions at both locations. Members of the research team in addition to the authors were Larry H. Ingraham, Christine Russell, Mark A. Vaitkus, Robert J. Ursano, Carol Fullerton, and Raymond Cervantes. Activities at Fort Campbell were observed during the first week after the crash and again during week four. Activities at Dover Air Force Base, including inside the mortuary, were observed for 3 day-long periods spread over the first 4 weeks after the crash. Observers functioned unobtrusively as much as possible, focusing on behaviors and events and recording observations in notebooks. Approximately 65 hours of observations were recorded at Dover during this period and 150 hours at Fort Campbell. These observations were assembled and integrated during field meetings of the research team held at Fort Campbell and team meetings held at Walter Reed Army Institute of Research following data collection.

Following this observation period, indepth interviews were conducted at both locations over the 2- to 6-month period after the crash. Specific individuals and groups known to have been intimately involved and affected by events were targeted for interview. The interview procedure followed a debriefing format, which encourages a chronological recounting of events as well as related thoughts, feelings, and actions of respondents.[7] Approximately 60 individuals from Dover were interviewed and 85 from Fort Campbell. These included both military and civilian community leaders, unit commanders, mental health workers, community support providers (for example, post Red Cross and Army Community Service workers), chaplains, medical personnel, morgue workers, casualty workers, widows, soldiers, and friends of the dead. See Wright,[5] Bartone,[8] and Ursano[9] for some of the original interview source material.

Dover Air Force Base

Dover Air Force Base, the Department of Defense port mortuary on the east coast, was selected as the site for processing of remains. The Gander crash occurred on Thursday; the first bodies arrived at Dover the following Monday. Body carrying cases continued to arrive for the next 3 weeks. Each flight carrying bodies from Gander was met by a full ceremonial honor guard to unload the flag-draped coffins. Once inside the mortuary, the cases were opened, and the contents carefully examined and catalogued. Each set of remains was then processed through a series of workstations in a morgue that had been specially configured for this task.

The attentions of three groups from outside the community converged on Dover. One was the news media. The Gander crash was a national news event, and some reporters went so far as to fly over the morgue in a hot-air balloon to take photographs of the operation. Next were various officials from the army, air force, and other government agencies based in Washington, DC. Many conflicting directives were issued by these outside officials who claimed authority in the situation. Initially there was some confusion because of the magnitude of the disaster itself, and thus, during those first days, time and energy of the Dover Air Force Base personnel were spent satisfying the demands of high-ranking visitors who came through to briefly observe the operation. Finally, many families and friends of the dead converged on Dover. Some travelled to the post and asked to view the remains of their loved one. Many telephoned seeking information. Fritz observed that such "convergence behavior"[10(p678)] was very common in disaster situations and often greatly complicates problems of coordination and control.

It is difficult for anyone not present to imagine the horror of the scene in the "body room" of the mortuary. In the words of one volunteer worker:

> We did not have enough bits and pieces for 256 people. . . . The entire back of the mortuary had transfer cases lined up. Every one of the transfer cases and body bags were opened. There were 50 remains there. There was a big wall with a blackboard that had charts on it. As they opened up the casket, they would look at the chart and give it a number and draw a picture of the torso on the board. They would scratch out on a torso what was missing. When a leg was found, they would go back and see which one of the torsos was missing a leg and see if it would match. It was very gruesome. We were standing there surrounded by gross remains. They had various degrees of completeness, and all of them were burned beyond recognition.

> There were so many of them, and we were right amongst them. It was very depressing. . . . In the first several days, there was a captain whose upper torso was intact. He was in the mortuary on a table for 2 months. We eventually found his legs and put them in a box with him.

Observation and interview data document common stress-related symptoms and problems among the morgue workers. These are described in more detail elsewhere.[5,9,11] The reactions most commonly observed and reported were trouble sleeping, frightening nightmares, depression, jumpiness, dizziness, shaking and trembling, fear of losing control, nausea, a sense of choking, washing compulsions, and heavy alcohol consumption. Problems appeared more common among volunteer morgue workers (who were also younger) than among pathologists and other medical professionals. Regarding eating problems, the following was reported by a supervisor of "body handlers" (volunteer morgue workers):

> The first night someone made the mistake of serving roast beef. Body handlers do not want to eat barbecued ribs. We eat right on the scene. I had to review the menu myself.

Even experienced professionals were not immune from such reactions:

> Dr. (X) of AFIP (Armed Forces Institute of Pathology) cannot eat barbecued chicken to this day. Dr. (Y) cannot eat barbecued ribs, and the dental surgeon in the (UNIT) cannot eat barbecued food.

Several cases of acute stress reaction in the morgue were so severe the workers had to be relieved by their supervisors. Over the next 6 months, there were three documented cases of post-traumatic stress disorder at Dover Air Force Base related to the Gander morgue operation. And although there is no definitive connection to the Gander disaster, a mini-epidemic of suicides and suicide attempts occurred among Dover community adolescents about 3 months after the crash.

Fort Campbell

The residents of Fort Campbell were physically far removed from the grim scenes of the Dover mortuary, a circumstance that contributed to an air of unreality in the community. Initial reactions were primarily disbelief and shock. Less than Dover, the post community still became an object of media attention. Families were of primary concern. There was a memorial service on Monday attended by President and Mrs. Reagan, the Secretary of the Army, and other dignitaries. The overwhelming sense was one of loss felt by the entire community, accompanied by an outpouring of concern for families and friends. Fort Campbell did not appear to experience the confusion in channels of authority and control seen in the early phase at Dover.

A sensitive, charismatic, and highly respected commanding general of the division and post asserted leadership and control from the beginning. He mobilized his staff with clear directions regarding what their actions should be. In several timely public appearances and news conferences, he shared his views and guidance, affirming his leadership role in the crisis. This pattern was repeated by key subordinate leaders so that a consistent message was broadcast to the post community. The essence of this message was as follows:

- We must first care for the grieving families.
- We must recover and pay homage to our dead comrades.
- We must experience and accept our own pain and help each other deal with it.
- We must direct our energies to the continuing mission with renewed commitment and dedication.

This message was reinforced by the example set by the leaders themselves.

Several leaders in the Fort Campbell community assumed critical roles in the mourning process, apparently solidifying the community in the aftermath of the Gander crash. For example, at the planned homecoming in the gymnasium where families were awaiting the arrival of soldiers, the brigade commander stood and spoke to the group. He communicated news of the crash in sometimes emotional tones and assured families that information would be passed on as soon as it became available. He focused attention on the importance of not being alone in grief and expressed empathy with those who had lost friends and family. At times, he wept openly. This willingness to express his own grief seemed to facilitate a healthy abreaction for both families and troops.

The presidential memorial service 4 days later provided additional examples of a phenomenon Ingraham[5] described as grief leadership, that is, behaviors and statements by key community leaders that serve to facilitate healthy coping with loss and grief among members of the group. In confronting grief associated with group loss, effective leaders take actions that have the effect of unifying the community in the mourning process. President and Mrs. Reagan joined the division commander and his wife in a televised memorial service at Fort Campbell. The division commander noted the value of the President's "sharing our sorrow" and walked with the President to greet and console bereaved families. President Reagan indicated that he represented the concerns of the American people and that the entire nation was grieving along with Fort Campbell.[5]

Several days later, a division memorial service was held on the Fort Campbell parade grounds. This service was significant because the entire Fort Campbell community, including adjacent townspeople, participated. The division commander pointedly remembered each "Fallen Eagle" by announcing his or her name, rank, and home state, along with a cannon salute for each. Nearly 3 months later, a special service was held in observance of the positive identification and burial of the final victim. The division commander decreed a 1-minute sounding of post sirens, followed by 2 minutes of silence to honor the 248 soldiers who died. Without fanfare, people stopped their cars and stood quietly with heads bowed.

The priority placed on caring for bereaved families was reflected in an innovative community intervention initiated by the local adjutant general's office on day two. By this time, it was clear that many family members of victims were travelling to Fort Campbell to attend memorial services and to manage administrative details related to the death. Instead of having family members search around the post for various agencies, a centralized family assistance center (FAC) was established for their convenience. Here, families could address any legal issues, provide necessary information to personnel and finance representatives, make decisions about funeral and burial matters, and also talk with chaplains, psychiatrists, and mental health workers who were on hand. Although it was a solemn place, the FAC became a focal point for sharing information, grieving, and providing and receiving psychological support.

Special telephone lines were installed to facilitate communication and information transfer. Both military and civilian volunteers staffed the center around the clock for the first week of its operation. Desks were arranged in a horseshoe shape, with each desk or station representing a separate agency helping the families. In addition, a quiet room was established in an area upstairs from the main activity of the FAC. Here, a psychiatrist, social worker, or mental health specialist was always available for the private counseling and support of individuals experiencing acute grief episodes or conflicts. This quiet room also became an important resource for exhausted or traumatized staff workers and provided an easy means for identifying individuals who had reached the limits of their endurance and those who might benefit from follow-up care.

Despite the powerful sense of pain and grief at Fort Campbell, there was a discernible community attitude of hope and rebuilding. Ordinarily strict interagency boundaries were relaxed as the post mounted a unified effort to assist families. Many regulations were amended or ignored to provide humane and sympathetic assistance to the bereaved. An enhanced sense of community solidarity was reported by many of those interviewed, as well as a greater sense of meaning in life. Many believed that their actions made a significant difference to suffering families. A similar sense of teamwork and solidarity was observed in the reconstituted unit, where fears that replacement soldiers would be rejected were seen to be unfounded. Instead, they were perceived as allies in the rebuilding of the social unit.[8] Six months after the crash, this unit received several performance awards won in competition with other units across the division. Although a variety of symptoms were reported by many respondents, including sleep disturbances, guilt, and alcohol abuse, these symptoms were usually transitory. No lasting ill-effects were apparent in the community as a whole.

Thus, despite the pain and sadness experienced at Fort Campbell following the Gander crash, there were some clear positive features to the community response. Most notable was the generalized sense of strengthened social cohesion and group solidarity. This reaction was especially apparent in the most severely affected battalion but was also observed throughout the community. Historically, this effect has been observed in other groups affected by disaster. For example, in summarizing a series of flood and tornado studies, Fritz[10] describes disasters as unifying forces that often foster mutual aid and cooperation in communities. Other investigators[12–14] have reported similar beneficial outcomes in social groups confronted by extreme stressful circumstances.

It was also Fritz who observed that disasters frequently "provide an unstructured social situation that enables persons and groups. . . . to introduce desired innovations into the social system."[10(p661)] Several innovative solutions were applied at Fort Campbell in the desire to "find something that works." Some have since been integrated into standard army procedures. The best example is the FAC, which was a creative and effective solution to an unusual set of problems. At one central location, with a minimum of bureaucratic hassles, family members could attend to the myriad details associated with death. The center coincidentally provided a locus around which mental health providers, psychiatrists, psychologists, social workers, chaplains, and enlisted specialists could concentrate their efforts to assist grieving families.

COMMUNITY RESPONSE TO DISASTER

An examination of the literature[6,15,16] on disasters reveals two widely divergent perspectives regarding the psychological effects of disasters on communities. One perspective emphasizes the negative, destructive impact on both individuals and social groups. The other perspective focuses more on the resilient quality of communities exposed to disaster and even allows for positive effects.

An example of the negative impact position is found in descriptions by Titchener and Kapp[17] and Erikson[18] regarding community responses to the Buffalo Creek flood. According to these investigators, this disaster had overwhelming destructive effects on the community. Homes were destroyed, families displaced, and the psychological sense of community that was once shared by neighbors in the valley was permanently damaged. This loss of sense of community appeared related to disabling psychiatric symptoms in over 90% of individuals interviewed.[17]

A contrasting position is taken by researchers who have observed a benign or even positive impact of disasters on individuals and communities. Most of the early National Opinion Research Center (NORC) studies supported such a view.[19,20] The Disaster Research Center (DRC), which grew out of the NORC, has since conducted many disaster studies that take the same position.[18,21,22] For example, one DRC report notes that up to 18 months after a tornado struck the town of Xenia, Ohio, there was an extremely low rate of mental illness.[23] Furthermore, a high proportion of respondents reported improved social relationships and personal growth as a result of the challenges they faced through the disaster.

Exponents of this perspective do not deny the existence of negative psychological effects of disasters for many people but argue that these effects are largely transitory. Which of these seemingly incompatible positions is correct regarding community responses to disaster? The question is an important one for those who want to provide effective psychiatric or mental health interventions. By comparing responses to the Gander disaster at Fort Campbell and Dover Air Force Base, we hope to identify some of the factors contributing to healthy or unhealthy reactions to such events at the community level.

Dover and Fort Campbell Comparison

While not equating the experiences of the Dover Air Force Base and Fort Campbell communities following the Gander disaster, a comparison of the two can suggest reasons why disasters may affect communities in different ways. At both locations, characteristics of the community as well as aspects of the disaster experience itself appear to have influenced responses.

First, for the community of Dover, the crash victims were strangers. This generated a sense of distance from the tragedy; they had little sense of psychological "ownership" over the loss. Although the Dover community sympathized with grieving army families and was certainly horrified by the number and condition of bodies, still the dead "belonged" to somebody else. Dover is an air force base, while the casualties were army soldiers from a distant location. Some mortuary workers described Dover as merely a way-station for the initial processing of bodies that belonged to Fort Campbell.

In contrast, the Fort Campbell community lost a significant portion of its own members. Here, the dead were real people, friends and neighbors rather than strangers. Scattered about the post were literally hundreds of friends, family members, cars, and homes belonging to the dead. The significant loss associated with the Gander disaster unquestionably belonged to Fort Campbell. For Dover, lack of a sense of ownership may have helped initially to establish a kind of community "disidentification" from the disaster, with some short-term prophylactic effects. In the long run, however, this very lack of ownership perhaps contributed to a deeper sense of meaninglessness and alienation. The community of Fort Campbell was shocked and hurt but able to place the loss in a framework of life and death, patriotic sacrifice, and dedication to "the mission." In contrast, the Dover Air Force Base community, while shocked and horrified by the magnitude of the loss, understood that supporting the mortuary was part of their job and their mission. It is clear that the nature of the disaster-related stress was different for the two communities. For Fort Campbell, the Gander disaster meant sudden large-scale death and loss of loved ones. For Dover, the disaster meant close exposure to badly burned and mutilated dead bodies.

Some chronic aspects of community life at Dover could conceivably enhance vulnerability to events like the Gander disaster. As one of the largest mortuary facilities in the world, Dover is called on to manage body recovery and identification operations in disasters and mass casualty events. For example, over 900 bloated and partially decomposed bodies were brought to Dover for processing following the mass-suicide of religious cult members at Jonestown, Guyana, in 1976.[24] In addition, the burned and fragmented bodies of 243 U.S. Marines were brought to Dover after the Beirut barracks bombing in 1983.[25] With this unusually gruesome history comes the communal knowledge that future disasters will mean additional mass casualty mortuary operations at the base. Living at Dover could be somewhat comparable with living near an active volcano or a nuclear reactor because there is a shared chronic sense of risk or dread. The fact that air operations are the primary business of the Dover base could also mean that aircraft disasters are especially disturbing to the community, as potent reminders of their own daily vulnerability to such events.

Another important difference between Dover and Fort Campbell following the Gander crash concerns leadership and lines of authority. In the early postcrash period, command-and-control channels at Dover became quite confused. Several outside officials with some legitimate authority arrived on site and asserted control. There was some dispute over whether the recovery and mortuary operation should be managed by the army or the air force. The usual functional boundaries between the community and outside groups seemed to be ruptured, at least for a time. Local (air force) commanders who had the greatest experience and expertise with mass casualty morgue operations were shunted to the side when it was determined to be an army operation. This may have contributed to a generalized and psychologically damaging sense of lack of control for Dover community members involved in mortuary operations (hundreds of air force volunteers helped) and an exaggerated fear of losing control over one's internal and external boundaries.

The leadership picture at Fort Campbell was markedly different. Not only were lines of authority clearly delineated, but also key leaders were highly visible and provided useful role models for their soldiers to follow. No outside authorities arrived to take charge. Even President Reagan during his visit deferred to the local army commanding general, while offering sympathy and support to the community. Community leaders were both task-oriented and psychologically sensitive. They clearly defined what needed to be done in the interest of community survival and recovery. Further, by their own behavior under duress, they modeled appropriate responses for the rest of the community. Through their words, gestures, and shared grief, they provided permission to the rest of the community to grieve. At the same time, these leaders acted responsibly in emphasizing the need for continued work and task management.

One important benefit of effective leadership in such crisis situations is to help reestablish a sense of control, predictability, and hope in the midst of confusion, chaos, and fear. Leaders at Fort Campbell tried to focus community attention on the opportunities to learn and grow provided by the disaster. A common theme was by having suffered through this tragedy together, we will be stronger and even better prepared for the national defense mission. This quality of positive leadership through disaster was less apparent at Dover.

Community Adaptation to Loss

In the early aftermath of the Gander crash, the Fort Campbell community seemed to revert to a more complete *gemeinschaft* form of social organization. The magnitude of the loss made normal functional divisions within the community seem unimportant because everyone was united in a shared sense of loss and mourning. For some days, the entire community focused on the same event, the violent death of 248 loved soldiers. Key community leaders stepped forward and, by speaking often of the common pain experienced and the need for survivors to support each other, reinforced this sense of community-based solidarity.

Correspondingly, formal roles and relationships in the Fort Campbell community shifted to more informal, implicit bonds based on mutual support in crisis. The shift in formal roles, the blurring of rigid organizational boundaries, and the relaxing of normal rules and regulations permitted several unusual and effective interventions following the crash.

Again, the ad hoc FAC provides a good example of and a metaphor for this phenomenon. It was quickly discovered that the standard organizational structuring of agencies on post, which reflects a division of labor according to function (more *gesellschaft* in quality), was not well-suited to the immediate postdisaster needs of the community. Consequently, a central location was established where representatives of various post agencies were available to assist families and the bereaved. The chaplains office, the mortuary affairs office, the Veterans Administration, the Red Cross, Army Mutual Aid, Army Community Services, the judge advocate general's office, the finance office, and mental health services all provided teams to the FAC.

Other innovative solutions that involved suspension of the standard interagency boundaries were observed. For example, to facilitate sharing of information and caring for the large number of victims' families, daily "skull-sessions" were held that included casualty affairs workers, personnel policy experts, and army legal department representatives. At these meetings, casualty workers could get quick and accurate answers to the many procedural questions raised by family members.

Strong and sensitive community leaders appear to be a necessary ingredient to the positive responses observed at Fort Campbell. As described above, these leaders focused the group on shared values, common goals, and the mutual experience of loss and bereavement. This perspective was reinforced through a series of memorial services that united the community, fostering a sense of integration and solidarity. In the following section, we summarize medical and psychiatric interventions that were applied and consider their effects in the context of a community united in grief.

MEDICAL AND PSYCHIATRIC INTERVENTIONS

In the aftermath of the Gander air disaster, the main goal of the mental health response was prevention of psychiatric problems through early supportive intervention. Of primary concern were the families of the victims, soldiers who were friends and comrades of the dead, and the various support personnel such as survivor assistance officers, FAC staff, chaplains, and leaders. Modes of psychiatric intervention applied were consultation and liaison psychiatry, mental health education, group therapy, and the identification and treatment of high-risk individuals.

Initially, there was some confusion and anxiety among the Fort Campbell mental health staff regarding what to expect and how to proceed. It was considered highly probable that the hospital mental health clinic would soon be overwhelmed with family members and soldiers experiencing acute grief reactions and related problems. A plan was thus implemented to staff the center 24 hours a day in anticipation of this increased patient load. In addition, the mental health clinic was renamed as a grief counseling center in an effort to make it less stigmatizing and more accessible to the community at large.

The expected flood of distressed individuals in fact never came, leading to a reorientation of mental health efforts in the direction of community outreach. The focus of these efforts was on consultation, outreach, support, and education about the grief process. The strategy was to take mental health services out of the hospital and to locations where affected individuals were gathering.

A three-member team was established to coordinate preventive psychiatric efforts. The division psychiatrist acted as the primary consultant and liaison to the community. The chief of the psychology service focused on mental health clinic readiness, and the chief of child and adolescent services worked with school officials and social work service to aid the affected children.

In keeping with the focus on early preventive interventions, a mental health team was quickly dispatched to the brigade gymnasium where families first received news of the crash. A second mental health team was later placed at the newly formed FAC, and a third team was stationed at the hospital's general medicine clinic to assist in the triage process and help identify any psychiatric problems. These teams were typically composed of two behavioral science specialists and one or more psychiatrists, psychologists, or social workers. It was understood that under the circumstances, grief and distress are normal reactions. The major effort of the teams was thus to identify and assist any soldiers, workers, or family members whose needs appeared extreme or who seemed unresponsive to support available from friends, family, and the FAC.

Special attention was also paid to surviving soldiers. To maximize identification of psychiatric problems through normal medical channels, a behavioral science specialist was stationed in each of the troop medical clinics around post. It is at these clinics that daily sick call occurs. Furthermore, a two-person grief counseling team was assigned to each army unit that lost soldiers in the crash. These teams provided informal classes and workshops on issues related to the grief process, including extensive question-and-answer periods. This approach proved an especially valuable mechanism not only for getting useful information to the soldiers, but for identifying high-risk individuals for more extensive follow-up care.

Of the various interventions tried, those offered under old structural boundaries (for example, mental health services provided in a hospital setting) proved less effective than those more in accord with a *gemeinschaft* community organization. Outreach efforts were most successful where good relationships across structural boundaries existed before the crash. For example, the active consultation role pursued by the division psychiatrist capitalized on an unusually strong command-consultation program already in place before the crisis. The psychiatrist was perceived as a trusted friend in the community, and his presence in the role of mental health expert following the crash was not surprising or threatening to community members. His ability to interact well with members of different post agencies, from administrative officers to chaplains, facilitated a relaxing of organizational boundaries that in turn permitted mental health teams to get involved in many postcrash tasks. This approach placed mental health personnel directly proximate to those in need of, but not always willing to actively seek out, services.

Another intervention strategy that appeared effective in the period of relaxed interagency boundaries was group debriefing. In the days and weeks following the crash, mental health teams visited affected army units to conduct a series of seminar-like debriefings on grief, loss, and related topics. Presented as nonthreatening information meetings, these sessions provided both cognitive and emotional avenues for managing grief, while avoiding the stigma sometimes attached to getting mental health assistance.

The FAC, initially created to centralize agencies and simplify administrative matters for families, soon developed into something broader in scope and function. In addition to helping with administrative details, FAC staff found themselves helping bereaved families with their emotions and grief surrounding the loss. The FAC evolved into a therapeutic setting in which family members (as well as staff) could express their grief in a supportive social environment. Community chaplains were especially helpful in this setting.

Alert mental health professionals used the opportunity presented by the FAC to place mental health services close to those in need. In addition to trained specialists who moved around the center, a special area was established where family members could grieve in private or with professional support. Unexpectedly, the mental health workers also became a valuable resource for FAC staff members who experienced their own grief reactions.

The grief leadership provided by leaders at various levels in the Fort Campbell community can also be usefully regarded as an effective intervention because it apparently facilitated healthy grief responses for many. By their own example of open, shared expression of grief, leaders consistently emphasized the importance of experiencing the sense of loss within a supportive social network, thereby avoiding a sense of isolation and despair. In addition, leaders provided critical avenues of communication, sharing information with the community as facts became available and local responses were organized.

Memorial services were often emotional events that reinforced the solidarity of the community in the grieving process. The family reception at the brigade gymnasium on the morning of the crash was the first and most spontaneous of these memorials. Under the leadership of the brigade commander, the value of grieving together as a community was reinforced. The same theme was played out in other memorial services held over the next few weeks.

Some agencies and individuals appeared unable to adjust from the highly specialized structures and roles that pertained before the crash. For example, mental health workers who refused to stray from the hospital clinics saw few grief-related cases. Those patients that were seen in the clinics typically had preexisting mental health problems. By rigidly maintaining their agency boundaries and emphasizing their distinctiveness from other groups, these healthcare providers missed an opportunity to provide valuable assistance to the community. Grieving individuals required confirmation of the normalcy of their responses rather than a suggestion of mental defectiveness. Unfortunately, many people still attach a stigma of weakness to seeking mental health services. When mental health teams were provided at community congregation points, this stigma was largely overcome.

SUMMARY AND CONCLUSION

This chapter has described the reactions of two communities to the same air disaster. The important dimensions distinguishing these two communities and accounting for their differential responses involve characteristics of the disaster situation, as well as more persistent or chronic features of the communities themselves. A sense of ownership as regards the disaster emerges as important in defining the general tone of community response. In addition, important are clear (and nonconflicting) lines of authority and leaders who can focus group attention on the work of recovery as well as the ongoing task responsibilities of the organization. Such leaders appear instrumental in imparting a sense of control in an atmosphere of chaos, coherence in the midst of confusion, and hope instead of despair. They help the community direct its energy toward "rising to the challenge" offered by the disaster and in learning useful lessons from the experience.

These findings suggest that the presence (or emergence) of effective leaders in community disasters may be a critical variable in defining how a community responds. Depending on the nature of the disaster, this variable could be more or less important. When entire communities are displaced and dispersed, for example, it might be less relevant. But even in a disaster as fragmenting as the Buffalo Creek flood, one can imagine that the presence of effective community leaders in the immediate aftermath might have galvanized the survivors and led to some very different long term effects.

In this chapter, we have identified some necessary, although probably not sufficient, factors in accounting for positive community responses to disaster. To recognize that disasters can have positive effects as well as negative ones is not to discount their potential destructiveness for individuals and groups. However, identifying these differences may be essential to an adequate understanding of community responses to disaster and thus to the planning of effective prevention and intervention strategies. This information can be used to help build psychological disaster plans for addressing the psychological needs of communities stricken by disaster. The documented experiences of the Fort Campbell community as it struggled to process the Gander tragedy should prove especially valuable to leaders and mental health workers who must be prepared to respond to future community disasters.

Understanding the dynamics of community response to disaster can also shed light on another major concern of military psychiatrists: How to prepare individuals and units to withstand the psychological stress of combat. In this regard, it is important to consider what valuable lessons might be taken from noncombat traumatic stressors, such as the Gander crash, that affect military units. By observing how individuals and groups respond to sudden, unexpected trauma outside of war, as well as by noting which interventions are helpful to recovery and which are not, we may be better prepared to reduce and prevent combat stress reactions, war-related post-traumatic stress disorders, and other psychiatric problems associated with exposure to combat.

REFERENCES

1. Sarason S. *The Psychological Sense of Community.* San Francisco: Jossey-Bass; 1988.
2. Tonnies F. *Community and Society.* Loomis C, ed. and translator. New York: Harper Torchbook; 1963.
3. Durkheim E. *The Division of Labor in Society.* New York: Macmillan; 1933.
4. Nisbet RA. *The Sociological Tradition.* New York: Basic Books; 1966.
5. Wright K, ed. *Human Response to the Gander Military Air Disaster.* Washington, DC: Walter Reed Army Institute of Research; 1987. Neuropsychiatry Division Report 88–5.
6. Quarantelli EL. An assessment of conflicting views on mental health: The consequences of traumatic events. In: Figley CR, eds. *Trauma and Its Wake.* New York: Brunnel/Mazel; 1985: 173–215.
7. Marshall SLA. *Bringing Up the Rear: A Memoir.* San Rafael, Calif: Presidio Press; 1979.
8. Bartone PT, Wright KM. Grief and group recovery following a military air disaster. *J Traumatic Stress.* 1990;3:523–539.
9. Ursano RJ, ed. *Exposure to Death, Disasters, and Bodies.* Bethesda, Md: Department of Psychiatry, Uniformed Services University of the Health Sciences; 1987.
10. Fritz CE. Disaster. In: Merton R, Nisbet RA, eds. *Contemporary Social Problems.* New York: Harcourt, Brace, and World; 1961: 651–694.
11. Ursano RJ, Ingraham L, Saczynski K, Russell C, Bartone PT, Cervantes RA. Update on military psychiatry: Psychiatric aspects of a tragedy. Presented at the 38th Institute on Hospital and Community Psychiatry, San Diego, Ca; 15 October 1986.
12. Bartone PT, Ursano RJ, Wright KM, Ingraham LH. The impact of a military air disaster on the health of assistance workers: A prospective study. *J Nerv Ment Dis.* 1989;177:317–328.
13. James W. On some mental effects of the earthquake. In: James W, ed. *Memories and Studies.* New York: Longmans, Green and Company; 1911.
14. Janis IL. *Air War and Emotional Stress.* New York: McGraw-Hill; 1951.
15. Figley CR, ed. *Trauma and Its Wake.* New York: Brunner/Mazel; 1985.

16. Tierney KJ. Disasters and mental health: A critical look at knowledge and practice. *U of Delaware*. 5–10 October 1986: 1–33.

17. Titchener JL, Kapp FT. Family and character change at Buffalo Creek. *Am J Psychiatry*. 1976;133(3):295–299.

18. Erikson K. Loss of communality at Buffalo Creek. *Am J Psychiatry*. 1976;133:302–305.

19. Fritz CE, Marks ES. The NORC studies of human behavior in disaster. *J Soc Issues*. 1954;10:26–31.

20. Marks ES, Fritz C, Bucher R, et al. *Human Reactions in Disaster Situations.* Chicago, Ill: National Opinion Research Center, University of Chicago; 1954.

21. Dynes RR. *Organized Behavior in Disaster.* Lexington, Mass: Heath Lexington Books; 1970.

22. Quarantelli EL. Human resources and organizational behaviors in community disasters and their relationship to planning. Columbus, Oh: Disaster Research Center, Ohio State University; 1982. Preliminary paper 76.

23. Disaster Research Center. Xenia survey data. Columbus, Oh: Disaster Research Center, Ohio State University; 1976. Internal memorandum.

24. Endleman R. *Jonestown and the Manson Family: Race, Sexuality, and Collective Madness.* New York: Psyche Press; 1993.

25. Russakoff D. First dead return to their soil. *Washington Post*. 30 October 1983:A32.

Chapter 19

SUMMATION

FRANKLIN D. JONES, M.D., F.A.P.A.*

*Colonel (ret), Medical Corps, U.S. Army; Clinical Professor, Uniformed Services University of the Health Sciences; Past President and Secretary and Current Honorary President of the Military Section, World Psychiatric Association

INTRODUCTION

Foremost among the peacetime activities of the military is the preparation to fight in defense of the nation. In that regard, the authors of this book have addressed the garrison military in terms of morale and cohesion, which involve family issues and burnout; liability to diseases; and mental illnesses that may manifest themselves as drug and alcohol abuse and homicides and suicides.

Clearly related to morale and cohesion are commanders acting ethically and in the best interests of their charges in accomplishing the mission. Readiness always requires appropriate training that may include the use of disasters and incidents of terrorism, rioting, and refugee management as material. The development of community mental health is an extension of the concept of readiness.

APPLICABILITY OF PRINCIPLES TO NONCOMBAT SETTINGS

Although developed empirically in the different settings, the practice of military psychiatry in the combat setting and in the garrison setting has a number of similarities, particularly when one is handling acute adjustment disorders. These practices include various elements of the proximity, immediacy, simplicity, expectancy, and centrality elements of combat psychiatry.

DEVELOPMENT OF ARMY COMMUNITY PSYCHIATRIC SERVICES

Halloran and Farrell[1] and Cohen[2] established mental hygiene consultation programs at replacement and training centers within the first years of United States' entry into World War II. Initially, these programs furnished a kind of orientation and "pep talk" for soldiers being sent overseas. Later, as the success in decreasing psychiatric casualties through such strengthening of morale became recognized, they spread to other settings and, by the end of the war, were an integral part of the mental health program of the army.

The continued conscription of young men after World War II and after the Korean conflict resulted in large numbers of unhappy soldiers who would much prefer to follow other pursuits. The Mental Hygiene Consultation Service became the preferred method of managing them.

Bushard[3] chronicled the empirical development of army community psychiatric services (the Mental Hygiene Consultation Service) during the decade following World War II. Cold War tensions had resulted in the continued need for drafted soldiers, many of whom preferred to be civilians. The early psychiatric services were little other than struggling outpatient clinics that were totally overwhelmed by the problems presented to them of large numbers of disaffected troops. Applying the usual psychiatric treatment techniques growing out of psychoanalytic theory in this situation produced results that were frequently discouraging. The usual conclusion was that, in view of the disparity between large referral load and psychotherapeutic talent available, little could be offered. Considering the large caseload and the brief period of the patient's stay on post, traditional psychotherapy was not feasible.

Eventually, a view of the soldier emerged in which he is seen as part of an interactional set with his environment. The dynamics involved relate not so much to oedipal traumas and disturbed biochemistry as to disturbed homeostasis in the soldier's social ecology. Adaptability was seen to relate to supports and circumstances that tend to prevent or strengthen the illness role. Depending on the balance achieved, one may see increased or decreased rates of ineffectiveness as measured by absent without leave (AWOL), venereal disease, sick call, and disciplinary action rates.

Civilian Settings

Usually it will be rare that the civilian psychiatric casualty has been exposed to the kind of conflict experienced by a combat soldier. Examples of persons exposed to hazardous occupations include police, firefighters, pilots, and so forth, but these are rare and do not involve legal or psychological stigmas as with the soldier.

The better analogy is the marriage partner, teacher, therapist (as in "professional burnout" syndrome), parent, supervisor, or other person who has responsibilities to a group or another person and who becomes demoralized in discharging those responsibilities. (See Chapter 3, Burnout in Military Personnel.)

In the workplace, psychological burnout can occur in those in stressful occupations such as the police, teaching, mental health workers, and so forth. Burnout is the civilian equivalent of combat fatigue and can be treated in similar fashion. Burnout seldom occurs in a cohesive group whose members can give psychological support to its members. Thus, prevention consists of maintaining group cohesion and morale, while treatment consists of establishing or reestablishing such bonds, sometimes after a period of rest from the job.

Many patients who are responding to crisis situations emanating from psychological antecedents will be given labels such as *adjustment reaction*, *depression*, or *anxiety neurosis* depending on presenting symptoms and therapeutic school. The comparability with the combat stress casualty is in the acceptance of a medical label as the solution to one's problems of living and one's inability to cope with them. This is not limited to psychiatric patients; in fact, it may be more common in other conditions; chronic low back and tension headache syndromes are frequent ailments prone to result in one's escape from the daily fray of work. Such organic conditions do not carry the psychiatric stigma, making them even more desirable as avenues of escape. Such persons are usually not malingering or consciously ineffective; rather, for them, the short-term rewards of the invalid or medical label outweigh the long-term rewards of mastery of the situation.

Training of Personnel

Training of personnel involves several important dimensions: technical proficiency, personality characteristics, strength and endurance, group cohesiveness, and stress inoculation. There is considerable overlap in all of these areas; for example, technical proficiency, which may require strength and endurance, leads to the personality characteristic of self-confidence, which along with technical proficiency produces a sense of mastery and increases one's value to the group, promoting group cohesion. All of these characteristics are positively associated with the ability to withstand combat stress.

Much of military training addresses all of these dimensions. Shared vigorous training not only increases strength and endurance and builds self-confidence but also increases group affiliation and cohesion.[4] Aware of the importance of cohesion, the military has kept personnel together in cohort units from basic training to deployment. In addition, efforts have been made to keep commanders with the same unit for longer periods to enhance not only horizontal (peers) but also vertical (hierarchical) cohesion (see Chapter 1).

Substance Abuse Problems

Although sporadic drug abuse problems, primarily in overseas deployment, have existed since World War I[5], they did not reach prominence until the Vietnam conflict.[6,7]

Treatment of substance abusers has varied considerably over time. Early approaches were to consider such casualties problems of a moral nature and later of a character defect with punishment as the primary intervention. It was only when such losses of manpower became significant in the Vietnam conflict that a nonpunitive, therapeutic approach was undertaken. By 1971, more soldiers were being evacuated from Vietnam for drug use than for war wounds.[8]

The main lessons from the U.S. experience in managing substance abuse in Vietnam are that treatment should be in country to prevent an evacuation syndrome and that the factors that prevent breakdown in general—cohesion, effective leadership, and good morale—may protect soldiers from substance abuse. For example, the Australians serving in Vietnam did not have significant personnel losses from substance abuse.[9,10] Australian forces were based on a regimental system with unit rather than individual rotations, and officers and troops had usually served together for long periods. This approach may have produced greater unit cohesion, a crucial difference from U.S. troops, and protected Australian troops from developing nostalgic problems of substance abuse and indiscipline.

Sexual Problems

Infectious diseases have plagued armies since ancient times. Venereal diseases (VDs) have been a major cause of lost soldier strength in wars of the 20th century. While modern medicine has markedly reduced the time lost and complications of VDs, it has not reduced the infection rates. Although malaria, hepatitis, and tuberculosis caused significant soldier attrition in Vietnam, the most common nostalgic disorder coming to medical attention was sexual intercourse with prostitutes leading to VDs. Although unlikely to have immediate effects on combat efficiency, the human immunodeficiency virus (HIV) poses severe problems in long-term prevention.

Prevention through education is a valid approach to VD even though some soldiers will risk infection no matter what the threat. Prevention should not be directed at preventing sexual intercourse, which is an unrealistic goal, but toward the use of readily available condoms.

Indiscipline

Indiscipline is a psychiatric issue because sociopsychological factors play a paramount role in its emergence. Furthermore, indiscipline and psychiatric breakdown merge almost imperceptibly as evacuation syndromes. For example, failure to take preventive hygiene measures in Korea allowed the development of frostbite in some cases. Similarly, failure to take the prophylactic chloroquine-primaquine pill in Vietnam allowed the infestation of malarial protozoans. In both cases, indiscipline rendered the soldiers unfit for duty.[11,12]

Indiscipline may range from relatively minor acts of omission to commission of serious acts of disobedience (mutiny) and even to murder (fragging). In an analysis and historical review, Rose[13] indicated that combat refusal has been a relatively frequent occurrence in most significant wars for which there are adequate data. Most indiscipline, of course, is more subtle than combat refusal and does not appear to be related to it. However, unavailability for combat is a frequent consequence of indiscipline. The main role of the psychiatrist is in prevention because the same conditions that give rise to neuropsychiatric casualties may produce indiscipline as another evacuation syndrome.

Terrorism

The U.S. Army maintains a special unit, Delta Force, at Fort Bragg, North Carolina, to combat terrorists. The need for such a unit with a unified command can be seen with the failure of a combined services attempt to rescue the 52 hostages in Iran.[14] Since Islamic terrorists have recently targeted the Central Intelligence Agency (CIA) and the World Trade Center in New York City, there will likely be an increased role in countering or responding to such threats.[15,16]

Since World War II (as, indeed, long before World War II), the Middle East has experienced essentially continual conflict. These conflicts have ranged from state-sponsored terrorism through low-intensity and guerrilla warfare to high-intensity and chemical warfare.[17] The significance of terrorist activities should not be minimized. In 1983, a single terrorist suicide attack killed 241 U.S. Marines on a peacekeeping mission in Beirut, producing nearly as many American deaths as the Spanish-American War.[18,19]

RESCUE OPERATIONS

Grenada

In October 1983, American forces invaded Grenada. Operation Urgent Fury was undertaken to ensure the safety of about 1,000 Americans, including 700 medical students, and to restore order as requested by Grenada's neighboring island countries. Most of the Americans killed in Grenada died from accidents although U.S. forces did meet stiff resistance from 600 well-armed and professionally trained Cuban soldiers.[20] Because elite forces (rangers, SEALs [SEa Air Land commandos in the U.S. Navy], and airborne units) made the assault, few psychiatric casualties were expected, and few occurred (3 so designated in 3,000 invading troops with 19 killed in action and 73 wounded in action).[20]

Dehydration and heat exhaustion casualties accounted for the majority of the preventable casualties. Fullerton[21] debriefed most of the commanders after combat had ended. He reported that one battalion suffered 29 heat casualties in a single day, but another battalion suffered only 2 heat casualties on the same day while both engaged in virtually identical tasks. The commander of the latter battalion had emphasized water discipline.

Some of the wounded soldiers suffered delayed post-traumatic stress disorders.[21,22] Mateczun and Holmes-Johnson[18] had an interesting opportunity to compare the psychological adjustment of Marines wounded in Grenada with those wounded in the Beirut massacre when casualties from both incidents arrived almost simultaneously at Bethesda

Naval Hospital. About 25 marines, more from Beirut than Grenada, were treated in a psychiatric consultation-liaison model with group therapy as the primary intervention. The group therapy was modeled after Marshall's[23] group debriefing technique; however, the Beirut casualties had less to recount because they were sleeping when the bomb exploded. Their memories centered on feelings of helplessness and fear of dying before rescuers could reach them. Survivor guilt was high among Beirut casualties but almost absent among Grenada casualties. Both groups had some symptoms of post-traumatic stress disorder (nightmares, intrusive thoughts, and anxiety), but Grenada casualties had high morale and a strong desire to return to the combat unit. In contrast, the Beirut casualties wanted to go home. These differences in symptoms are attributable to the different forms of combat. In Beirut, the marines had no clear enemies or mission, and some viewed themselves as vulnerable targets; however, American forces in Grenada had a clear mission with a known enemy and had numerical and logistical superiority.

The Persian Gulf War

When Iraq invaded Kuwait and threatened the West's oil supply lifeline, the United States formed a coalition with other forces to rescue Kuwait and end the aggression. Operations Desert Shield and Storm were the largest deployment of U.S. forces since Vietnam.[24] The 540,000-member U.S. forces had 148 killed in action and 467 wounded.[25] Of these casualties, 35 were killed and 78 wounded in fratricidal ("friendly fire") incidents. Iraq's military is estimated to have lost between 30,000 and 100,000 killed and 100,000 to 300,000 wounded. There were an estimated 60,000 to 70,000 Iraqi prisoners of war by war's end.[25]

Neuropsychiatric casualties were relatively few. During the deployment phase (Operation Desert Shield), some soldiers anticipating deployment sought psychiatric care, usually for anxiety symptoms but sometimes for somatic symptoms. During the fighting phase (Operation Desert Storm), combat stress casualties were minimal.[26]

Nostalgic casualties were few because the host country (Saudi Arabia), in keeping with Muslim tradition, did not allow importation of alcoholic beverages or prostitution. Accidents reportedly were one-third the rate of other U.S. forces because of the absence of alcohol.[27] However, casualties secondary to substance abuse may have occurred when soldiers attempted to make homemade alcohol. Only a few drug-related incidents occurred including that of an air force pharmacist who used and distributed drugs illegally. After the liberation of Kuwait, U.S. forces assisted Kurdish and Shiite refugees displaced by the fighting.[28]

Somalia

In 1992, President Bush ordered U.S. troops to assist in the distribution of food to starving Somalis. The Secretariat of the United Nations also wished to disarm local warlords and restore representative government, resulting in a state of undeclared war. There have been few reports of psychiatric casualties among American military personnel in Operation Restore Hope to Somalia despite sporadic combat casualties, including 18 American soldiers dead and 75 wounded in an ill-fated attempt to capture a local warlord in October 1993.[29] In part, this may be due to the humanitarian nature of the mission, the use of volunteer forces, and the very low rate of surgical casualties. Febo[30] reported that there was a very liberal evacuation policy so that over 700 soldiers had been evacuated with complaints such as headaches, backaches, and so forth. Some of these cases may have been masked psychiatric casualties.

FUTURE ROLES OF THE MILITARY

While defense of the nation through readiness for combat is the *raison d'etre* of a military, many other roles have been played in the past and will be played in the future. These roles have included peacekeeping (currently underway in the Sinai and Macedonia)[31,32] often with other United Nations forces, refugee management and relocation (as occurred in the influx of Cuban refugees and Haitians and Bosnians),[33–35] rescue operations (as occurred in Grenada and Somalia), large-scale rioting (as occurred in Chicago, Washington, D.C., and Los Angeles),[36–38] assistance in disasters (as occurred with Hurricanes Hugo and Andrew and with the 1993 Mississippi River flooding),[39–41] and interdiction of drug trafficking (as occurred in South America and as a cooperative effort with the Justice and Treasury Departments[42]). Recently, military forces have taken a proactive stance, interdicting commercial refugees from Haiti and China.

New roles for the military may include resocialization of offenders of the criminal justice system. Experimental programs based on basic training approaches and run by former military personnel are being tried by some jurisdictions. It is reasonable to expect that the military itself could assume such responsibilities if not engaged in other pressing activities.[43]

SUMMARY AND CONCLUSION

As events in the past decade have demonstrated, there is an ongoing need for a strong U.S. military. The military missions have ranged from major military deployments and high-technology combat to small-scale police actions. The U.S. Army Medical Department must remain flexible in supporting these missions. The principles of military psychiatry, while the bedrock of treatment, will require adaptation to ameliorate the stress of combat on the soldier.

REFERENCES

1. Halloran RD, Farrell MJ. The function of neuropsychiatry in the Army. *Am J Psychiatry*. 1943;100:14–20.
2. Cohen RR. Mental hygiene for the trainee. *Am J Psychiatry*. 1943;100:62–71.
3. Bushard BL. The U.S. Army's mental hygiene consultation service. In: *The Symposium on Preventive and Social Psychiatry*. Washington, DC: GPO; 1957: 431–443.
4. Belenky GL, Kaufman LW. Cohesion and rigorous training: Observations of the Air Assault School. *Milit Rev*. 1983;63:24–34.
5. Froede RC, Stahl CJ. Fatal narcotism in military personnel. *J Forensic Sci*. 1971;16(2):199–218.
6. Holloway HC. Epidemiology of heroin dependency among soldiers in Vietnam. *Milit Med*. 1974;139:108–113.
7. Jones FD, Johnson AW. Medical and psychiatric treatment policy and practice in Vietnam. *J Soc Issues*. 1975;31(4):49–65.
8. Stanton MD. Drugs, Vietnam, and the Vietnam veteran: An overview. *Am J Drug Alcohol Abuse*. 1976;3(4):557–570.
9. Spragg G. Psychiatry in the Australian military forces. *Med J Aust*. 1972;1:745–751.
10. Spragg G. Australian forces in Vietnam. Presented at the Combat Stress Seminar; 20 July 1983; Washington, DC.
11. Jones FD, Crocq L, Adelaja O, et al. Psychiatric casualties in modern warfare: I. Evolution of treatment. In: Pichot P, Berner P, Wolf R, Thau K, eds. *Psychiatry: The State of the Art*. Vol 6. New York: Plenum; 1985: 459–464.
12. Jones FD, Johnson AW. Medical and psychiatric treatment policy and practice in Vietnam. *J Soc Issues*. 1975;31(4):49–56.
13. Rose E. The anatomy of mutiny. *Armed Forces Society*. 1982;8(4):561–574.
14. Kyle JH, with Eidson JR. *The Guts To Try: The Untold Story of the Iran Hostage Rescue Mission by the On-Scene Desert Commander*. New York: Orion Books; 1990.
15. Miller AC. Gunman kills 2 CIA employees at agency's gate. *Los Angeles Times*. 26 January 1993. Vol 112:A1.
16. Wright R, Ostrow RJ. Incident may signal new round of terrorist action (bombing of NYC's World Trade Center). *Los Angeles Times*. 28 February 1993. Vol 112:A1.

17. Taheri A. *Holy Terror: Inside the World of Islamic Terrorism.* Bethesda, Md: Adler and Adler; 1987.

18. Mateczun J, Holmes-Johnson E. The psychiatric care of the combat-injured and clinical differences between Beirut and Grenada casualties. In: Mangelsdorff AD, King JM, O'Brien DE, eds. *Proceedings, Fourth Users' Workshop on Combat Stress: Lessons Learned in Recent Operational Experiences.* Fort Sam Houston, Tex: U.S. Army Health Services Command; 1985: 180–206.

19. Department of Defense. *Selected Manpower Statistics, 1992.* DoD, Washington Headquarters Service. Washington, DC: GPO; 1993. GPO Stock No. 1993–720–091/80107.

20. Adkin M. *Urgent Fury: The Battle for Grenada.* Lexington, Mass: Lexington Books; 1989.

21. Fullerton T. A soldier's view of combat medicine in Grenada. Presented at the Psychiatric Grand Rounds, Walter Reed Army Medical Center; 14 November 1984; Washington, DC.

22. Belenky GL. Talking with U.S. casualties from Grenada. Presented at the Chief's Roundtable, Division of Neuropsychiatry, Walter Reed Army Institute of Research; 5 December 1983; Washington, DC.

23. Marshall SLA. *Bringing Up the Rear: A Memoir.* San Rafael, Calif: Presidio Press; 1979.

24. Department of Defense. *Conduct of the Persian Gulf War: Final Report to Congress.* Washington, DC: GPO; 1992.

25. Gunby P. Another war . . . and more lessons for medicine to ponder in aftermath. *JAMA.* 1991;266(5):619–621.

26. Gunby P. Mental health professionals find fewer problems than expected in Desert Storm. *JAMA.* 1991;265(5):559–560.

27. Gunby P. Service in strict Islamic nation removes alcohol, other drugs from major problem list. *JAMA.* 1991;265(5):560,562.

28. Gerstenzang J, Meisler S. US, Iran may thaw relations to aid refugees. *Los Angeles Times.* 24 April 1991. Vol 110:A1.

29. Richburg KB. US envoy to Somalia urged policy shift before 18 GIs died. *Washington Post.* 11 November 1993: A39,44.

30. Febo M. *U.S. Army Psychiatry.* Bethesda, Md: Report to the Psychiatry Committee of the Society of Medical Consultants to the Armed Forces; 6 November 1993.

31. Segal DR, Harris JJ, Rothberg JM, Marlowe DH. Paratroopers as peacekeepers. *Armed Forces and Society.* 1984;10(4):487–506.

32. Sciolino E. US says it will send 300 troops to Balkan Republic to limit strife (peacekeeping force in Macedonia to include 700 Scandinavian troops). *New York Times.* 11 June 1993. Vol 142:A1.

33. Cruz P, Febo M, Jones FD. Cuban refugee camps: Psychological perspectives. 1986. Syllabus.

34. Pine A. US moves to stifle Haitian exodus. *Los Angeles Times.* 16 January 1993. Vol 112:A12.

35. US Congress. Senate Committee on Armed Services. Current military operations: Hearings before the Committee on Armed Services, US Senate, 103rd Congress, 1st Session, 6 August, 4, 7, 12–13 October 1993. Washington, DC: GPO; 1994.

36. Grimshaw AD. *Racial Violence in the United States.* Chicago: Aldine Publishing Company; 1969.

37. US Kerner Commission. *Report of the National Advisory Commission on Civil Disorders.* New York: Bantam; 1968.

38. Boesel D, Rossi PH, eds. *Cities Under Siege: An Anatomy of the Ghetto Riots. 1964–1968.* New York: Basic Books; 1971.

39. Hevesi D. Troops ordered to Virgin Islands after hurricane sets off looting. *New York Times*. 21 September 1989. Vol 139:A1.

40. Healy M, Stolberg S. Hurricane relief blows in winds of change for military. *Los Angeles Times*. 11 September 1992. Vol 111:A24.

41. Parrett C, Melcher NB, James RW. *Flood Discharges in the Upper Mississippi River Basin, 1993.* Washington, DC: GPO; 1993.

42. *Wall Street Journal*. Pentagon is ordered to set plans for drug interdiction. *Wall Street Journal*. 19 September 1989:A3.

43. Winter EL, Heugel AJ, Leven DD. Train nonviolent offenders at former bases. (Letter to the editor). *New York Times*. 24 January 1992. Vol 141:A14.

ACKNOWLEDGEMENTS

This book owes much to too many people to enumerate them all, but some whose efforts may not have been recognized elsewhere must be mentioned. LTG Charles Pixley, then the Army Surgeon General, assigned the author and first editor (FDJ) to Walter Reed Army Institute of Research (WRAIR) in 1981, and his successors, LTG Bernhard Mittemeyer, LTG Quinn Becker, LTG Frank Ledford and LTG Alcide LaNoue continued the assignments, making the undertaking and development of the project possible.

An atmosphere of inquiry and intellectual ferment was provided by the members of the Combat Stress Work Group (1981-1983), which included many distinguished foreign visitors: COL Pinchas Harris, LTC Shabtai Noi, and COL Reuven Gal, Ph.D., Israel; LTC Nikic, M.D., Yugoslavia; COL Carlos Collazo, M.D., Argentina; Brigadier General Olukayode Adelaja, M.D., Nigeria; General Louis Crocq, M.D., France; LTC Yeng Hoi Fong, M.D., Chief Medical Officer, Singapore Armed Forces; and others. Also contributing were former WRAIR members: the late COL Albert Julius Glass, M.D.; the late David McK. Rioch, M.D.; Edwin Weinstein, M.D.; COL Frederick Tyner, M.D.; COL Frederick Manning, Ph.D.; and COL Mike Camp, M.D.; and current members of WRAIR: COL Gregory Belenky, M.D.; Fred Hegge, Ph.D.; and many others. Special thanks are given for the contributions of the late William Datel, Ph.D. of WRAIR. Many of the ideas presented are distilled from their knowledge and experience.

The editors are particularly indebted to David Marlowe, Ph.D., Chief, Department of Military Psychiatry, WRAIR, for providing numerous educational experiences, not the least of which were his own spirited exigeses of complex material and his review of some of the productions. In a similar vein, COL Frederick Manning, Ph.D., LTC Faris Kirkland, Ph.D., and COL Larry Ingraham, Ph.D. applied their considerable analytical skills to much of the material.

We also wish to acknowledge the contribution of Ronald Koshes, M.D., who edited a number of chapters and also contributed to several chapters as first or later author. Donald Jenkins, Ph.D. and his successor, COL Ronald Bellamy, M.D., provided invaluable support for several authors and for the project as a whole. Dr. Bellamy also provided important editorial assistance and guidance. COL James Stokes of the Army Medical Department Center and School (Fort Sam Houston, Texas), in addition to being a chapter coauthor, rendered invaluable editorial assistance in the Herculean task of reviewing all the chapters for doctrine. His direct contribution of material added immeasurably to the completeness and interest of this volume.

We also owe thanks to the many individuals who reviewed drafts, suggested resource materials and, in general, gave us the support necessary to complete this project: COL David Armitage, M.D.; COL (Ret) Mike Bain, M.D.; COL (Ret) Stu Baker, M.D.; Doug Bey, M.D.; COL James Collins, M.D.; COL Manuel Febo, M.D.; Don Ferguson, Ph.D.; COL Richard Fragala, M.D.; LTC Terry Fullerton, Ph.D.; COL (Ret) Harry Holloway, M.D.; COL Steve Hursh, Ph.D.; COL (Ret) Craig Llewellyn, M.D.; COL (Ret) Matt Parrish, M.D.; COL Norman Ream, M.D.; MAJ E. Cameron Ritchie, M.D.; MG James Rumbaugh, M.D.; and CAPT (Ret) Robert Strange, M.D.

The enlisted members of the Department of Military Psychiatry rendered outstanding logistical and moral support (yes, SGT Nathan Williams, we mean the coffee pot and photocopying). Special thanks are due to SGT Lena Rapp who helped manage the project as it grew in size and scope. Likewise, our thanks to Joy Ann Rohan-Phillips and Louisette Vega, summer interns who contributed to the final organization and preparation of the manuscripts. Our thanks also to Ms. Caren Carney, Mr. Richard Howard, Mr. Richard Oldakowski, Mrs. Iris Hunt, and Mrs. Anna Robinson for their various contributions during the early days of this effort. Our profound thanks to Mrs. Betty Bugash, who cheerfully took on the enormous task of typing and retyping many of the original drafts in the years before we had computers.

—The Specialty Editors

ACRONYMS AND ABBREVIATIONS

A

AA: Alcoholics Anonymous
ACAP: Army Career and Alumni Program
ACOA: Adult Children of Alcoholics
ADAPCP: Alcohol and Drug Abuse Prevention and Control Program
AIDS: acquired immunodeficiency syndrome
APA: American Psychiatric Association
AWOL: absent without leave

B

BAC: blood alcohol concentration
BAS: battalion aide station

C

CA: Cocaine Anonymous
CAGE: Have you tried to **C**ut down? Are people **A**ngry when you drink? Do you feel **G**uilty about drinking? Do you take an **E**ye-opener in the morning?
CDC: Centers for Disease Control
CIA: Central Intelligence Agency
CIWA-A: Clinical Institute Withdrawal Assessment for Alcohol
CMHA: community mental health activities
CMHS: community mental health services
CMTC: Combat Maneuver Training Center
COHORT: cohesion, operational readiness, and training
CRO: carded for record only
CSC: combat stress control
CSR: combat stress reaction

D

DoD: Department of Defense
DRC: Disaster Research Center
DSM III–R: *DSM Diagnostic and Statistical Manual of Mental Disorders* (3rd ed., revised)
DT: delirium tremen

F

FAC: family assistance center
FALN: Fuerza Allianza Libertad Nacional
FBI: Federal Bureau of Investigation
FTX: field training exercise

H

HIV: human immunodeficiency virus

I

3ID: Third Infantry Division
ICD: International Classification of Diseases
ICD–CM: International Classification of Diseases-Clinical Modification
IDF: Israeli Defence Force
IM: intramuscular

J

JRTC: Joint Readiness Training Center

K

KIA: killed in action

L

LSD: lysergic acid

M

MAST: Michigan Alcoholism Screening Test
MBI: Maslach Burnout Inventory
MEDEX: medical exercise
MHCS: mental hygiene consultation services
MILES: Multiple Integrated Laser Engagement System
MOPP: mission-oriented protective posture
MTT: mobile training team

N

NA: Narcotics Anonymous
NATO: North Atlantic Treaty Organization
NCO: noncommissioned officer
NCOIC: noncommissioned officer in charge
NORC: National Opinion Research Center
NTC: National Training Center
NYPD: New York Police Department

O

OPFOR: opposing force

P

PCP: phencyclidine
PIES: proximity, immediacy, expectancy, and simplicity
POC: patient operations center
PTSD: post-traumatic stress disorder

R

ROTC: Reserve Officers' Training Corps
RTF: residential treatment facility
RVN: Republic of Vietnam

S

SEALS: SEa Air Land commandos in the U.S. Navy
Sp4: Specialist 4th Class
SPRINT: special psychiatric rapid intervention team
SWAT: special weapons and tactics

T

TB: tuberculosis

U

UCR: *Uniform Crime Reports*
UN: United Nations

V

VD: venereal disease

W

WIA: wounded in action
WRAIR: Walter Reed Army Institute of Research

INDEX

A

B

E

F

G

Q

R

U

V

W

X

Y

Z

☆U.S. GOVERMENT PRINTING OFFICE : 2003 301-869